Neurology and Neurobiology

---

1 • **Cytochemical Methods in Neuroanatomy,** Victoria Chan-Palay and Sanford L. Palay, *Editors*

2 • **Basic Mechanisms of Neuronal Hyperexcitability,** Herbert H. Jasper and Nico M. van Gelder, *Editors*

3 • **Anorexia Nervosa: Recent Developments in Research,** Padraig L. Darby, Paul E. Garfinkel, David M. Garner, and Donald V. Coscina, *Editors*

4 • **Clinical and Biological Aspects of Peripheral Nerve Diseases,** Leontino Battistin, George A. Hashim, and Abel Lajtha, *Editors*

5 • **The Physiology of Excitable Cells,** Alan D. Grinnell and William J. Moody, Jr., *Editors*

6 • **Developing and Regenerating Vertebrate Nervous Systems,** Penelope W. Coates, Roger R. Markwald, and Alexander D. Kenny, *Editors*

7 • **Glutamine, Glutamate, and GABA in the Central Nervous System,** Leif Hertz, Elling Kvamme, Edith G. McGeer, and Arne Schousboe, *Editors*

8 • **Catecholamines,** Earl Usdin, Arvid Carlsson, Annica Dahlström, and Jörgen Engel, *Editors*. Published in three volumes: *Part A: Basic and Peripheral Mechanisms; Part B: Neuropharmacology and Central Nervous System—Theoretical Aspects; Part C: Neuropharmacology and Central Nervous System—Therapeutic Aspects*

9 • **Development of Visual Pathways in Mammals,** Jonathan Stone, Bogdan Dreher, and David H. Rapaport, *Editors*

10 • **Monoamine Innervation of Cerebral Cortex,** Laurent Descarries, Tomás R. Reader, and Herbert H. Jasper, *Editors*

11 • **The Neurobiology of Zinc,** C.J. Frederickson, G.A. Howell, and E.J. Kasarskis, *Editors*. Published in two volumes: *Part A: Physiochemistry, Anatomy, and Techniques; Part B: Deficiency, Toxicity, and Pathology*

12 • **Modulation of Sensorimotor Activity During Alterations in Behavioral States,** Richard Bandler, *Editor*

13 • **Behavioral Pharmacology: The Current Status,** Lewis S. Seiden and Robert L. Balster, *Editors*

14 • **Development, Organization, and Processing in Somatosensory Pathways,** Mark Rowe and William D. Willis, Jr., *Editors*

15 • **Metal Ions in Neurology and Psychiatry,** Sabit Gabay, Joseph Harris, and Beng T. Ho, *Editors*

16 • **Neurohistochemistry: Modern Methods and Applications,** Pertti Panula, Heikki Päivärinta, and Seppo Soinila, *Editors*

17 • **Two Hemispheres—One Brain: Functions of the Corpus Callosum,** Franco Leporé, Maurice Ptito, and Herbert H. Jasper, *Editors*

18 • **Senile Dementia of the Alzheimer Type,** J. Thomas Hutton and Alexander D. Kenny, *Editors*

19 • **Quantitative Receptor Autoradiography,** Carl A. Boast, Elaine W. Snowhill, and C. Anthony Altar, *Editors*

20 • **Ion Channels in Neural Membranes,** J. Murdoch Ritchie, Richard D. Keynes, and Liana Bolis, *Editors*

21 • **PET and NMR: New Perspectives in Neuroimaging and in Clinical Neurochemistry,** Leontino Battistin and Franz Gerstenbrand, *Editors*

22 • **New Concepts in Cerebellar Neurobiology,** James King, *Editor*

23 • **The Vertebrate Neuromuscular Junction,** Miriam M. Salpeter, *Editor*

24 • **Excitatory Amino Acid Transmission,** T. Philip Hicks, David Lodge, and Hugh McLennan, *Editors*

25 • **Axonal Transport,** Richard S. Smith and Mark A. Bisby, *Editors*

26 • **Respiratory Muscles and Their Neuromotor Control,** Gary C. Sieck, Simon C. Gandevia, and William E. Cameron, *Editors*

27 • **Epilepsy and the Reticular Formation: The Role of the Reticular Core in Convulsive Seizures,** Gerhard H. Fromm, Carl L. Faingold, Ronald A. Browning, and W.M. Burnham, *Editors*

28 • **Inactivation of Hypersensitive Neurons,** N. Chalazonitis and Maurice Gola, *Editors*

29 • **Neuroplasticity, Learning, and Memory,** N.W. Milgram, Colin M. MacLeod, and Ted L. Petit, *Editors*

30 • **Effects of Injury on Trigeminal and Spinal Somatosensory Systems**, Lillian M. Pubols and Barry J. Sessle, *Editors*

31 • **Organization of the Autonomic Nervous System: Central and Peripheral Mechanisms**, Franco R. Calaresu, J. Ciriello, Canio Polosa, and Leo P. Renaud, *Editors*

EFFECTS OF INJURY ON TRIGEMINAL AND SPINAL SOMATOSENSORY SYSTEMS

EFFECTS OF INJURY ON TRIGEMINAL AND SPINAL SOMATOSENSORY SYSTEMS

Proceedings of a Satellite Symposium of the XXX Congress of the International Union of Physiological Sciences Held at Timberline Lodge, Oregon, July 20–23, 1986

Editors

Lillian M. Pubols

Neurological Sciences Institute
Good Samaritan Hospital
and Medical Center
Portland, Oregon

Barry J. Sessle

Faculty of Dentistry
University of Toronto
Ontario, Canada

ALAN R. LISS, INC., NEW YORK

Address all Inquiries to the Publisher
Alan R. Liss, Inc., 41 East 11th Street, New York, NY 10003

Printed in the United States of America

Library of Congress Cataloging-in-Publication Data

Effects of injury on trigeminal and spinal somatosensory systems.

(Neurology and neurobiology ; v. 30)
Includes bibliographies and index.
1. Senses and sensations—Research—Methodology. 2. Afferent pathways—Wounds and injuries—Animal models. 3. Trigeminal nerve—Wounds and injuries—Complications and sequelae. 4. Spinal cord—Wounds and injuries—Complications and sequelae. I. Pubols, Lillian M. II. Sessle, Barry J., 1941–
III. Series. [DNLM: 1. Peripheral Nerves—injuries. 2. Receptors, Sensory—injuries. 3. Spinal Cord Injuries. 4. Trigeminal Nerve—injuries.

W1 NE337B v.30 / WL 500 E27]
QP431.E35 1987 599′.0188 87-3173
ISBN 0-8451-2732-2

Contents

Contributors

A. Vania Apkarian, Department of Neurosurgery, SUNY Health Science Center, Syracuse, NY 13210 **[313,511,513]**

Jan Arvidsson, Department of Anatomy, Karolinska Institutet, Stockholm, Sweden **[143,159]**

Samir F. Atweh, Department of Internal Medicine, Faculty of Medicine, American University of Beirut, Beirut, Lebanon **[281]**

R. Baranowski, Department of Physiology, University College, London, England **[115]**

K.I. Baumann, Department of Physiology, Faculty of Medicine, The Chinese University of Hong Kong, Shatin, New Territories, Hong Kong **[29]**

Karen J. Berkley, Department of Psychology, Florida State University, Tallahassee, FL 32306-1051 **[429]**

Jean-Marie Besson, Unité de Recherches de Neurophysiologie Pharmacologique, INSERM U 161, Paris 75014, France **[331]**

Helmut Blumberg, Neurologische Klinik, Universität Freiburg, Freiburg 7800, Federal Republic of Germany **[85]**

James G. Broton, Faculty of Dentistry, University of Toronto, Toronto, Ontario, Canada **[189,525]**

Paul B. Brown, Department of Physiology, West Virginia University Medical Center, Morgantown, WV 26506 **[273,289,461]**

Michael J. Buckley, Department of Neurology, Northwestern University Medical School, Chicago, IL 60611 **[527]**

Elizabeth Bullitt, Departments of Physiology and Neurosurgery, University of North Carolina, Chapel Hill, NC 27514 **[499]**

Kim J. Burchiel, Department of Neurological Surgery, University of Washington, Veterans Administration Hospital, Seattle, WA 98108 **[77,485]**

Harold Burton, Departments of Anatomy and Neurobiology, Washington University School of Medicine, St. Louis, MO 63110 **[437]**

Margaret R. Byers, Department of Anesthesiology and Biological Structure, University of Washington, Seattle, WA 98195 **[3]**

James N. Campbell, Department of Neurosurgery, Johns Hopkins School of Medicine, Baltimore, MD 21205 **[383]**

The numbers in brackets are the opening page numbers of the contributors' articles.

Robert C. Canfield, Department of Restorative Dentistry, School of Dentistry, University of Washington, Seattle, WA 98195 **[151,509]**

Mary Carlson, Department of Psychiatry, Washington University School of Medicine, St. Louis, MO 63110 **[437]**

José Castro-Lopes, Institute of Histology and Embryology, Faculty of Medicine, Porto 4200, Portugal **[159]**

S.B. Cheng-Chew, Department of Physiology, Faculty of Medicine, The Chinese University of Hong Kong, Shatin, New Territories, Hong Kong **[29]**

Nicolas L. Chiaia, Department of Anatomy and Pediatrics, University of Medicine and Dentistry of New Jersey, Piscataway, NJ 08854 **[49]**

Eric H. Chudler, National Institute of Dental Research, National Institutes of Health, Bethesda, MD 20892 **[339]**

M. Cline, Department of Neurology, Good Samaritan Hospital and Medical Center, Portland, OR 97210 **[389]**

Richard E. Coggeshall, University of Texas Medical Branch, Marine Biomedical Institute, Galveston, TX 77550 **[69]**

Bruce A. Cohen, Department of Neurology, Northwestern University Medical School, Chicago, IL 60611 **[527]**

Antonio Coimbra, Institute of Histology and Embryology, Faculty of Medicine, Porto 4200, Portugal **[159]**

Brian Y. Cooper, Department of Neuroscience and Center for Neurobiological Sciences, University of Florida College of Medicine, Gainesville, FL 32610 **[419,517]**

Bert Csillik, Department of Anatomy, University Medical School, Szeged H-6701, Hungary **[175]**

Y. Dateoka, Department of Oral Anatomy, Oral-Maxillofacial Surgery, Hiroshima University School of Dentistry, Hiroshima, Japan **[501]**

Marshall Devor, Department of Zoology, Life Sciences Institute, Hebrew University of Jerusalem, Jerusalem 91904, Israel **[215]**

Jack Diamond, Department of Neurosciences, McMaster University, Hamilton, Ontario, Canada **[43]**

Willie K. Dong, Department of Anesthesiology, School of Medicine, University of Washington, Seattle, WA 98195 **[3,339]**

Jonathan O. Dostrovsky, Department of Physiology, Faculty of Medicine and Faculty of Dentistry, University of Toronto, Toronto, Ontario, Canada **[197]**

R. Dotson, Department of Neurology, Veterans Administration Medical Center, Portland, OR 97201 **[389]**

N. Fujitsuka, Department of Physiology, Nagoya University School of Medicine, Nagoya 466, Japan **[481]**

Michael E. Goldberger, Department of Anatomy, Medical College of Pennsylvania, Philadelphia, PA 19129 **[261,399]**

Kay-Michael Gottschaldt, Neurobiologie, Max-Planck-Institut für Biophysikalische Chemie, D-3400 Göttingen, Federal Republic of Germany **[487]**

Gunnar Grant, Department of Anatomy, Karolinska Institutet, Stockholm, Sweden **[159]**

Brian H. Hallas, Department of Neuroscience, New York College of Osteopathic Medicine, Old Westbury, NY 11568 **[205]**

W. Hamann, Department of Physiology, Faculty of Medicine, The Chinese University of Hong Kong, Shatin, New Territories, Hong Kong **[29]**

P.J. Hand, Department of Animal Biology, School of Veterinary Medicine, University of Pennsylvania, Philadelphia, PA 19104 **[371]**

H. Handwerker, II Physiological Institute, Universität Heidelberg, Heidelberg 1, Federal Republic of Germany **[477]**

Ronald L. Hayes, Department of Surgery, Medical College of Virginia, Virginia Commonwealth University, Richmond, VA 23298-0001 **[411]**

Michael A. Henry, Department of Oral Biology, University of Florida College of Dentistry, J. Hillis Miller Health Center, Gainesville, FL 32610 **[151,509]**

B. Heppelmann, Department of Physiology, University of Würzburg, Würzburg, Federal Republic of Germany **[19]**

M.K. Herbert, Department of Physiology, University of Würzburg, Würzburg, Federal Republic of Germany **[19]**

Paul R. Hess, Department of Anatomy and Pediatrics, University of Medicine and Dentistry of New Jersey, Piscataway, NJ 08854 **[49]**

Harumitsu Hirata, Neurological Sciences Institute, Good Samaritan Hospital and Medical Center, Portland, OR 97209 **[289]**

Charles J. Hodge, Jr., Department of Neurosurgery, SUNY Health Science Center, Syracuse, NY 13210 **[313,511,513]**

G. Rex Holland, Faculty of Dentistry, University of Alberta, Edmonton, Alberta, Canada **[11,493]**

James W. Hu, Department of Physiology, Faculty of Medicine and Faculty of Dentistry, University of Toronto, Toronto, Ontario, Canada **[189,197]**

Ainsley Iggo, Department of Preclinical Veterinary Sciences, University of Edinburgh, Edinburgh, Scotland **[133]**

F. Ito, Department of Physiology, Nagoya University, School of Medicine, Nagoya 466, Japan **[481]**

Hiroshi Itoga, Department of Physiology, Nihon University, School of Dentistry, Chiyoda-ku, Tokyo 101, Japan **[515,521]**

Koichi Iwata, Department of Physiology, Nihon University, School of Dentistry, Chiyoda-ku, Tokyo 101, Japan **[515,521]**

Suhayl J. Jabbur, Department of Physiology, Faculty of Medicine, American University of Beirut, Beirut, Lebanon **[281]**

Mark F. Jacquin, Department of Neuroscience, New York College of Osteopathic Medicine, Old Westbury, NY 11568 **[49,205,503]**

Wilfrid Jänig, Physiologisches Institut, Universität Kiel, Kiel D-2300, Federal Republic of Germany **[85]**

Chung-Bii Jenq, University of Texas Medical Branch, Marine Biomedical Institute, Galveston, TX 77550 **[69]**

Lonnie R. Johnson, Department of Surgical Dentistry, School of Dentistry, University of Colorado, Denver, CO 80262 **[151,509]**

M.W. Jones, Department of Neurosurgery, SUNY Health Science Center at Syracuse, Syracuse, NY 13210 **[513]**

Terrell E. Jones, Department of Anatomy, The Milton S. Hershey Medical Center, Pennsylvania State University, Hershey, PA 17033 **[61,479]**

S.L. Juliano, Department of Anatomy, USUHS, Bethesda, MD 20814 **[517]**

J.H. Kaas, Department of Psychology, Vanderbilt University, Nashville, TN 37240 **[347]**

Katherine Kalil, Department of Anatomy and Neurosciences, Training Program, University of Wisconsin, Madison, WI 53706 **[355,529]**

Yoichi Katayama, Department of Neurosurgery, Nihon University, Tokyo 173, Japan **[411]**

Yoriko Kawakami, Department of Anesthesiology, School of Medicine, University of Washington, Seattle, WA 98195 **[339]**

Joyce Keifer, Neurosciences Training Program and Department of Anatomy, University of Wisconsin, Madison, WI 53706 **[529]**

Andrew M. Kelahan, Department of Neurology, Northwestern University Medical School, Chicago, IL 60611 **[527]**

Herbert P. Killackey, Departments of Psychobiology and of Anatomy and Neurobiology, University of California, Irvine, CA 92717 **[363]**

Bradley G. Klein, Department of Neuroscience, New York College of Osteopathic Medicine, Old Westbury, NY 11568 **[49,205]**

H. Richard Koerber, Department of Neurobiology and Behavior, SUNY, Stony Brook, NY 11794 **[249,505]**

Gabriele-Monika Koschorke, Department of Physiology, University of Heidelberg, Heidelberg, Federal Republic of Germany **[93]**

Natsu Koyama, Department of Physiology, Medical College of Shiga, Seta, Otsu 520-21, Japan **[305]**

Harald Kräft, Neurobiologie, Max-Planck-Institut für Biophysikalische Chemie, D-3400 Göttingen, Federal Republic of Germany **[487]**

L. Kruger, Department of Anatomy, Brain Research Institute, UCLA School of Medicine, Los Angeles, CA 90024 **[297]**

Sally N. Lawson, Department of Physiology, The Medical School, University of Bristol, Bristol, England **[125]**

Yvonne Lenz, Faculty of Dentistry, University of Toronto, Toronto, Ontario, Canada **[189]**

Christiana M. Leonard, Department of Neuroscience and Center for Neurobiological Sciences, University of Florida College of Medicine, Gainesville, FL 32610 **[419]**

M.S. Leung, Department of Physiology, Faculty of Medicine, The Chinese University of Hong Kong, Shatin, New Territories, Hong Kong **[29,483]**

Alan R. Light, Department of Physiology, University of North Carolina at Chapel Hill, Chapel Hill, NC 27514 **[467]**

S.J.W. Lisney, Department of Physiology, The Medical School, University of Bristol, Bristol, England **[107]**

A. Low, Department of Physiology, Monash University, Clayton, Victoria 3168, Australia **[477]**

B. Lynn, Department of Physiology, University College, London, England **[115]**

W. Magerl, II Physiological Institute, Universität Heidelberg, Heidelberg 1, Federal Republic of Germany **[477]**

P. Marchettini, University of Milano, Milan, Italy **[389]**

Howard Markus, Department of Zoology, University of Toronto, Toronto, Ontario M5S 1A1, Canada **[507]**

Robert J. Martin, Department of Neurosurgery, SUNY Health Science Center, Syracuse, NY 13210 **[313]**

Steven Martini, Department of Neurosurgery, SUNY Health Science Center, Syracuse, NY 13210 **[313]**

Bruce Matthews, Department of Physiology, The Medical School, University of Bristol, Bristol, England **[11]**

P.A. McKinley, Department of Kinesiology, UCLA, Los Angeles, CA 90024 **[519]**

Lorne M. Mendell, Department of Neurobiology and Behavior, SUNY, Stony Brook, NY 11794 **[249,505]**

Richard A. Meyer, Applied Physics Laboratory, Johns Hopkins University, Laurel, MD 20707 **[383]**

D.E.R. Meyers, Laboratory of Neural Control, National Institutes of Health, Bethesda, MD 20205 **[227]**

Richard D. Mooney, Department of Anatomy and Pediatrics, University of Medicine and Dentistry of New Jersey, Piscataway, NJ 08854 **[49,503]**

Bryce L. Munger, Department of Anatomy, The Milton S. Hershey Medical Center, Pennsylvania State University, Hershey, PA 17033 **[61,479]**

Hiroyuki Muramatsu, Department of Physiology, Nihon University School of Dentistry, Chiyoda-ku, Tokyo 101 Japan **[515,521]**

Marion Murray, Department of Anatomy, Medical College of Pennsylvania, Philadelphia, PA 19129 **[261]**

Robert G. Nagele, Department of Anatomy and Pediatrics, University of Medicine and Dentistry of New Jersey, Piscataway, NJ 08854 **[49]**

Matti V. Närhi, Department of Physiology, University of Kuopio, Kuopio, Finland **[3]**

Yasuo Nishikawa, Department of Physiology, Medical College of Shiga, Seta, Otsu 520-21, Japan **[305]**

J. Ochoa, Department of Neurology, Good Samaritan Hospital and Medical Center, Portland, OR 97210 **[389]**

Edward R. Perl, Department of Physiology, School of Medicine, University of North Carolina, Chapel Hill, NC 27514 **[297,499]**

Marc Peschanski, Unité de Recherches de Neurophysiologie Pharmacologique, INSERM U 161, Paris 75014, France **[331]**

A. Pini, Department of Physiology, University College, London, England **[115]**

Bruce Pomeranz, Departments of Zoology and Physiology, University of Toronto, Toronto, Ontario, Canada **[239,507]**

A. Pratt, Department of Physiology, Monash University, Clayton, Victoria 3168, Australia **[477]**

Lillian M. Pubols, Neurological Sciences Institute, Good Samaritan Hospital and Medical Center, Portland, OR 97209 **[289]**

Srinivasa N. Raja, Department of Anesthesiology, Johns Hopkins School of Medicine, Baltimore, MD 21205 **[383]**

Diane D. Ralston, Department of Anatomy, University of California, San Francisco, CA 94143 **[321]**

Henry J. Ralston III, Department of Anatomy, University of California, San Francisco, CA 94143 **[321]**

D.D. Rasmusson, Department of Physiology and Biophysics, Dalhousie University, Halifax, Nova Scotia, Canada B3H 4H7 **[523]**

William E. Renehan, Department of Neuroscience, New York College of Osteopathic Medicine, Old Westbury, NY 11568 **[49,205,503]**

Robert W. Rhoades, Department of Anatomy and Pediatrics, University of Medicine and Dentistry of New Jersey, Piscataway, NJ 08854 **[49,503]**

Peter P. Robinson, Department of Physiology, Birmingham University Medical School, Birmingham, England **[11,489,493]**

J.P. Rosenfeld, Department of Psychology, Northwestern University, Evanston, IL 60201 **[525]**

Lisa C. Russell, Department of Neurological Surgery, University of Washington, Veterans Administration Hospital, Seattle, WA 98108 **[77,485]**

Nayef E. Saadé, Department of Natural Sciences, Faculty of Sciences, Lebanese University, Beirut, Lebanon **[281]**

Karl Sanders, Department of Physiology, University of Heidelberg, Heidelberg, Federal Republic of Germany **[93]**

H.-G. Schaible, Department of Physiology, University of Würzburg, Würzburg, Federal Republic of Germany **[19]**

S.-C. Scheu, National Yang-Ming Medical College, Taipei, Taiwan, Republic of China **[371]**

R.F. Schmidt, Department of Physiology, University of Würzburg, Würzburg, Federal Republic of Germany **[19]**

Barry J. Sessle, Department of Physiology, Faculty of Medicine and Faculty of Dentistry, University of Toronto, Toronto, Ontario, Canada **[189,197,451]**

Y. Shigenaga, Department of Oral Anatomy, Oral-Maxillofacial Surgery, Hiroshima University School of Dentistry, Hiroshima, Japan **[501]**

T. Shimosato, Department of Oral Anatomy, Oral-Maxillofacial Surgery, Hiroshima University School of Dentistry, Hiroshima, Japan **[501]**

Etsuo Shohara, Faculty of Dentistry, University of Toronto, Toronto, Ontario, Canada **[189]**

J.L. Smith, Department of Kinesiology, UCLA, Los Angeles, CA 90024 **[519]**

P.J. Snow, Department of Anatomy, University of Queensland, St. Lucia, Queensland 4067, Australia **[227]**

R.T. Stevens, Department of Neurosurgery, SUNY Health Science Center at Syracuse, Syracuse, NY 13210 **[511,513]**

William D. Stofer, Department of Physiology, University of Pittsburgh, Pittsburgh, PA 15261 **[499]**

Henry H. Stonnington, Department of Rehabilitation Medicine, Medical College of Virginia, Virginia Commonwealth University, Richmond, VA 23298-0001 **[411]**

Tomosada Sugimoto, 2nd Department of Oral Anatomy, Faculty of Dentistry, Osaka University, Osaka 565, Japan **[167]**

Rhyuji Sumino, Department of Physiology, Nihon University School of Dentistry, Chiyoda-ku, Tokyo 101, Japan **[515,521]**

Aiko Suzuki, Department of Physiology, Nihon University School of Dentistry, Chiyoda-ku, Tokyo 101, Japan **[521]**

L. Swyter, Department of Kinesiology, UCLA, Los Angeles, CA 90024 **[519]**

Ann Marie Szczepanik, Department of Anatomy and Pediatrics, University of Medicine and Dentistry of New Jersey, Piscataway, NJ 08854 **[49]**

J. Szolcsanyi, II Physiological Institute, Universität Heidelberg, Heidelberg 1, Federal Republic of Germany **[477]**

K. Tabuchi, Department of Oral Anatomy, Oral-Maxillofacial Surgery, Hiroshima University School of Dentistry, Hiroshima, Japan **[501]**

Julia K. Terzis, Microsurgical Research Department, Eastern Virginia Medical School, Norfolk, VA 23501 **[37,491]**

Richard J. Traub, Department of Neurobiology and Behavior, SUNY, Stony Brook, NY 11794 **[249]**

Y. Tsuiki, Department of Oral Anatomy, Oral-Maxillofacial Surgery, Hiroshima University School of Dentistry, Hiroshima, Japan **[501]**

K. Tsuru, Department of Oral Anatomy, Oral-Maxillofacial Surgery, Hiroshima University School of Dentistry, Hiroshima, Japan **[501]**

B.G. Turnbull, Department of Physiology and Biophysics, Dalhousie University, Halifax, Nova Scotia B3H 4H7, Canada **[491,523]**

Christiane Vahle-Hinz, Physiologisches Institut, Universität Würzburg, D-8700 Würzburg, Federal Republic of Germany **[487]**

Charles J. Vierck, Jr., Department of Neuroscience, College of Medicine, University of Florida, Gainesville, FL 32610 **[419,429,499,517]**

J.T. Wall, Department of Psychology, Vanderbilt University, Nashville, TN 37240 **[347]**

Susan Warren, Department of Psychiatry, Washington University School of Medicine, St. Louis, MO 63110 **[437]**

R.A. Westerman, Department of Physiology, Monash University, Clayton, Victoria 3168, Australia **[477,495]**

Lesnick E. Westrum, Department of Neurological Surgery, School of Medicine, University of Washington, Seattle, WA 98195 **[151,509]**

R. Widdop, Department of Pharmacology, Monash University, Clayton, Victoria 3168, Australia **[477]**

W.D. Willis, Marine Biomedical Institute, University of Texas Medical Branch, Galveston, TX 77550-2772 **[373]**

P. Wilson, Department of Anatomy, University of Queensland, St. Lucia, Queensland 4067, Australia **[227]**

Liang-Fang Wu, Department of Anatomy, Medical College of Pennsylvania, Philadelphia, PA 19129 **[261]**

Jan Ygge, Department of Anatomy, Karolinska Institutet, Stockholm, Sweden **[159]**

Toshikatsu Yokota, Department of Physiology, Medical College of Shiga, Seta, Otsu 520-21, Japan **[305]**

Manfred Zimmermann, Department of Physiology, University of Heidelberg, Heidelberg, Federal Republic of Germany **[93,495]**

Preface

This volume summarizes the proceedings of a satellite symposium of the XXXth Congress of the International Union of Physiological Sciences held at Timberline Lodge, Oregon from July 20 through 23, 1986. The symposium was jointly sponsored by the Oral Physiology Commission and Somatosensory Commission of the International Union of Physiological Sciences. It was organized to promote interaction between investigators working on the effects of injury to somatosensory systems representing the orofacial region (trigeminal systems), and their counterparts working on systems representing other body regions (spinal systems), and to facilitate the application of research in this area to clinical situations. Presentations at this meeting, while focussing upon somatosensory systems, dealt with the broad themes of peripheral and central neural regeneration, pathophysiological effects of injury to the nervous system, and mechanisms underlying recovery and alteration of function following such injury. The program consisted of four sessions involving slide presentations, two workshops, and one poster session. The first three slide sessions on morphological and physiological studies were organized by anatomical levels, with trigeminal-related and spinal-related lectures intermingled within each session. The final slide session dealt specifically with Pathophysiology and Behavior, but all participants were encouraged to relate their findings to clinical and pathophysiological phenomena.

The program was designed to encourage discussion of controversies and gaps in our knowledge. Ample time was allotted for discussion, and slide session chairmen were asked to provide critical summaries of the discussions. These summaries appear at the end of each of the first four sections of this volume. The two concurrent workshops dealt with Mechanisms of Plasticity, and New Methodologies and Future Directions. The first topic is the source of many of the controversies in the field. The second relates to ways in which these and other controversies might be resolved, and gaps in knowledge filled. The workshop chairmen have summarized for this volume the informal presentations and discussions which took place in the workshops.

A special effort was made to involve new investigators in this symposium, as a means of promoting their interest in the field. New investigators were invited to present poster demonstrations of their work. The poster abstracts are reprinted in the final section of this volume.

In keeping with the spirit of free and open exchange which prevailed at the symposium, the contributions to the proceedings have not been subjected to external scientific review. However, the slide session and workshop chairmen have summarized the discussions in detail, and have added their own evaluative comments. The reader should take careful note of these summaries, and should exercise critical judgement concerning strengths and weaknesses of individual claims and conclusions.

The editors would like to thank Dr. Ainsley Iggo and Dr. Ronald Dubner, chairmen of the Somatosensory Commission and the Oral Physiology Commission of IUPS, respectively, for inviting us to organize this symposium. We gratefully acknowledge financial support for the symposium from the Somatosensory Commission of IUPS, from the Good Samaritan Hospital and Medical Center, and from the National Institute of Dental Research of the U.S. National Institutes of Health (Grant # 1 R13 DEO7843). We wish to express our deep appreciation to Dr. Patricia Bryant of the National Institute of Dental Research, and to Dr. Christine Phillips of the National Institute of Neurological and Communicative Disorders and Stroke for their advice and encouragement in planning this symposium. We would also like to acknowledge the outstanding secretarial and technical help of Joyce Gregory, Sue Dawson, Maggie Zimet, Jackie Bolen, Rod Iwata, and Lynn Simmons, and the assistance during the conference of Cecelia Yu, Sherry Provencal, Dr. Harumitsu Hirata, and Dr. Benjamin H. Pubols, Jr.

Lillian M. Pubols
Barry J. Sessle

I
RECEPTORS AND PERIPHERAL NERVE

Effects of Injury on Trigeminal and Spinal Somatosensory Systems, pages 3–10

RESPONSE OF DENTAL SENSORY RECEPTORS TO INJURY OF DENTIN AND PULP

Margaret R. Byers, Matti V. Närhi, Willie K. Dong

Dept. of Anesthesiology, (M.R.B., W.K.D.) and Biol. Structure (M.R.B.), Univ. of Washington, Seattle, WA, 98195, USA; Dept. of Physiol. (M.V.N.), University of Kuopio, SF70211, Finland

INTRODUCTION

Numerous studies have shown that the pulp-dentin border area of tooth cusps contains many trigeminal somatosensory receptors, which form plexuses of free endings in peripheral pulp and which can extend free nerve fibers 100-150 µm into dentinal tubules (for review: Fearnhead, 1961; Frank, 1968; Byers, 1984). Recent work suggests that the myelinated fibers in teeth innervate dentin and cause sharp pain sensations, whereas the unmyelinated C-fibers primarily innervate pulp and cause dull ache sensations (Närhi et al, 1982; Närhi, 1985 a,b; Trowbridge, 1985). In addition, the fastest conducting fibers from teeth are A-beta mechanoreceptors which may be specialized to detect high frequency vibration at non-noxious intensities (Dong et al, 1985).

We have studied the effects of drilling and drying dentinal cavities on the structure of somatosensory receptors in pulp and dentin, using autoradiographic labeling techniques in adult dogs and rats. Previous studies in human teeth by Brännström have shown that when dentin cavities are drilled and air dried, the underlying pulp is disrupted and odontoblasts are aspirated into dentin (Brännström, 1963, 1981). In an electron microscopic study, some nerve fibers were found to be pulled 100 µm farther into dentin than normal (Lilja et al., 1982); however, these changes did not necessarily alter the sensitivity of dentin (Brännström and Astrom, 1964).

In order to investigate further the acute reactions to dentin injury, we have drilled and stimulated dentin of adult dog and rat teeth in which the trigeminal somatosensory receptors were already labeled by 24 hours axonal transport of ^{3}H-protein. Chronic reactions of the nerve fibers were studied at 5-7 days after injury to rat molars in which the nerve fibers were labeled during the last 24 hours. In some of the rat molars that had been injured for 5-7 days, there was formation of new reparative dentin or various degrees of pulpal inflammation; in these teeth we could thus study neural reactions to pathological pulp reactions, as well as to dentin injury. Preliminary reports of this work have been presented (Byers and Närhi, 1986; Närhi, et al, 1986).

METHODS

The methods for this work are explained in detail elsewhere (Byers, 1980; Byers and Dong, 1983; Byers et al., 1986). Briefly, cavities were drilled to varying depths in dentin, acid etched to open the dentin tubules, air dried for 15-60 seconds, and covered with resin. Dentin was injured just prior to fixation, or 5-7 days earlier. In two anesthetized dogs (15-20 kg) and 14 adult rats (350-400 g), one trigeminal ganglion was exposed by hemidecerebration, and concentrated (10-25 µCi/µl) ^{3}H-proline plus ^{3}H-leucine (Amersham) was injected at several sites in the maxillary and mandibular divisions. After 24 hours of axonal transport, the animals were anesthetized and perfused with aldehyde fixative. Excised teeth were decalcified and processed for LM-autoradiography or EM-autoradiography by standard procedures.

RESULTS

The acute reaction of somatosensory receptors to dentin injury was greater for deeper than for shallow cavities. In dog teeth, some labeled nerve endings were pulled away from their normal innervation zone as far as 1.0 mm into dentin. Less than 50% of the normal dentinal innervation remained (Fig. 1), and most of the aspirated nerve fibers and pulp cells accumulated as debris at the base of the cavity. The dentin exposure and drying had more extensive effects on rat molars due to their small size and thin dentin. Cavities that came close to pulp caused loss of innervation, dispersion of labeled debris and pulp disruption (Fig. 2A-B). Shallower cavities pulled odontoblasts and labeled nerves partway into dentin, with odontoblasts moving farther and more easily (Fig. 2C-D). Nerve fibers that were only pulled 100 µm farther into dentin than normal often survived and could be labeled by axonal transport 5-7 days later.

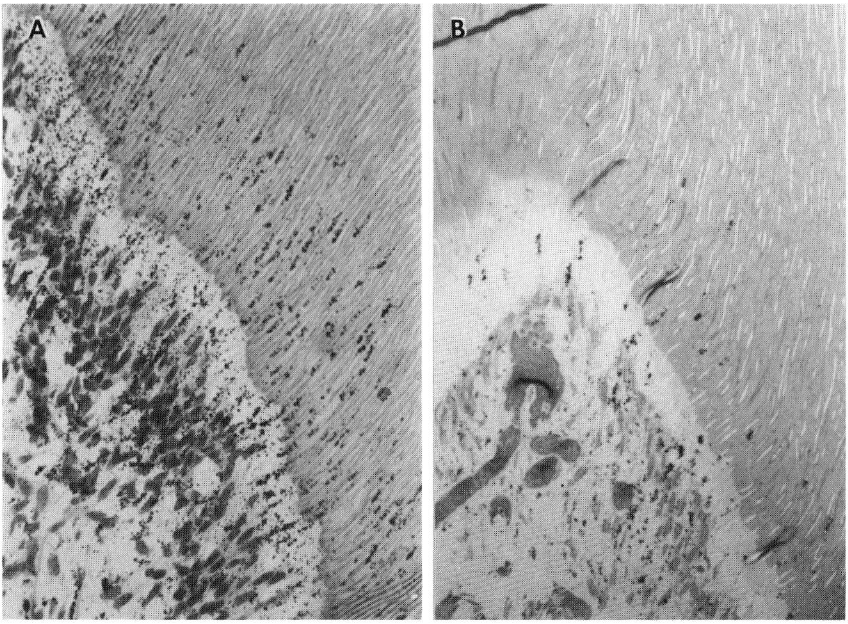

Figure 1. Dog teeth: acute reaction. A. Normal innervation. B. Dentinal innervation has been aspirated away from inner dentin and the pulp is disrupted at the cusp tip. 260x.

In 4 of 9 rat molars injured 5-7 days earlier, new reparative dentin had formed under the cavity sealing off exposed dentin. The labeled nerve fibers had relocated to form dense dentinal arbors in the uninjured mid-crown areas (Fig. 3).

In 3 of 9 rat molars injured 5-7 days earlier, pulpal inflammation was extensive, filling the affected cusp in two cases, and most of the tooth in the third. Labeled sensory fibers were absent from dentin and pulp near necrotic and severely inflammed pulp, but in moderately inflamed areas, labeled pulpal innervation could be found (Fig. 4). The apparent neural retraction away from inflamed cusps did not produce relocation to surviving root dentin; relocation to dentin was only found when some normal coronal areas remained.

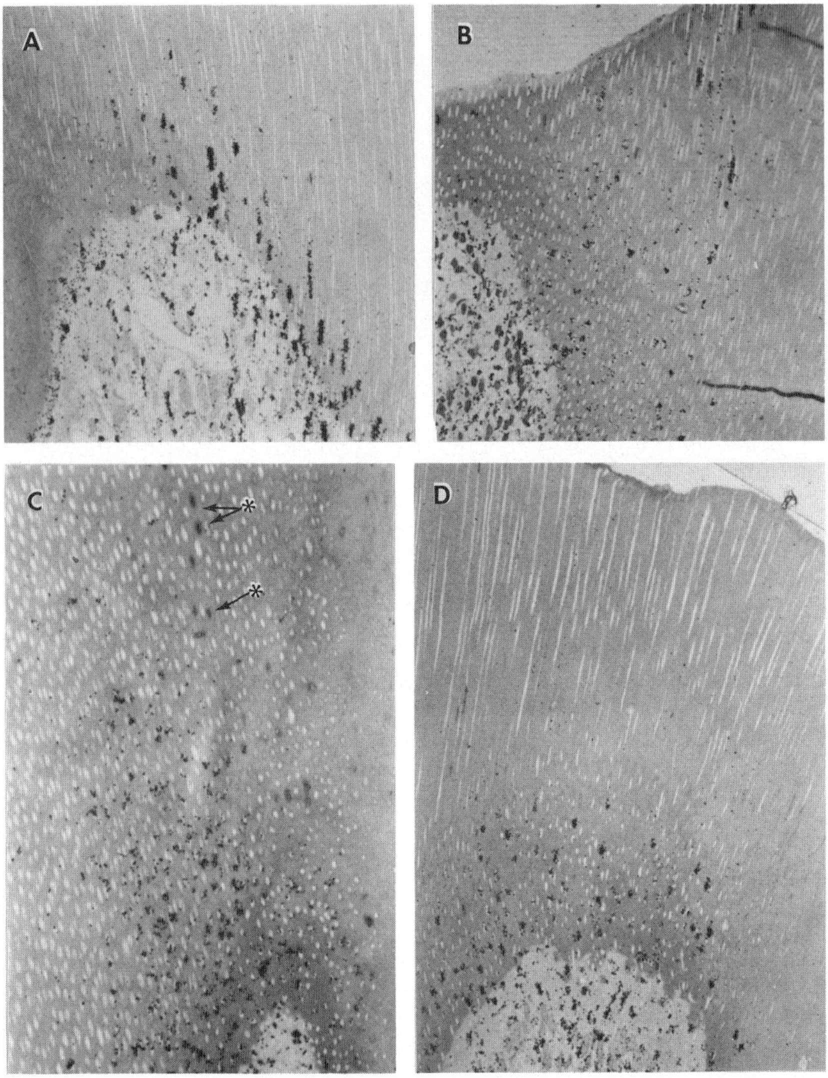

Figure 2. Rat molar: acute reaction. A. Normal innervation. B. Deep acute cavity with movement of label far into dentin. C. Shallow acute cavity with odontoblast nuclei (*) aspirated farther into dentin than nerve label. D. Control molar drilled after fixation, with no movement of pulp cells or nerve label. 260x.

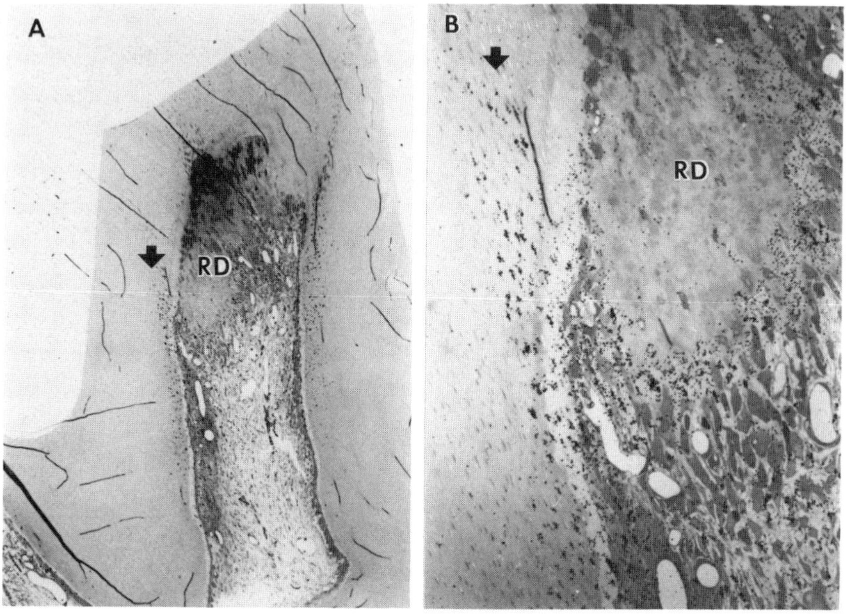

Figure 3. Rat molar cusp drilled 7 days before fixation. Reparative dentin (RD) has formed to seal off a damaged pulp zone (dark stain, *). The sensory innervation of dentin (arrow) has been lost from the affected cusp tip and relocated to mid-crown areas. A: 55x B: 260x.

DISCUSSION

We have shown that injury of dentin causes aspiration and loss of somatosensory receptors in the underlying dentin and adjacent pulp. If aspiration is gentle, some nerve fibers survive and are found farther into dentin. Shallow cavities caused much less damage than deep ones, and might only have affected fast-conducting sensory neurons that end in dentin and not the pulpal C-fibers. For deep cavities, many more nerve endings were damaged and the peripheral pulp was also affected. Specific labeling of normal or surviving nerve fibers was confirmed by EM-autoradiography.

Odontoblasts responded to deep dentinal injury by making reparative dentin. Consequently, surviving axons were blocked from reinnervating their original receptive field. The axons responded to this loss of target tissue by regenerating into neighboring intact dentin. When reparative dentin formation was

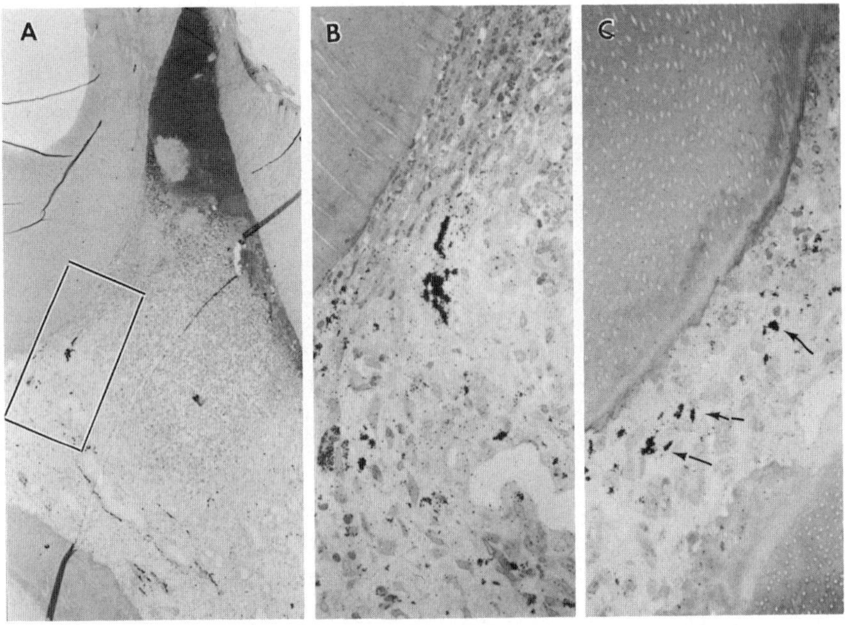

Figure 4. Rat molar cusp drilled 7 days before fixation. Entire cusp is filled with necrotic and inflamed tissue; A&B. Labeled fibers are only in pulp below affected cusp. C. Mild inflammation: some labeled fibers (arrows) remain in pulp. A: 55x B&C: 260x.

extensive, this relocation of regenerating fibers resulted in innervation of cervical coronal dentin (normally innervated sparsely) but not root dentin.

Earlier studies of nerve regeneration into denervated rat molars found that reinnervation of pulp and cusp dentin had begun within 6-7 days after transsection of the inferior alveolar nerve (Berger et al., 1983; Berger and Byers, 1983). Thus, by one week after injury to nerve fibers in dentin and coronal pulp, much regeneration will have occurred. When inflammation was present, dentinal innervation was missing from mildly and severely affected regions, whereas some pulp innervation remained in areas of mild inflammation. This neural pattern is interesting considering the hypersensitivity that inflammation can induce.

Neural regeneration involves different metabolic and axonal transport mechanisms than does normal maintenance of nerve endings

(McDougal, 1984). It is likely that the loss of receptor arbors due to injury or inflammation and their regeneration demonstrated here would cause metabolic changes in the sensory perikaryon. Such changes might also affect the central nerve terminals, as suggested by the altered morphology of CNS terminals of primary afferents following tooth extraction in cats (Johnson et al., 1983), or peripheral nerve injury (Aldskogius et al, 1985). However, the extent to which the tooth injuries described here may affect the CNS has not yet been determined. During normal aging in rats, relocation of sensory fibers to deeper coronal zones is found, apparently in response to the slow erosion of molar crowns with induced reparative dentin formation (Byers et al, 1982). Whether such normal alterations in peripheral dental innervation affect the CNS also remains to be studied.

Acknowledgement: We thank Kelly Mecifi, Laurie Maechler, Dianne Calkins, Marie Doman, and Carol Rubenstein for expert technical help. Supported by NIH grants DE00099, DE05159, DE05130, and Academia Finland.

REFERENCES

Aldskogius H, Arvidsson J and Grant G (1985). The reaction of primary sensory neurons to peripheral nerve injury with particular emphasis on transganglionic changes. Brain Res. Rev. 10:27-46.

Berger RL, Byers MR and Calkins DF (1983). Dental nerve regeneration in rats. I. Electrophysiological studies of molar sensory deficit and recovery. Pain 15:345-357.

Berger RL and Byers MR (1983). Dental nerve regeneration in rats II. Autoradiographic studies of nerve regeneration to molar pulp and dentin. Pain 15:359-375.

Brännström M (1963). Dentin sensitivity and aspiration of odontoblasts. J. Am. Dent. Assoc. 66:366-370.

Brännström M (1981). "Dentin and Pulp in Restorative Dentistry." Dental Therapeutics AB, Nacka, Sweden.

Brännström M and Astrom, A (1964). A study in the mechanism of pain elicited from the dentin. J. Dent. Res. 43:619-625.

Byers MR (1980). Development of sensory innervation in dentin. J. Comp. Neurol. 191:413-427.

Byers MR (1984). Dental sensory receptors. Int. Rev. Neurobiol. 25:39-94.

Byers MR and Dong WK (1983). Autoradiographic location of sensory nerve endings in dentin of monkey teeth. Anat. Rec. 205:441-454.

Byers MR and Närhi MV (1986). Acute and chronic cavities alter rat tooth odontoblasts and innervation J. Dent. Res. 65:726.

Byers MR, Gerlach RS and Berger RL (1982). Development of sensory receptor structure and function in rat molars. In. "Anatomical, Physiological and Pharmacological Aspects of Trigeminal Pain" (B. Matthews and R. Hill, Eds). Experta Medica, Amsterdam, pp. 15-26.

Byers MR, Närhi MV and Dong WK (1986). Sensory innervation of pulp and dentin of adult dog teeth demmonstrated by autoradiography: comparison of coronal, cervical, intercuspal, septal, radicular and reparative dentin. Submitted to Anat. Rec.

Dong WK, Chudler EH and Martin RF (1985). Physiological properties of intradental mechanoreceptors. Brain Res. 334:389-395.

Fearnhead RW (1961). The neurohistology of human teeth. Proc, R. Soc. Med., 54:877-884.

Frank RM (1968). Ultrastructural relationship between the odontoblast, its process, and the nerve fibre. In "Dentine and Pulp: Their Structure and Reactions" (N.B.B. Symons, Ed.). Livingstone, Edinburgh, pp. 115-146.

Johnson LR, Westrum LE and Canfield RC (1983). Ultrastructural study of transganglionic degeneration following dental lesions. Exp. Brain Res. 52:226-234.

Lilja J, Nordenvall K-J, and Brännström M (1982). Dentin sensitivity, odontoblasts and nerves under desiccated or infected experimental cavities. Swedish Dent. J. 6:93-103.

McDougal DB (1984). Transport of transmitter-related enzymes: changes after injury. In. "Axonal Transport in Neuronal Growth and Regeneration" (J. Elum and P. Cancalon, Eds.). Plenum, New York, pp. 105-118.

Närhi MV (1985a). Dentin sensitivity: a review. J. Biol. Buccale 13:75-96.

Närhi MV (1985b). The characteristics of intradental sensory units and their responses to stimulation. J. Dent. Res. 64:564-571.

Närhi M, Jyväsjärvi E, Hirvonen, T and Houpaniemi, T (1982). Activation of heat-sensitive nerve fibres in the dental pulp of the cat. Pain 14:317-326.

Närhi MV, Byers MR and Dong WK (1986). Effects of dentinal stimulation on morphology of dog intradental nerves. J. Dent. Res. 65:726.

Trowbridge HO (1985). Intradental sensory units: Physiological and clinical aspects. J. Endo. 11:489-498.

Effects of Injury on Trigeminal and Spinal Somatosensory Systems, pages 11–18

REINNERVATION OF DENTINE FOLLOWING PERIPHERAL NERVE SECTION IN THE CAT

Bruce Matthews, G. Rex Holland, and Peter P. Robinson

Dept. of Physiology, Univ. of Bristol, England
Faculty of Dentistry, Univ. of Alberta, Canada
Dept. of Physiology, Univ. of Birmingham, England

INTRODUCTION

The experiments to be described, which are in progress, are being carried out to identify at the ultrastructural level the nerves in dentine, determine if these nerves are part of the receptor system which responds to mechanical stimulation of dentine, and establish whether denervated dentine can become reinnervated.

The tubules in both human and cat dentine appear to contain no vital cellular material in the outer half to two-thirds of their length (reviews: Holland, 1985; Matthews, 1985). In the inner dentine, many tubules contain a single process which fills the tubule and has a simple internal structure, the only prominent organelles being microtubules and microfilaments. These processes are assumed to be extensions of the odontoblast cells which line the pulpal surface of the dentine (Holland, 1985). Other tubules in the inner dentine have one or more smaller processes in addition to an odontoblast process. Some of these smaller processes have a similar ultrastructural appearance to that of the odontoblast processes, but others contain mitochondria and/or microvesicles (Holland, 1981). It is known from the light microscope studies of Fearnhead (1957, 1961), that dentine contains some nerve terminals and it has therefore been assumed that some of the small processes seen in the electronmicroscope are the terminals of nerves. None of the cell processes in dentine is associated with a Schwann cell or a myelin sheath.

Labelled leucine and proline injected into the trigeminal ganglion of rats, cats and monkeys are transported along axons to the inner dentine, where EM autoradiography indicates that the labelled material is associated with some of the small processes in the tubules (Byers, 1977; Byers and Dong, 1983), thus providing further evidence that these are nerves. However, it is not known for how long after injection the labelled material is confined to nerves, and the possibility that it might have entered other cells secondarily cannot be excluded.

Denervation of the teeth has been used in an attempt to identifiy the nerves in cat dentine. Arwill et al. (1973) found no small processes in the dentinal tubules of teeth 2-4 weeks after denervation but they did not record the numbers of tubules or the precise areas of the dentine which they examined and since some areas of normal dentine contain no small processes (Holland, 1981), the significance of their result is in doubt, particularly since Frank et al. (1972) found small processes two months after denervation.

The sensitivity of dentine to stimulation in man and certain experimental animals (Matthews, 1985) suggests that it is innervated although the lack of cellular material in the outer ends of the tubules suggests that there must be some intermediate step between stimulus and receptor which is involved in the transduction mechanism.

A report on the results of part of this study has been published (Holland et al., 1986).

METHODS

The left inferior alveolar nerve was sectioned at the level of the anterior border of the masseter muscle in nine young adult cats. The cut ends of the nerves were carefully replaced in apposition. Two animals were allowed to recover for 56 hours, one each for 4, 5, 7 and 9 weeks and the remaining 3 for 12 weeks.

At the ends of these periods, the animals were re-anaesthetized, electrophysiological experiments were carried out, and they were perfused for electronmicroscopy.

In most of the animals, the threshold of the jaw-opening reflex to stimulation of the pulp of the denervated canine was determined and compound action potentials were recorded both from the inferior alveolar nerve central to the site of section during electrical stimulation of the denervated canine, and from the tooth during stimulation of the nerve. The tip (0.5mm) of the canine was removed with a bur and the exposed dentine was etched with acid to ensure that the ends of the tubules were unblocked. A cap was cemented over the tip of the tooth. The cap contained a Ag/AgCl electrode which, together with a similar electrode in a cavity near the neck of the tooth was used both for stimulating and for recording from nerves in the teeth (Kollmann and Matthews, 1982). It was also used to keep the exposed dentine covered with Ringer. Responses can be recorded from normal teeth with such electrodes during mechanical stimulation of the exposed dentine with a smooth glass probe (tip diam. 0.5mm) under Ringer.

At 12 weeks, recordings were also made from single fibres dissected from the nerve central to the original lesion. Recordings were made during the application of a variety of different stimuli but only the responses to mechanical stimulation will be considered here. The methods used were similar to those described previously.

The head of each animal was perfused through the carotids with 5% glutaraldehyde in phosphate buffer containing 2.7% dextran, and post-fixed in 5% glutaraldehyde overnight. Both the lower canine teeth were removed, the tooth on the unoperated side acting as control. They were decalcified in a solution of 4% EDTA with 1% glutaraldehyde. Only the teeth from the 56 hour and 12 week animals have been examined at present. The crowns of these teeth were cut transversely into 1mm thick discs with a razor blade and the discs osmicated and embedded in Araldite. Sections of the dentine were cut at right angles to the long axis of the tubules, stained with uranyl acetate and lead citrate, and examined in the electron microscope. Each section was related in position to the tip of the pulp. The number of processes in each of a sample of tubules in the predentine and adjacent calcified dentine was counted.

RESULTS

Electrophysiology

Compound action potentials could not be recorded from a denervated tooth during stimulation of the inferior alveolar nerve central to the lesion, or vice versa, until 5 weeks after denervation. This was also the first time that a jaw opening reflex could be elicited by stimulating the same tooth.

Responses to mechanical stimulation of the dentine were recorded from the tooth electrodes 12 weeks after denervation but not earlier. Also at 12 weeks, 2 of 38 single pulpal units which were isolated from the inferior alveolar nerve central to the original lesion, responded to mechanical stimulation. In both cases, each action potential recorded from the nerve filament corresponded with a unitary potential in the tooth record.

Histology

All the tubules in the predentine of control teeth contained at least one process and those with multiple processes contained one large process and one or more smaller processes. An example of such a tubule in calcified dentine is shown in Fig. 1. The proportion of tubules in the predentine with more than one process varied according to the region of the tooth from which the sample was taken. It was highest in the predentine at the level of the pulp cornu, where it was approximately 83% (range: 58.2 to 93.5% in individual animals) and fell progressively down the side of the crown to 6.5% (range: 0 - 19.1%) 3mm below the tip of the pulp. Below this level tubules vary rarely have more than one process.

Fifty six hours after nerve section, all but a very small proportion of the tubules in the predentine contained just one large process. The few small, secondary processes which survived were all in one tooth. Some tubules contained unrecognizable extracellular debris, which was assumed to be from degenerating secondary processes.

After 12 weeks, large numbers of tubules in the pre

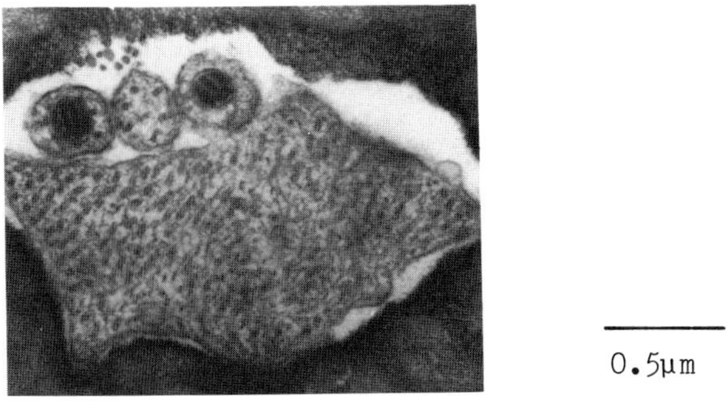

Fig.1 A tubule containing multiple processes from the calcified dentine of a control tooth.

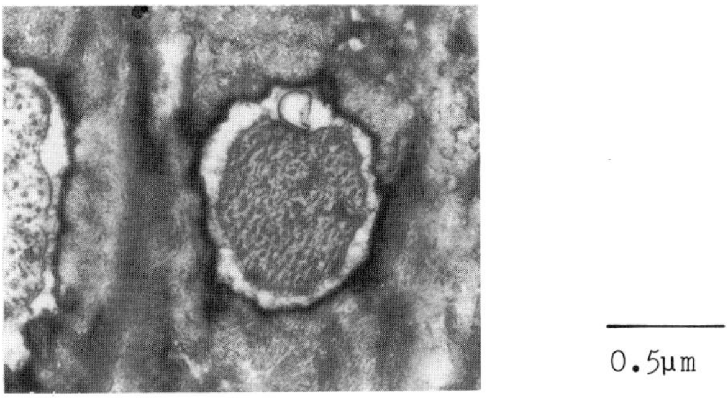

Fig.2 A tubule from the calcified dentine of a tooth which was denervated 56 hours previously.

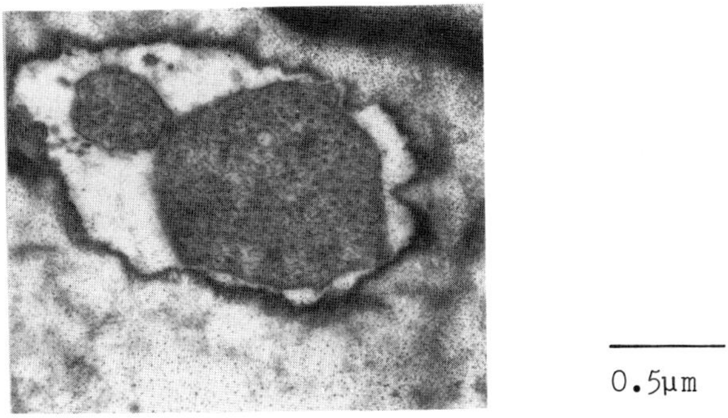

Fig.3 A tubule from the calcified dentine of a tooth that was denervated 12 weeks previously.

dentine (21%, 55% and 46% in the 3 teeth) again had more than one process in them, although fewer than in the control teeth. As in the control teeth, the proportion became less the further down the crown the samples were taken and was 0 in two of the three teeth 3mm below the pulp cornu.

In the calcified dentine, none of the tubules sectioned 100µm above the level of the pulp cornu in control teeth had more than one process. This was in contrast to the very high proportion in the pre-dentine just below this level and shows that the secondary processes extend no more than 100µm into the dentine in this region. In sections taken lower down the tooth, where some of the tubules would have been sectioned less than 100µm from the pulp, the proportion of the tubules with at least one process which had more than one in them (Fig. 1), fell from 37% at the level of the pulp cornu to 1% 3mm lower down the tooth.

In a sample of tubules from calcified dentine in teeth that had been denervated 56 hours previously, 6390 tubules had only one process (Fig. 2) and just one (near the pulp cornu) had two. The proportion had increased 12 weeks after denervation: at the level of the pulp cornu the corresponding figures were 1085 and 108, and 3mm lower down the crown, 584 and 6. Fig. 3 shows an example of a tubule with more than one process 12 weeks after denervation.

DISCUSSION

The histological observations agree with the findings of Arwill et al. (1973) and provide strong evidence that all the small processes in dentinal tubules are nerves.

The only other explanation for the disappearance of the small processes 56 hours after denervation could be that there was a rapid loss of some other type of cell due to the removal of a trophic effect. Although there is evidence for the loss of around 25% of taste buds 2 days after denervation (State and Dessouky, 1977) and of Merkel cells from cutaneous tactile corpuscles after 4 days (English et al., 1983), some Merkel cells show only minor ultrastructural changes after 48 hours (Palmer, 1965). There appears to be little evidence on the detailed ultrastructural changes which take place in nerve terminals and associated cells in the first 2 days after denervation but it seems unlikely that cell processes other than of nerves could have been lost so completely after 56 hours. The few small processes that remained can be accounted for by the small proportion of nerves in cat tooth pulp that are derived from sources other than the inferior alveolar nerve (Robinson, 1980).

The small processes were distributed unevenly in the dentine of normally innervated teeth; extending no more than 100μm into the tubules and being confined mostly to the region close to the cornu of the pulp. This is similar to the distribution of labelled leucine and proline transported axonally from the trigeminal ganglion in the cat (Byers and Matthews, 1981).

Twelve weeks after denervation, nerve terminals had re-entered many of the tubules. Furthermore, their distribution was very similar to that in normal teeth. Thus, if the target tissue has a role in regulating the regeneration or sprouting of nerves, it seems that the odontoblast, which is the only other cell in the dentine, must play a part in that mechanism and there may be differences in this respect between the odontoblasts in different regions of the tooth. Since there are no Schwann cells around the terminal 100-200μm of these nerves in the outer pulp and the dentinal tubules, the last stage of their regeneration will not have been guided by these cells.

The results suggest that the return of the responses of the nerves to mechanical stimulation may coincide with the arrival of the regenerating nerve terminals in the tubules, but the data on this is as yet incomplete.

ACKNOWLEDGEMENT

Supported by the Medical Research Council.

REFERENCES

Arwill T, Edwall L, Lilja J, Olgart L, Svensson,S-E (1973). Ultrastructure of nerves in the dentinal-pulp border zone after sensory nerve and autonomic nerve transection in the cat. Acta odont scand 31:273-281.

Byers MR (1977) Fine structure of trigeminal receptors in rat molars. In Anderson DJ, Matthews B (eds): "Pain in the Trigeminal Region," Amsterdam: Elsevier/North Holland, pp. 13-24.

Byers MR, Dong WK (1983). Autoradiographic location of sensory nerve endings in dentin of monkey teeth. Anat Rec 205:441-454.

Byers MR, Matthews B (1981). Autoradiographic demonstration of ipsilateral and contralateral sensory nerve endings in cat dentin, pulp and periodontium. Anat Rec 201:249-260.

English KB, Kavka-Van Norman D, Horch K. (1983). The effects of chronic denervation in type I cutaneous mechanoreceptors (Haarscheiben). Anat Rec 207:79-88.

Fearnhead RW (1957). Histological evidence for the innervation of human dentine. J Anat 91:267-277.

Fearnhead RW (1961). The neurohistology of human dentine. Proc Roy Soc Med 54:877-884.

Frank RM, Sauvage C, Frank P. (1972). Morphological basis of dental sensitivity. Int dent J 22:1-19.

Holland GR (1981). The incidence of dentinal tubules containing more than one process in the cuspal dentin of cat canine teeth. Anat Rec 200:437-442.

Holland GR (1985). The odontoblast process: form and function. J dent Res 64(spec. issue):499-514.

Holland GR, Matthews B, Robinson PP (1986). An electrophysiological and morphological study of the innervation and reinnervation of cat dentine. J Physiol (in press).

Kollmann W, Matthews B (1982). Responses of intradental nerves to thermal stimulation of teeth in the cat. In Matthews B, Hill RG (eds): "Anatomical, Physiological and Pharmacological Aspects of Trigeminal Pain," Amsterdam: Excerpta Medica, pp. 51-65.

Matthews B (1985). Peripheral and central aspects of trigeminal nociceptive systems. Phil Trans Roy Soc B 308:313-324.

Palmer P (1965) Ultrastructural alterations of Merkel cells following denervation. Anat Rec 151:396-397.

Robinson PP (1980) An electrophysiological study of the pathways of pulpal nerves from mandibular teeth in the cat. Archs oral Biol 25:825-829.

State FA, Dessouky HI (1977) Effect of length of distal stump of transected nerve upon the rate of degeneration of taste buds. Acta Anat 98:353-360.

Effects of Injury on Trigeminal and Spinal Somatosensory Systems,
pages 19–27

MORPHOLOGICAL AND PHYSIOLOGICAL CHARACTERISTICS OF THE INNERVATION OF CAT'S NORMAL AND ARTHRITIC KNEE JOINT.

B. Heppelmann, M.K. Herbert, H.-G. Schaible, R.F. Schmidt

Department of Physiology, University of Würzburg, Röntgenring 9, D-87 Würzburg, FRG

I Morphology of the innervation of the knee joint.

Articular nerves. The knee of the cat is mainly supplied by the medial (MAN) and posterior (PAN) articular nerves. The MAN contains some 200 myelinated and 450 unmyelinated afferents plus 500 unmyelinated efferents. The PAN is composed of about 270 myelinated afferents, 410 unmyelinated afferent and 520 unmyelinated efferent units (Langford and Schmidt 1983). The distribution of the diameters of the myelinated afferents in MAN is unimodal ranging from 1 to 14 um with a maximum at 3 to 4 um (Fig. 1B). In the PAN the distribution of the diameters of myelinated fibres is bimodal with maxima at 3 to 4 um and 8 to 9 um (Fig. 1C). The distribution of the diameters of unmyelinated units in MAN is unimodal in the range from 0.1 um to 1.4 um (Fig.1A). Thus the majority of the afferent units in joint nerves are fine myelinated and unmyelinated terminating in "free nerve endings".

Receptive endings. An effort is made to reconstruct the terminations of the articular fine afferents, using electron microscopy. The example shown after in Fig. 1D is one of the terminals of a fine myelinated unit whose diameter in the last myelinated segment was about 2 µm. The fiber became unmyelinated and lost its perineural sheath after 8 µm. The fiber ran parallel to the long axis of a small venous vessel, and split up into 4 branches. All terminations were located in the connective tissue surrounding blood vessels. One ending was found beneath a fat cell. The distance to the blood vessels varied between 1 and 30 µm. The axons were incompletely surrounded by Schwann cells, so that in places the axon terminals were covered only by basal lamina. All terminals contained clusters of mitochondria, clear and dense core vesicles. The terminal region expanded to about 4 µm in length and 2 µm in diameter.

II Physiology of the innervation of the knee joint.

1) Mechanosensitivity of afferent fibres from normal and inflamed joints.

The response properties of single fine afferent units in MAN and PAN were studied (for Methods and literature see Schaible and Schmidt, 1983a,

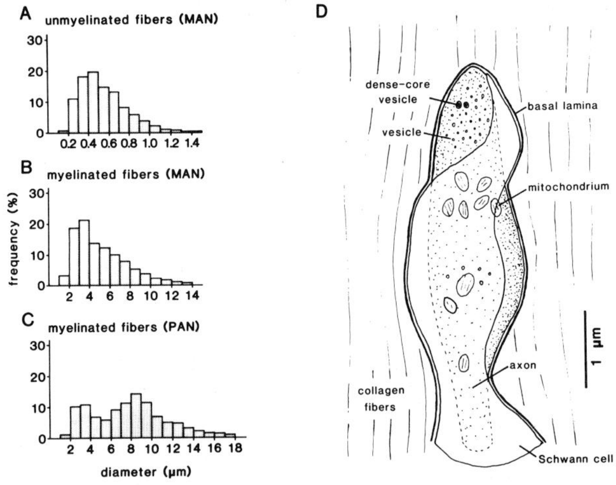

Figure 1. A-C: Diameter distribution of the axons in MAN and PAN. D: Reconstruction of a group III fiber ending.

1983b, 1984, 1985). Emphasis was on the changes in discharge behaviour induced by an acute experimental arthritis. In normal joints the population of afferents is composed of units with different mechanosensitivities. It ranges from responsiveness to innocuous stimuli up to unresponsiveness even to noxious stimulation.

In the MAN of normal joints four different categories of afferents could be distinguished according to their reponses to passive movements (Schaible and Schmidt 1983b, 1984). Units of category 1 were activated by movements in the working range of the joint. Afferent units of category 2 were only weakly excited by such movements but responded clearly to movements against the resistance of the tissue. Their activity may signal that the joint leaves its normal working range. Units of category 3 reacted only to movements against the resistance of the tissue. We assume that these fibres are purely nociceptive. Finally units of category 4 were not activated by any movement. Their activation seems to depend on additional factors (see below). Fig. 2 (upper row) illustrates which percentages of the various fiber groups in MAN were classified as belonging to the categories 1 to 4.

Units in PAN could also be grouped into these 4 categories. But, surprisingly, the vast majority of the group IV fibres did not respond to mechanical stimulation (local pressure and movements) at all (Grigg et al. 1986). We conclude that many of the unmyelinated afferents in PAN have no mechanosensitive function in the normal joint.

Resting activity was found in some of the fibres form normal joints. The spontaneously active units belonged mostly to the categories 1 and 2.

To study the discharges of afferent units from inflamed joints we induced an acute experimental arthritis. It had two major consequences:

an increased mechanosensitivity and resting activity (Schaible and Schmidt 1985). Fig. 2 (lower row) illustrates the percentages of the group II, III and IV afferents in MAN classified as above. Obviously, the afferents of the categories 2 to 4 (predominantly in the group III and IV fibre range) were sensitized by the inflammation and had shifted to category 1. Thus inflammation lowers the threshold of units which in the normal joint respond preferentially or exclusively to noxious movements and it induces mechanosensitivity in previously unsensitive units. The same happened in the PAN: during inflammation for a much higher percentage of group IV units a receptive field could be localized in the joint (Grigg et al. 1986). We have evidence that also those groups III and IV units which have primarily low threshold may become more sensitive during the arthritis.

Resting activity was generally higher in units from inflamed joints: e.g. in MAN 75 % of the group III and 83 % of the group IV units from

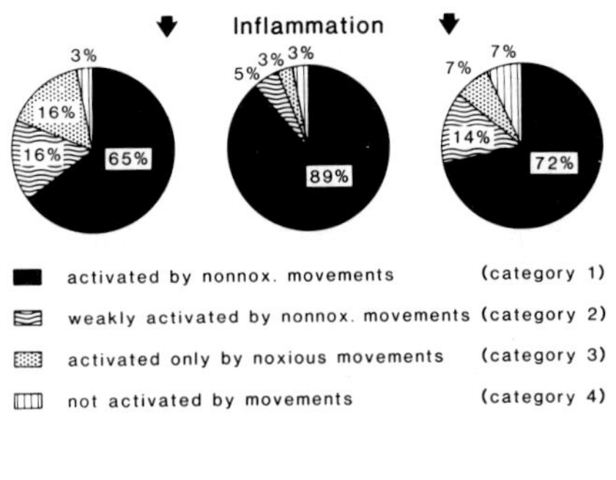

Figure 2. Responses of group II (c.v. 20-60 m/s) group III (c.v. 2.5-20 m/s) and group IV (c.v.<2.5 m/s) units to passive movements.

inflamed joints (versus 35 % of the group III and 36 % of the group IV units from normal joints) showed resting discharges which often had a higher frequency than in units from normal joints (Schaible and Schmidt 1985).

The sensitization of units with low or not detectable mechanosensitivity in the normal joint and the increased resting discharges may be the afferent base for the movement evoked and spontaneous arthritic pain.

2) Chemosensitivity of afferent fibres from normal and inflamed joints.

Chemosensitivity as revealed by close i.a. injection is typical for groups III and IV afferents (Methods in Kanaka et al. 1985). On the background of the results described above for units from inflamed joints it was tested whether inflammatory mediators are capable to induce afferent activity as observed in units from inflamed joints. Further we looked whether the mediators modulate spontaneous activity in the units from the arthritic knee.

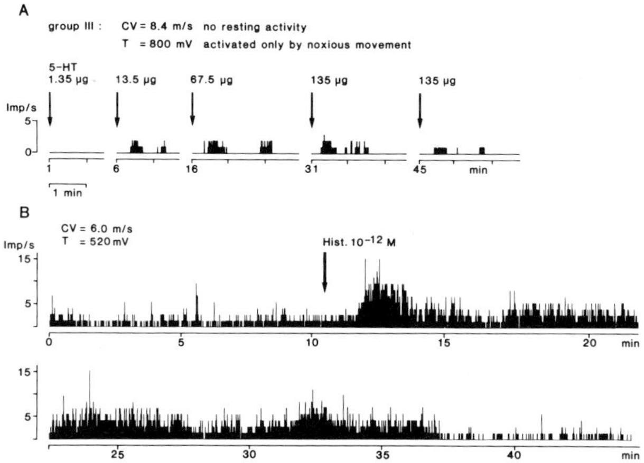

Figure 3. A: Responses of a group III unit to injection of 5-HT. B: Responses of a group III unit from an inflamed joint to histamine.

Afferent units from the normal and inflamed joints were excited by histamine, 5-hydroxytryptamine (5-HT), bradykinin and prostaglandins. All these substances are released or synthesized in inflammatory processes (Garcia Leme 1979, Moncada et al. 1979). These mediators had in common to excite groups III and IV units but not group II ones.

5-HT. In normal joints 5-HT excited 10 of 23 group III and 8 of 11 group IV units. Sixteen of the responding afferents belonged to the categories 1-3. Fig. 3A shows the response in a group III unit to injection of 5-HT. Increase of the dosage evoked stronger responses. On the other hand, repetition of the injections led to a pronounced tachyphylaxis against 5-HT. In normal joints the duration of excitation did not exceed 90 s. The responses were obtained with threshold doses of 1.35 up to 135 ug in most units 13.5 ug were effective. In inflamed joints 5-HT excited 11 of 14 group III and 5 of 14 group IV units. In a few units the excitatory action lasted 6 to 10 minutes and tachyphylaxis was weak.

Bradykinin. In a dosage from 0.026 to 26 ug bradykinin excited 11 of 13 group III and 14 of 15 group IV units sampled in MAN from normal joints. Fine afferent units of all 4 categories were activated. Latency and duration of the effects were comparable to those of 5-HT. In spite of tachyphylaxis to repeated injections dose response curves could be demonstrated (Kanaka et al. 1985).

Prostaglandins. In MAN from normal joints PGE_2 excited 10 of 12 group III and 7 of 10 group IV units of all 4 categories. In contrast to 5-HT and bradykinin, PGE_2 induced or increased activity for long periods of time (up to 10 min or more) in some units. Threshold dose for single injection varied from 0.06 to 30 ug. Dose response curves could be demonstrated. In addition, PGE had sensitizing effects for the action of bradykinin, i.e. responses to bradykinin were increased after an intermittent injection of PGE. In 5 of 8 group III units the responses to movements were influenced by PGE: in low threshold units reactions to movements were increased, in high threshold units reactions to movements in the working range were induced (Heppelmann et al. 1985). In MAN from inflamed joints PGE reversed the depressing effects of ASA and indomethacin on the ongoing and movement evoked activity of single units (Heppelmann et al. 1986).

Histamine. In contrast to the other substances this mediator excited in the dosage of 10^{-12} to 10^{-3} M only those groups III and IV units which had ongoing activity: Whereas 15 of 21 units displaying resting activity could be excited, 12 of 13 without resting discharges were insensitive. The higher the level of resting discharges the lower the effective dose of histamine. Effects were longlasting with a slow onset. An example is illustrated in Fig. 3B. In most cases tachyphylaxis was very pronounced. No differential effect could be observed in units from normal and inflamed joints, and also none between group III and IV ones.

These data show that the population of the chemosensitive units (groups III and IV) matches with the population of units sensitized by an experimental arthritis. This supports the assumption that inflammatory mediators may be an important factor in changing the response behavior of afferent units during inflammation. Because of the short duration of the responses and the tachyphylaxis it is improbable that 5-HT and bradykinin play a major role in sensitization. Prostaglandins may be better candidates because of their longlasting excitatory and sensitizing effects. For histamine a critical role in the sensitization is unlikely since it affects only units with resting activity.

References

Garcia Leme J (1979). Bradykinin-System. In Vane JR, Ferreira SH (eds): Handbook Exp. Pharm. 50/I Inflammation, Berlin: Springer, pp 464 - 522.

Grigg P, Schaible H-G, Schmidt RF (1986). Mechanical sensitivity of group III and IV afferents from posterior articular nerve in normal and inflamed cat knee. J. Neurophysiol. 55: 635-643.

Heppelmann B, Pfeffer A, Schaible H-G, Schmidt RF (1986). Effects of acetylsalicylic acid (ASA) and indomethacin on single groups III and IV units from acutely inflamed joints. Pain, in press.

Heppelmann B, Schaible H-G, Schmidt RF (1985). Effects of prostaglandins E1 and E2 on the mechanosensitivity of groups III afferents from normal and inflamed cat knee joints. In Fields HL, Dubner R, Cervero R (eds): Advances in Pain Research and Therapy, Vol. 9, New York: Raven, pp 91 - 101.

Kanaka R, Schaible H-G, Schmidt RF (1985). Activation of fine articular afferent units by bradykinin. Brain Res. 327: 81 - 90.

Langford LA, Schmidt RF (1983). Afferent and efferent axons in the medial and posterior articular nerves of the cat. Anat. Rec. 206: 71 - 78.

Moncada S, Ferreira SH, Vane JR (1979). Pain and inflammatory mediators. In Vane JR, Ferreira SH (eds): Handbook of Exp. Pharm. 50/I Inflammation, Berlin: Springer, pp 588 - 616.

Schaible H-G, Schmidt RF (1983a). Activation of groups III and IV sensory units in medial articular nerve by local mechanical stimulation of knee joint. J. Neurophysiol. 49: 35 - 44.

Schaible H-G, Schmidt RF (1983b). Responses of fine medial articular nerve afferents to passive movements of knee joint. J. Neurophysiol. 49: 1118 - 1126.

Schaible H-G, Schmidt RF (1984). Mechanosensibility of joint receptors with fine afferent fibres. In Creutzfeldt O, Schmidt RF, Willis WD (eds): Sensory-Motor Integration in the Nervous System, Exp. Brain Res. Suppl. 9: 284 - 297.

Schaible H-G, Schmidt RF (1985). Effects of an experimental arthritis on the sensory properties of fine articular afferent units. J. Neurophysiol. 54: 1109 - 1122.

Effects of Injury on Trigeminal and Spinal Somatosensory Systems, pages 29–36

RESPONSIVENESS OF S.A.I. RECEPTORS IN DEGENERATIVE SKIN CONDITIONS AND AGEING IN THE RAT AND THE CAT

Baumann, K.I., Cheng-Chew S.B., Hamann, W., & Leung, M.S.
Department of Physiology, Faculty of Medicine, The Chinese University of Hong Kong, Shatin, New Territories, HONG KONG.

INTRODUCTION

Viscoelastic properties of surrounding tissues are known to affect the stimulus response characteristics of mechanoreceptors (Nakajima & Onodera, 1969; Husmark & Ottoson, 1971; Baumann, 1978; Pubols, 1982a,b). The present study is concerned with the viscoelasticity of the skin and how it affects the responsiveness of slowly adapting type I (s.a.I) cutaneous mechanoreceptors. Receptors of this type consist of a cluster of tactile or Merkel cells at the epidermo-dermal border. Each cluster is in close contact with a terminally enlarged branch of a myelinated nerve fibre (Iggo & Muir, 1969). The hypothesis tested here is that in the course of ageing, during vitamin A deficiency as well as chronic exposure to neomycin, changes in the responsiveness of s.a.I. receptors are an expression of changed skin compliance.

METHODS

Vitamin A deficiency was induced in Sprague-Dawley rats by rearing the animals from weaning up to an age of 9-11 months on a vitamin A deficient (v.A.d.) diet (Purina) until acute electrophysiological experiments were performed. Animals were kept in individual cages. Matched controls were pair-fed with the same diet supplemented with vitamin A (Baumann et al., 1986a).

Chronic administration of aminoglycosides produces necrosis

in hair cells of the inner ear. Hair cells and Merkel cell receptors are both very sensitive mechanoreceptors with several common design features. Six week old rats were given 100 mg/kg of neomycin (i.m.) daily for 21 days. Acute experiments were performed at ages between 3-4 months (Baumann et al., 1984). The control animals of the neomycin experiment were the group of young animals in the ageing experiments and the control group of the v.A.d. rats served as ´adult´ population (Baumann et al., 1986b).

The rats were anaesthetized with urethane (20% w/v, 6 ml i.p.) for electrophysiological recordings from nerve fibres of clunium nerves supplying touch corpuscles in the skin of the proximal hind limb. Single-unit recordings were made during trains of 30 constant force stimuli rising within 100 ms to a force of 20 mN at which level it was kept for 1.9 s. Stimuli were applied through a probe of 1 mm diameter (spherical tip) attached to a Statham (UC 2) force transducer and Bruel & Kjaer ´minishaker´ (type 4810). During the interstimulus intervals of 700 ms, a contact force of 0.5 mN was maintained which was below threshold for the receptors. The indentation was measured, and the difference between the positions of the probe at the end and just before a stimulus was defined as stroke amplitude (Baumann et al., 1986b).

Recordings were also made from nerve fibres in the saphenous nerve supplying touch corpuscles in the skin of the anterior aspect of the lower leg of cats anaesthetized with pentobarbitone. Every 30 seconds a standard constant force stimulus of 20 mN was given. Nervous responses and displacements were recorded. Neomycin was infused (at a dose of 2.5 mg/min for 5 or 10 minutes) through a catheter in the circumflex femoris artery allowing high concentrations of neomycin at the receptor site without interfering with the normal blood supply (Baumann et al., 1986c).

RESULTS AND DISCUSSION

Figure 1A shows the stroke amplitudes necessary to maintain a plateau force of 20 mN during individual stimuli in trains of 30. Displacements are plotted against ordinal number of stimulus for young, adult, vitamin A deficient rats as well as rats treated chronically with neomycin.

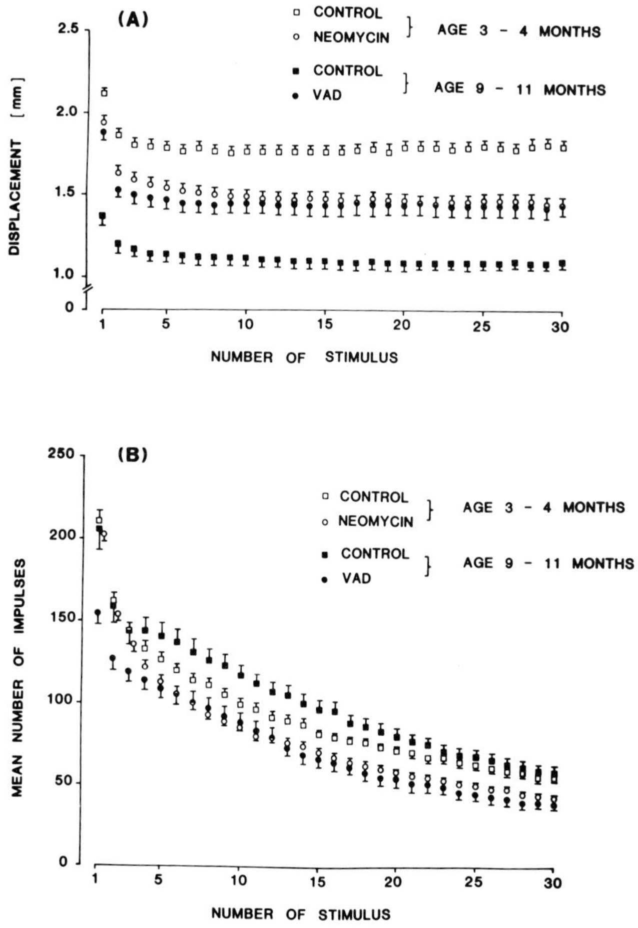

Fig. 1: A) Stroke amplitudes required to maintain a force of stimulation of 20 mN plotted against ordinal number of stimulus for 4 groups of rats: young control group (9 rats, 15 units, 51 runs), young neomycin treated group (11 rats, 28 units, 85 runs), adult control group (6 rats, 15 units, 45 runs), and adult vitamin A deficient (VAD) group (6 rats, 19 units, 59 runs).
B) Responsiveness in mean number of nerve impulses per stimulus to trains of 20 mN constant force stimuli plotted against ordinal number of stimulus. Same groups as in A).

The higher the stroke amplitude, the softer the skin, including the underlying tissue, or, in other terms, the greater the compliance. A large proportion of the compliance is likely to be determined by the dermis and underlying tissue, as the epidermis is very thin. The s.a.I. receptors investigated were all positioned on the upper thigh, a relatively soft part of the body.

Each of the individual groups of results shows an initial drop in the stroke amplitude. This is likely to be due to extrusion of tissue fluid which is not given enough time to diffuse back during the relatively short interstimulus intervals ('creep recovery'; Pubols, 1982b).

The different groups also appeared to be arranged according to magnitude of stroke amplitudes. The group with the lowest compliance was the adult control group (filled squares). Stroke amplitudes from v.A.d. animals and from (young) rats treated with neomycin settled at an intermediate displacement value of about 1.5mm. By far the largest displacements were required by the young control rats (open squares).

If changes in responsiveness are governed only by the compliance of the skin, there should be a matching change in the nervous responses. The lowest compliance should produce the highest response - in this case the adult control rats. On the other hand the young control rats should have the lowest number of nervous impulses. Figure 1B shows the actual nervous responses. Whilst some of these results comply with the hypothesis of "the higher the compliance the lower the response", others clearly do not. The adult control rats (filled squares) with the hardest skin are at the top of the response curves for nearly all 30 stimuli. However, the position of the young control rats in this graph does not fit this hypothesis. In spite of their high compliance, most nervous responses were significantly higher than those obtained in the v.A.d. rats ($p \leq 0.05$ for stimuli no. 1 to 5 and 13 to 19) or those of the neomycin treated rats ($p \leq 0.05$ for stimuli no. 5 to 30).

Direct damage to the afferent nerve is an unlikely explanation for the present results. Plate 1 shows electronmicroscope pictures of Merkel cell nerve fibre complexes in normal and vitamin A deficient rats. Nerve

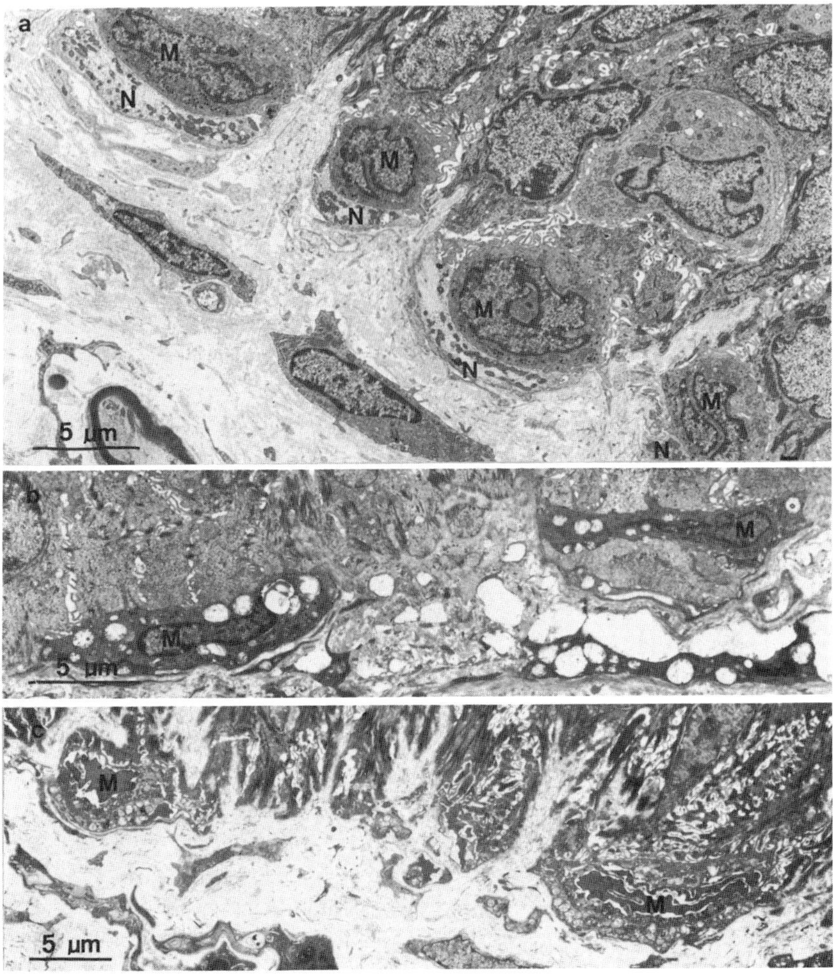

Plate I: Electron micrographs of touch corpuscles showing degenerative changes of Merkel cells.

(a) Normal Merkel cells (M) from rat with the presence of dense-cored granules in the cytoplasm and the associated neurite terminals (N).

(b) Merkel cells (M) from a vitamin A deficient rat. Mitochondria are swollen, and disintegrating cristae are commonly seen in the lucent matrix.

(c) Merkel cells (M) from cat s.a.I receptor 4 hours after infusion of 50 mg neomycin. Cells show signs of degeneration which include highly contracted nuclei and appearance of large numbers of light and empty vesicles.

fibres appeared unchanged while degenerative changes in Merkel cells were found. Most noticeable was destruction of mitochondria in Merkel cells as well as in nerve terminals. Ultrastructural changes after chronic injection of neomycin were less obvious, while no specific differences between young and adult rats were observed.

Recently, for a number of secondary sensory receptors, there has been increasing evidence supporting the presence of an inositol based second messenger system. The receptors concerned are vertebrate cones (Lewin, 1986), the Limulus photoreceptor (Brown et al., 1984), and receptors in the acoustico lateral line system (Schacht,1976; Yanagisawa et al., 1984). In this second messenger system, stimulation results in the splitting of phosphatidylinositol 4,5-bisphosphate into diacylglycerol and inositol 1,4,5-trisphosphate. This substance facilitates the release of Ca^{++} from intracellular stores. Dephosphorylation to inositol and at the same time phosphorylation of diacylglycerol allows reconstruction of phosphatidylinositol in the cell membrane.

At the rephosphorylation level this process is susceptible to lack of energy-rich phosphates and therefore hypoxia. Furthermore, turnover of membrane phosphatidylinositol can be affected by aminoglycosides like neomycin. Also, the enzyme inositol 1-phosphatase can be inhibited by lithium, resulting in backlog-accumulation of precursor molecules (for review, see Berridge, 1984). Thus, application of neomycin or lithium can be used as a test for the phosphoinositol hypothesis.

Experiments were carried out on cats involving close arterial infusion of neomycin. Recordings were made from the saphenous nerve supplying s.a.I receptors in the skin of the lower leg (Baumann et al., 1986c). Mean number of nervous impulses in response to standard stimuli of 20 mN force every 30 s decreased within a few minutes after an infusion of 2.5 mg/min neomycin was given. Five minutes of neomycin infusion (total dose 12.5 mg neomycin) depressed responsiveness to 62 ± 7 % of the control level while after 10 minutes of infusion (total dose 25 mg neomycin) only 45 ± 5 % of the control responses were obtained. At the same time, no significant changes in the mechanical parameters of stimulation were observed. Impaired nervous conduction is an unlikely explanation for the observed reduction in responsiveness. Topically applied neomycin in a concentration of 350 mg/l to a desheathed nerve did not change the shape of the A-component of electrically evoked compound action potentials (Chan et al., 1985). Thus, it appears that neomycin exerts a direct action on the receptor in a way consistent with the hypothesis of a phosphoinositol based second messenger system.

Preliminary results from experiments on rats with chronic injection of lithium are also in support of an action on an inositol based second messenger system. Similar to the effects of Li^+ at the neuromuscular junction (Crawford, 1974) there was an initial increase in responsiveness of s.a.I receptors of these rats. However, due to the side effects of Li^+ further experiments may have to be done in vitro.

In conclusion, compliance of the skin can certainly not be ruled out as a major factor determining the responsiveness of s.a.I receptors. At the same time, interference with cellular mechanisms of the receptor itself appears to be an effective way to reduce responsiveness during degenerative skin conditions. One mechanism that may be relevant in this context is the phosphoinositol based second messenger system.

REFERENCES

Baumann T (1978). Viscoelastic properties of the type I mechanoreceptor in hairy skin of the cat. (M.S. Thesis), Ithaca, NY: Cornell University.

Baumann KI, Cheng-Chew SB, Hamann W, Leung MS (1984). Tactile responses after neomycin and during vitamin A deficiency in rats. In Hamann W, Iggo A (eds): "Sensory Receptors Mechanisms," Singapore: World Scientific Publishing Co., pp. 253-261.

Baumann KI, Cheng-Chew SB, Hamann W, Leung MS (1986a). Responsiveness, mechanics and ultrastructure of slowly adapting type I mechanoreceptors in vitamin A deficient rats. J Physiol 371:339-349.

Baumann KI, Hamann W, Leung MS (1986b). Mechanical properties of the skin and responsiveness of slowly adapting type I mechanoreceptors in rats at different ages. J Physiol 371: 329-337.

Baumann KI, Hamann W, Leung MS (1986c). Reduced responsiveness of touch (SA I) receptors in the cat following close arterial infusion of neomycin. Brain Res 377: 160-162.
Berridge MJ (1984). Inositol trisphosphate and diacylglycerol as second messengers. Biochem J 220: 345-360.
Brown JE, Rubin LJ, Ghalayini AJ, Tarver AP, Irvine RF, Berridge MJ, Anderson RE (1984). Myo-inositol polyphosphate may be a messenger for visual excitation in Limulus photoreceptors. Nature 311:160-163.
Crawford AC (1974). Lithium ions and the release of transmitter at the frog neuromuscular junction. J Physiol 246: 109-142.
Chan WS, Cheng-Chew SB, Hamann W, Ng KC (1985). Acute exposure of myelinated nerve fibres to neomycin. Neurosci Lett Suppl 20: S41.
Husmark I, Ottoson D (1971). The contribution of mechanical factors to the early adaptation of the spindle response. J Physiol 212: 577-592.
Iggo A, Muir AR (1969). The structure and function of a slowly adapting touch corpuscle in hairy skin. J Physiol 200: 763-796.
Lewin R (1986). Unexpected progress in photoreception. Science 227:500-503.
Nakajima S, Onodera K (1969). Adaptation of the generator potential in the crayfish stretch receptors under constant length and constant tension. J Physiol 200: 187-204.
Pubols BH Jr (1982a). Factors affecting cutaneous mechanoreceptor response. I. Constant-force versus constant-displacement stimulation. J Neurophysiol 47: 515-529.
Pubols BH Jr (1982b). Factors affecting cutaneous mechanoreceptor response. II. Changes in mechanical properties of skin with repeated stimulation. J Neurophysiol 47: 530-543.
Schacht J (1976). Biochemistry of neomycin ototoxicity. J Acoust Soc Amer 59: 940-944.
Yanagisawa K, Yoshioka T, Katsuki Y (1984). Sound transducer mechanism and phospholipids in the hair cell of the ear. In Hamann W, Iggo A (eds): "Sensory Receptor Mechanisms," Singapore: World Scientific Publishing Co., pp. 109-116.

Effects of Injury on Trigeminal and Spinal Somatosensory Systems, pages 37–42

REINNERVATION OF GLABROUS SKIN IN PRIMATES

Julia K. Terzis

Microsurgical Research Center
Eastern Virginia Medical School
Norfolk, Virginia 23501

INTRODUCTION

The properties of cutaneous mechanoreceptors serving the glabrous skin of the baboon hand have been examined in normal and regenerating nerves. Following a crush injury to the ulnar nerve, the reinnervated mechanoreceptors regained response properties that allowed them to be assigned to the same submodalities found in normal skin (Dykes & Terzis, 1979). Following ulnar nerve transection and repair, the return to normality is much slower due to the misalignment of the regenerating axons at the suture site (Terzis & Dykes, 1980).

In these experiments, the right and left ulnar and median nerves in three adult female baboons (Papio anubis) were surgically transected and repaired using one of four microsurgical nerve repair procedures. To compare epineurial and perineurial nerve repair techniques, the left and right median nerves were utilized. The left and right ulnar nerves were transected and repaired to compare a tension repair to a nontension repair using a sural nerve graft.

METHODS

Nerve regeneration and cutaneous reinnervation were assessed electrophysiologically between 7 and 10 months following surgery. Animals were initially sedated with Ketamine, and surgical levels of anesthesia were maintained for the duration of each recording session with i.v. injections of pentobarbitol. Cutaneous reinnervation was examined using single fiber dissection and recording techniques described in detail elsewhere (Dykes & Terzis, 1979). The presence of active fibers was determined by delivering electrical stimuli to the nerve proximal to the repair site. Fiber latencies were measured from oscilloscope tracings, and the surface of the hand was then searched using glass probes. These mechanically stimulated fibers were then classified by their modality and submodality on the basis of their response. The receptive field (RF) of each cutaneous fiber was mapped using threshold and 2 gm stimuli applied with calibrated nylon filament aesthesiometers.

In each experiment, rapid adapting (RA) and slowly adapting (SA) fibers were examined for their response properties when stimulated with an electromechanical stimulator at the most sensitive area of that fiber's RF. For SA fibers, the responses to skin indentations (94 mu to 725 mu) were collated by a microprocessor and averaged over 3 to 5 trials at each stimulus intensity used. RA fibers were examined for their sensitivity to vibratory stimuli (2 Hz to 250 Hz). For each frequency tested, the amplitude of the stimulus was varied until the minimum displacement required to elicit an entrained response was determined. The stimulus-response and tuning curves for the SA and RA were constructed and compared to normal fibers from a previous experiment (Dykes & Terzis, 1979).

To assess nerve regeneration, compound action potentials (CAP's) were recorded at the end of the experiment, proximal and distal to the repair. Skin and nerve biopsies were obtained for histological analysis.

RESULTS AND DISCUSSION

A total of 843 single fibers were recorded in these experiments. Of these, approximately 29% were classified as cutaneous mechanoreceptors, and 20% as innervating deep tissues. The remaining fibers which were nonresponsive to the usual stimuli, were termed "No Drive" fibers; see Table 1.

TABLE 1. Fiber Populations

TYPE REPAIR		FIBER TYPE (No. FIBERS) SKIN	DEEP	NO DRIVE	MISC.	TOTAL
Epineurial	n	64	37	63	3	167
	%	38	22	38	2	100
Perineurial	n	71	38	79	5	193
	%	37	20	41	3	101
Graft	n	60	55	85	5	205
	%	29	27	41	2	99
Tension	n	46	35	190*	7	278
	%	17	13	68	2	100
TOTAL	n	241	165	417	20	843
	%	29	20	49	2	100

*significant

The proportions of skin, deep and "No Drive" fibers obtained following either epineurial or perineurial nerve repair were very similar (χ^2 = 1.0881; d.f. = 3; $0.7<P<0.8$). For both types of repair, approximately 37 to 38% were classified as cutaneous and a breakdown of these fibers is represented in Table 2. SA fibers were the most common type of cutaneous receptor recorded in these repairs (61 - 67%), while RA fibers accounted for 27 to 36%. Differences in the proportions of these fiber types were not, however, significant.

The proportions of fiber types recorded following the graft and tension repairs were highly dissimilar (Table 1). The most significant difference here was the preponderance of fibers in the tension group which could not be driven by mechanical stimulation (χ^2 = 37.0846; d.f. = 3; $P<<0.0005$). The proportions of cutaneous and deep modalities were approximately equal for both nerve repair groups. However, the proportions of RA, SA and Pacinian (Pc) fibers were not equal (Table 2), in that a significantly greater number of Pc fibers were recorded in the tension group (χ^2 = 9.457; d.f. = 2; $P<0.01$). The increase of "No Drive" fibers in the tension group possibly indicates an overall failure in the number of fibers that successfully crossed the repair. The increase of Pc fibers is of additional interest as few Pc fibers were found in earlier reinnervation studies (Dykes & Terzis, 1979; Terzis & Dykes, 1980).

TABLE 2.

(A) Cutaneous Fiber Population for Epineurial and Perineurial Repair

TYPE REPAIR		FIBER TYPE (No. FIBERS)			
		RA	Pc	SA	TOTAL
Epineurial	n	23.0	2.0	39.0	64.0
	%	35.9	3.1	60.9	99.0
Perineurial	n	19.0	4.0	48.0	71.0
	%	26.8	5.6	67.6	100.0
TOTAL	n	42.0	6.0	87.0	135.0
	%	31.1	4.4	64.4	99.9

(B) For Tension and Graft Repair

TYPE REPAIR		FIBER TYPE (No. FIBERS)			
		RA	Pc	SA	TOTAL
Graft	n	32.0	1.0	27.0	60.0
	%	53.3	1.7	45.0	100.0
Tension	n	15.0	8.0*	23.0	46.0
	%	32.6	17.4	50.0	100.0
TOTAL	n	47.0	9.0	50.0	106.0
	%	44.3	8.5	47.2	100.0

*significant

Figure 1 presents the threshold distributions for normal fibers recorded in a previous study (Dykes et al., 1984) and fibers recorded from the epineurial and perineurial repair groups. Figure 1 also includes the threshold data recorded from the graft and tension repair groups. In the normal nerve, most cutaneous fibers (63%) had thresholds less than 300 mg, and 87% had thresholds less than 1 gm. This skewed unimodal distribution was dramatically altered to a bimodal distribution in all nerve repair groups. While the proportion of higher threshold fibers was greatest in the tension repair group (40%) this difference was not found to be significant.

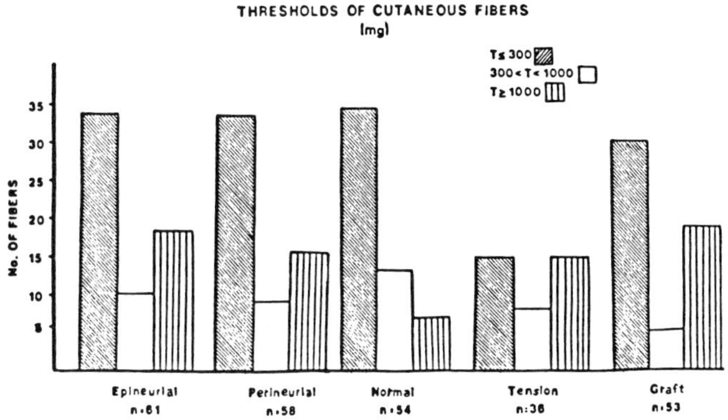

Figure 1. Fiber Thresholds

When the normal RF's of RA and SA fibers are mapped the RF's are found to have oval or circular boundaries and a single point of maximum sensitivity (Dykes & Terzis, 1979). Following cutaneous reinnervation, virtually all of the 184 RA and SA fiber RF's exhibited abnormal properties, ie., irregular contours and ectopic foci of maximum sensitivity. Approximately 26% of these RF's exhibited more dramatic changes, ranging from the presence of multiple foci within the RF to fibers innervating discrete, spatially separate, multiple areas of the skin. The distribution of these highly abnormal RF's was not, however, significant. Additionally, the responses of 22

RA and 28 SA fibers were studied using an electromechanical stimulator. The resulting stimulus-response curves (SA) and tuning curves (RA) from all four repair groups were compared to each other and to normal curves and no statistically significant differences were found. However, there appeared to be a tendency for regenerated RA fibers to tune to lower frequencies than normal fibers but to require higher stimulus displacements. While this shift might represent a change in the transduction mechanism of RA receptors, it is conceivable that such shifts could also result from denervation related changes in the viscoelastic properties of the skin that may have altered mechanical filtering.

While histologic data and electrophysiological recordings yielded no significant differences between repair groups, the basic trends of the data collected in this study show a marked decrease in the regeneration/reinnervation potential tension repair group. This is evident by the increase in the "No Drive" fibers in which statistical differences were found and also by the overall increase in the threshold of mechanical excitation in the fibers of the tension group. Both of these observations lead to the conclusion that repairs done under tension have poorer prognosis and less regeneration potential than alternate repair techniques.

REFERENCES

Dykes, RW, Terzis, JK (1979). Reinnervation of glabrous skin in baboons: properties of cutaneous mechanoreceptors subsequent to nerve crush. J Neurophysiol 42: 1461-1478.

Dykes, RW, Terzis, JK, Turnbull, BG (1984). Properties of mechanoreceptive fibers serving skin grafts transferred to the hands of adult baboons (Papio anubis). J Physiol 357: 1-22.

Terzis, JK, Dykes, RW (1980). Reinnervation of glabrous skin in baboons: properties of cutaneous mechanoreceptors subsequent to nerve transection. J Neurophysiol 44: 1214-1225.

Effects of Injury on Trigeminal and Spinal Somatosensory Systems, pages 43–48

PLASTICITY AND STABILITY IN THE SENSORY INNERVATION OF SKIN

Dr. Jack Diamond

Department of Neurosciences, McMaster University
1200 Main St. W., Hamilton, Ontario
Canada L8N 3Z5

The skin constitutes the major sensory interface between the central nervous system (CNS) and the external environment of the organism. In this capacity it is provided with a complex innervation that nevertheless can be reduced to two dominant roles. Firstly, it subserves a continuous sensing of the environment by the organism, evoking essentially "reactive" behaviors. Secondly, by virtue of the active participation of the organism, the cutaneous innervation makes possible a more prospective assessment of the environment, whose features can be systematically examined by a nervous system programmed for exploratory behavior. In general, we can expect the second of these major sensory functions of skin to be especially prominent in more advanced species. Our findings indicate that both plasticity and stability are present in the innervation of skin and, interestingly, those modalities especially (though not exclusively) employed in exploratory behavior appear to have a relatively stable neural basis, while those that underlie the more passive sensing of the environment have a more plastic character.

The two generalized modalities are (i) light touch and pressure, signalled by large fast-conducting myelinated axons, and (ii) nociception signalled by fine myelinated and unmyelinated axons. The axons of the first group are readily activated by stroking the skin with a fine bristle, and the low-threshold mechanosensory receptive field of a nerve can be accurately mapped by recording the afferent impulses evoked by such a stimulus. How stable are these fields? This was tested in two ways, firstly by denervating adjacent skin to see whether it would evoke collateral sprouting from the remaining nerves, and secondly by crushing a remaining nerve to evoke its regeneration, then measuring electrophysiologically the extent to which it functionally reinnervated the denervated skin. The results were strikingly different between lower and higher vertebrates. In salamanders, collateral sprouting of a spared nerve occurred into denervated skin, and this sprouting was largely confined to the "parent" dermatome of the nerve (Macintyre and Diamond, 1981). However, in adult rabbits (Jackson and Diamond, 1983) and rats (Jackson and Diamond, 1984) no collateral sprouting of low-threshold mechanosensory nerves was detected (see also Nurse et al., 1984). In these experiments the cut nerves were prevented from regenerating into skin, so the failure of the axons to sprout was not because the denervated skin had become reoccupied by its former nerves. This was an important point, because in fact these low-threshold nerves were able to regenerate readily, and both in salamanders and mammals could then functionally reinnervate not only the skin they previously supplied, but often that formerly innervated by the other nerves whose regeneration had been prevented.

One possibility these experiments did not exclude however was that sprouting might occur within a partially denervated receptive field of a nerve (we had looked only at adjacent denervated skin). We have examined this possibility in recent studies of single touch domes in rat skin (Diamond et al., 1984); these domes are mechanosensory structures of 200-300 μm diameter that contain 50-100 of the specialized sensory cells known as Merkel cells (Nurse et al., 1983). A mechanical prodder of 16 μm tip diameter was used to map the innervation within a single dome (the "domains") of each of a pair of axons supplying the dome. The two domains often overlapped significantly. In preliminary experiments, we have found that when one axon is eliminated, the other fails to sprout over the period of at least a few months (a 50 μm shift in the remaining domain border would have been detected); however if the remaining axon were crushed and allowed to regenerate, it would easily reinnervate both its own and the foreign domain.

Thus, sprouting and regeneration can have very contrasting properties. We later demonstrated this for the nociceptive nerves in an even more dramatic fashion.

To examine nociceptive nerves, we used both behavioral and morphological techniques. In the rat, the extensive cutaneus trunci muscle (CTM), which connects to the dermis of the dorsal and flank skin, is reflexly activated by either pinching the skin or by brief application to it of a hot probe (Nixon et al., 1984; Doucette et al., 1983); the bilateral contraction of the CTM is seen as a distinct furrowing of the skin, even in the anesthetized animal. Using essentially the same sprouting paradigm as was employed in the examination of the low-threshold nerves in adult rats, a quite different result was now obtained. Firstly, over the 2-4 weeks following its "isolation" a remaining mechano-nociceptive field was found to expand extensively into the surrounding denervated skin. This expansion was shown by correlative electrical and morphological techniques to be attributable to the sprouting of Aδ axons from the isolated nerve (Nixon et al., 1984). Recently, we completed similar studies of C fibers in the dorsal cutaneous nerves (DCNs), that also drive the CTM reflex (Doucette and Diamond, in preparation). These fibers include those responsible for heat-nociception, since both they and the heat-nociceptive response of the back skin are eliminated by administration of capsaicin to neonatal rats (Doucette et al., 1983). Interestingly, the pinch-sensitive Aδ axons seemed unaffected by the capsaicin treatment. The heat-nociceptive field of an isolated DCN expands into the surrounding denervated skin approximately pari-passu the (large) mechano-nociceptive one. We used both the Evans blue extravasation test for sensory C fibers and electronmicroscopy to correlate this expansion with the sprouting of C fibers from the remaining nerve.

Central changes may have occurred consequent to the initial nerve sections in our experiments, but we find it difficult to see how these could have contributed to the observed field expansions, since only when expansion occurred was the skin surrounding the initially isolated field observed to contain nerves (Nixon et al., 1984; Doucette and Diamond, in preparation). However, plasticity within the CNS is certainly documented (see this volume), although not always associated with correlative studies of the peripheral innervation, and we are alert to the seductive quality of objective evidence in causing an apparent neglect of possible alternative mechanisms, even when these have yet to be described.

A surprising finding is that a modest amount of impulse activity in both the Aδ axons (Nixon et al., 1984) and the C fibers (Doucette and Diamond, in preparation), within an intact DCN causes their subsequent sprouting into surrounding denervated skin to be significantly accelerated. Utilizing tetrodotoxin as a blocking agent we showed that the impulses needed to be conducted centrally for this "precocious sprouting" to be evoked; the phenomenon did not occur when impulses were allowed to conduct only antidromically toward the skin. The effect of the impulses was to reduce the latency to onset of sprouting, which began almost a week sooner than that following the denervation alone; once begun however, the sprouting continued at approximately its usual rate. A report of findings apparently not in accord with these results (Greenfield and Devor, 1981) seems to have been based on an inadequate protocol (Nixon et al., 1984). The possible advantages to the organism of this phenomenon relate to the likelihood that trauma leading to partial denervation of skin is likely also to evoke activity in surviving axons; a precocious sprouting of these would speed up the provision of a trophic support to the deprived skin, in addition to the reestablishment of nociceptive function in it.

In the light of all these findings on nociceptive nerves, the limitation of plasticity (to only regenerate growth) in the low-threshold skin innervation is surprising. We may suppose however that the maintenance of the "local sign" character of these highly discriminating nerves is of major importance to the organism. Thus, although gross trauma might lead to the creation of "blind spots" in low-threshold sensibility, this might be less dangerous to the organism than the potential errors in precise localization consequent to sprouting of remaining low-threshold nerves into neighbouring skin areas. The ability, however, of high-threshold nerves to sprout into these regions and thus signal potentially harmful conditions would more than offset their relatively poorly localizing character. This interpretation of our findings leaves out however the fact that regeneration of low-threshold nerves can occur readily into foreign denervated skin. We are currently investigating whether arrays of regenerating nerves reimpose territorial delineations into the cutaneous innervation, and whether an initial loss of local sign character by any one is corrected subsequently.

Finally, we now have an indication of the stimulus that causes the sprouting of intact Aδ and C nociceptive nerves (Diamond et al., 1986); this sprouting was totally prevented by daily administration of anti-serum to nerve growth factor (anti-NGF), and resumed rapidly when treatment was discontinued. Thus in the adult organism NGF may well participate in the continuous regulation of nociceptive cutaneous fields (and by extrapolation, we suggest, of the terminal fields of any neurons, including those in the CNS, that resemble peripheral sensory neurons in being NGF-dependent during primary development and able to sprout in the adult). Surprisingly however, regeneration of these same nociceptive axons seemed quite unaffected by an anti-NGF treatment regime well in excess of that needed to block sprouting. Thus, although the potential importance of regeneration is beyond question, it seems to have a relatively unregulated character, possibly driven by non-specific influences, in contrast to sprouting which appears to be the more regulated, physiologically significant, phenomenon.

Acknowledgements

Much of the work described in this report was supported by the MRC (Canada) and the MS Society of Canada. Drs. Linda Mills and Anne Foerster made valuable comments on the text, for which I am most grateful. Ms. Shelley Gormley worked hard, at short notice, to make its printing possible.

References

Diamond, J., Coughlin, M., Holmes, M. and Macintyre, L. (1986) Anti-NGF discriminates between sprouting and regenerating axons: a role for NGF in the adult mammalian nervous system? Soc. Neurosci. Abs. In press.

Diamond, J., Yasargil, G.M., Macintyre, L. and Doucette, R. (1984) Integrity of mechanosensory domains within shared touch domes of rats. J. Physiol. (Lond.) 358:27P.

Doucette, R. and Diamond, J. The normal and precocious sprouting of heat nociceptors in the skin of adult rats. In preparation.

Doucette, R., Theriault, E. and Diamond, J. (1983) Identification of cutaneous fiber groups responsible for signalling noxious heat and noxious mechanical stimuli in the rat. Soc. Neurosci. Abs. 9:780.

Doucette, R., Theriault, E. and Diamond, J. Regionally selective elimination of cutaneous thermal nociception in rats by neonatal capsaicin. In preparation.

Greenfield, Z. and Devor, M. (1981) Collateral reinnervation of rat hindlimb does not depend on repeated sensory testing. Neurosci. Lett. 25:305-309.

Jackson, P.C. and Diamond, J. (1983) Failure of intact cutaneous mechanosensory axons to sprout functional collaterals in skin of adult rabbits. Brain Res. 273:277-283.

Jackson, P.C. and Diamond, J. (1984) Temporal and spatial constraints on the collateral sprouting of low-threshold mechanosensory nerves in the skin of rats. J. Comp. Neurol. 226:336-345.

Macintyre, L. and Diamond, J. (1981) Domains and mechanosensory nerve fields in salamander skin. Proc. Roy. Soc. Lond. B 211:471-499.

Nixon, B.J., Doucette, R., Jackson, P. and Diamond, J. (1984) Impulse activity evokes precocious sprouting of nociceptive nerves into denervated skin. Somatosen. Res. 2:97-126.

Nurse, C.A., Mearow, K.M., Holmes, M., Visheau, B. and Diamond, J. (1983) Merkel cell distribution in the epidermis as determined by quinacrine fluorescence. Cell Tiss. Res. 228:511-524.

Nurse, C.A., Macintyre, L. and Diamond, J. (1984) Reinnervation of the rat touch dome restores the Merkel cell population reduced after denervation. Neurosci. 13:563-571.

Effects of Injury on Trigeminal and Spinal Somatosensory Systems, pages 49–60

DEVELOPMENT AND LESION INDUCED REORGANIZATION OF THE PERIPHERAL PROJECTIONS OF THE TRIGEMINAL GANGLION IN RAT

Robert W. Rhoades, Richard D. Mooney, Nicolas L. Chiaia, Ann Marie Szczepanik, Paul R. Hess, William E. Renehan, Bradley G. Klein, Robert G. Nagele and Mark F. Jacquin
Departments of Anatomy and Pediatrics, University of Medicine and Dentistry of New Jersey, Piscataway, New Jersey 08854 (R.W.R., R.D.M., N.L.C., A.M.S., P.R.H. and R.G.N.) and Department of Neuroscience, New York College of Osteopathic Medicine, Old Westbury, New York, 11568 (W.E.R., B.G.K. and M.F.J.).

INTRODUCTION

Many investigators (see especially Van der Loos and Woolsey, 1973; Belford and Killackey, 1979, 1980; Durham and Woolsey, 1984; Bates and Killackey, 1985) have demonstrated the utility of the rodent's infraorbital nerve and its major target, the mystacial vibrissae follicles, for the study of peripheral influences upon the development of patterns in the central nervous system. Less attention has been paid to the normal development of the peripheral projections of this nerve and the manner in which they may be altered by damage during early postnatal life. We will briefly review data which address these two issues.

DEVELOPMENT OF INFRAORBITAL PROJECTIONS TO THE PERIPHERY

Thymidine labelling studies (Forbes and Welt, 1981) have demonstrated that trigeminal ganglion cells in rat undergo their final divisions between the 11th and 13th embryonic days. Silver staining experiments (Erzurumlu and Killackey, 1983) have shown further that maxillary (and thus infraorbital) axons reach the periphery by the 13th embryonic day. By the time the rat is born, the topography of ganglionic projections observed in the adult (Welt, 1982; Arvidsson, 1982; Math et al., 1984) is largely present (Erzurumlu and Killackey, 1983; Klein et al., 1986; Fig. 1). Interestingly, this has occurred

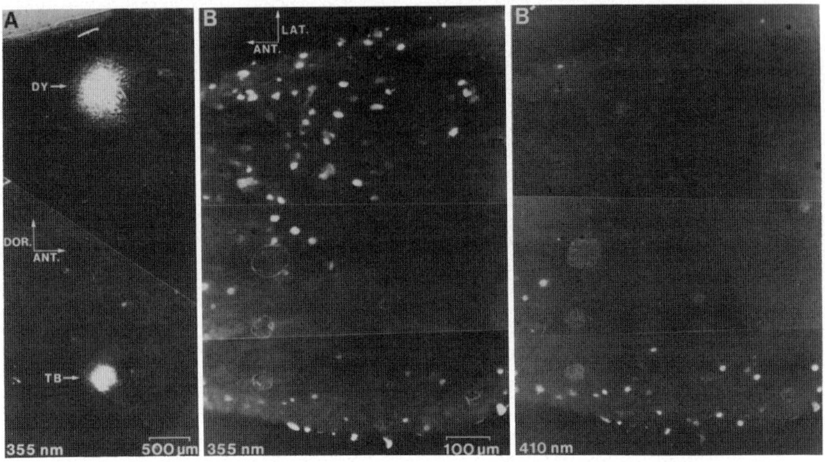

Figure 1. A is an episcopic fluorescence montage which shows an injection of diaminindino yellow (DY) into follicle A-1 and true blue (TB) into E-1 in a newborn rat. B is a montage of a horizontal section through the trigeminal ganglion taken with a 355 nm filter package. TB labelled cells are visible laterally and DY labelled neurons can be seen medially. B' shows the same section taken with a 410 nm filter. The DY labelled cells fluoresce more brightly and the TB labelled neurons are much dimmer.

at a time when the infraorbital nerve contains approximately 10,000 more fibers than it will in an adult animal (Renehan and Rhoades, 1984).

LESION INDUCED REORGANIZATION OF INFRAORBITAL PROJECTIONS

Neonatal transection of the infraorbital nerve results in the death of a considerable number of trigeminal ganglion cells. Several groups (eg. Savy et al., 1981; Waite and Cragg, 1982) have used indirect methods to estimate the number of infraorbital neurons which survive such damage and we (Chiaia et al., 1986) have addressed this question directly by labelling the nerve with HRP in adult animals proximal to the point of the neonatal transection. In these experiments, we labelled an average of 4,392 ganglion cells (sd.=1,316) in 4 neonatally nerve damaged animals. Survival of those ganglion cells which remain after neonatal transection of the infraorbital nerve does not appear to depend upon reformation of contacts with peripheral targets. We (Chiaia et al., 1986) have examined this possibility by cutting the infraorbital nerve on the day of birth an resectioning it at weekly intervals until the time of a terminal anatomical experiment. We verified that the remaining infraorbital ganglion cells in these rats did not project back to the vibrissal pad by injecting DY into it prior to depositing HRP into the nerve itself proximal to the point at which the transections were carried out. No double labelled cells were found. In addition, the average number of ganglion cells labelled by our HRP injections (Fig. 2) in these animals was 4,244 (sd.=864) and this did not differ significantly from the value obtained in rats which sustained a single transection on the day of birth.

There is considerable evidence that damage to peripheral nerves may result in sprouting of undamaged axons at the periphery. In adult mammals, this is probably true for high threshold mechanoreceptors (Weddell et al., 1941; Devor et al., 1979), but it also appears to be the case for low threshold fibers in perinatal animals (Jackson and Diamond, 1984).

We have recently begun to examine the possibilty that neonatal infraorbital nerve damage may result in "misrouting" of axons at the level of the ganglion. This investigation was prompted by two observations. First, in experiments where HRP was applied to the regenerate infraorbital nerve after neonatal transection, a small number of fibers were observed in mandibular sensory nerves (Fig. 3). We never observed such labelling after application of HRP to the infraorbital nerve in normal adult rats. Secondly, single unit recording from the trigeminal ganglion of neonatally nerve damaged animals revealed a small number of cells which could be activated by electrical stimulation of the regenerate infraorbital nerve and which also had peripheral receptive fields that were restricted to non-infraorbital territory such as the auriculotemporal sinus hair (Jacquin et al., 1987). Both of these observations suggested that a given ganglion cell

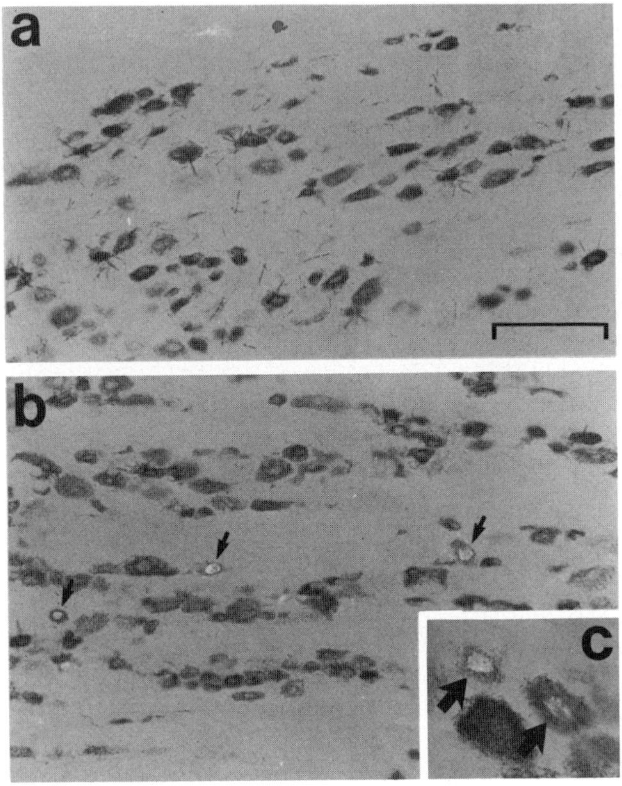

Figure 2. a is a combined fluorescence-brightfield photomicrograph of a portion of a section through the trigeminal ganglion of an animal which sustained multiple transections of the infraorbital nerve prior to a DY-HRP labelling experiment (see text for details). Note that, while HRP labelled cells are visible, no double labelled neurons can be seen. b illustrates similar data from a rat in which the nerve was transected only once on the day of birth. Several double labelled cells (denoted by arrows) are visible. c depicts two such cells at a higher magnification. The calibration is 100 μm for a and b and 30 μm for c.

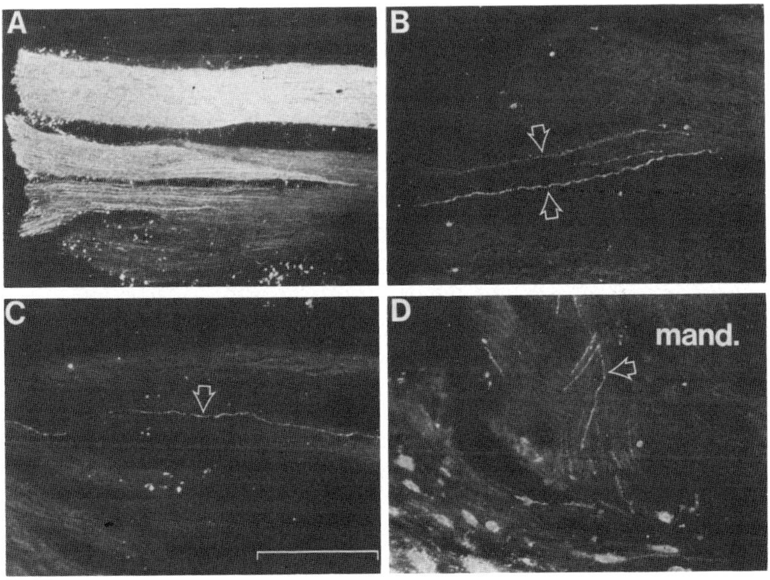

Figure 3. A is a polarized darkfield montage that depicts the location of an HRP injection into the regenerate infraorbital nerve of a rat subjected to transection of this trigeminal branch on the day of birth. B and C illustrate HRP labelled axons in mandibular sensory branches (arrows) and D shows several of these fibers coursing from the mandibular (mand.) to the ophthalmic maxillary portion of the ganglion.

might project into multiple trigeminal branches in a neonatally nerve damaged rat.

We have confirmed and extended these two observations with multiple retrograde labelling techniques. In a first set of experiments, we injected TB in non-infraorbital peripheral fields and DY directly into the infraorbital nerve in adult rats subjected to neonatal transection of this trigeminal branch. These injections invariably produced a small number (120-415) of double labelled cells in the ophthalmic-maxillary portion of the ganglion (Fig. 4a). We verified the fact that this labelling arose as a result of ganglion cells with axons in different trigeminal branches and not simply from labelling of infraorbital axons that may have sprouted in the periphery by carrying out one additional experiment. Here, DY was injected into the regenerate nerve and it was then recut just distal to the point of the tracer injection one day later. After the transection, TB was then injected into non-infraorbital peripheral fields. This procedure also produced double labelled cells (Fig. 4b).

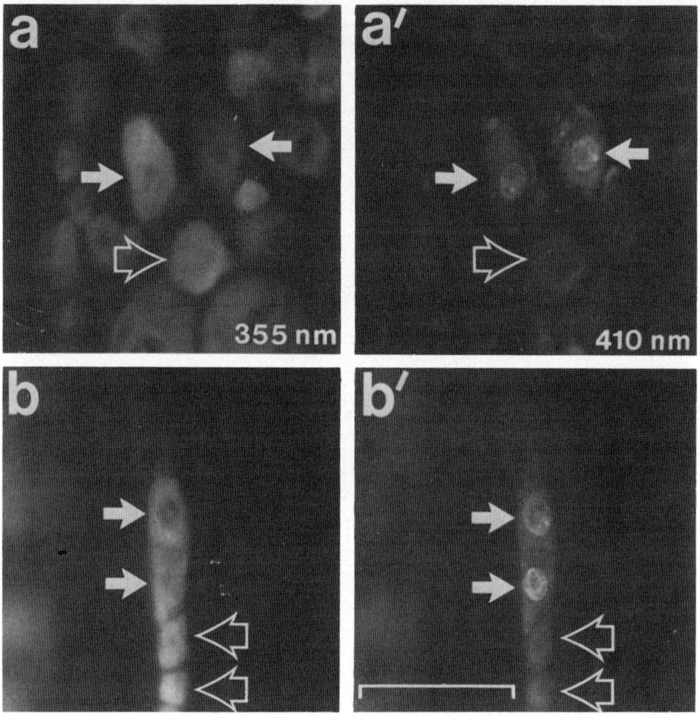

Figure 4. Episcopic fluorescence photomicrographs showing the results of the double labelling experiments described in the text. a and a' show double labelled cells (solid arrows) observed in the single stage double labelling experiment. The open arrow denotes a cell labelled only with TB. b and b' illustrate similar labelling from a two-stage double labelling experiment. Conventions are as in a. The calibration is 50 μm.

These results, and those obtained in the electrophysiological and HRP tracing experiments, thus provide three independent lines of evidence which indicate that neonatal transection of the infraorbital nerve does result in the development of supernumerary axon collaterals by a small number of trigeminal ganglion cells. Importantly, this result probably does not reflect the maintenance of normally transient "exuberant" projections (eg. Land and Lund, 1979). Multiple retrograde labelling experiments in normal neonates (Klein et al., 1986) have revealed only a very small (<20) number of double labelled cells in these animals.

We have also used multiple retrograde labelling methods to evaluate the topographic organization of the regenerate infraorbital projection to the vibrissae follicles (Klein et al., 1985). Here, we have compared, within a given ganglion, the distributions of the neurons which innervate follicles A-1 and E-1. Unlike the case in either the normal adult (Math et al., 1984) or neonate (Klein et al., 1986; see above), the ganglion cells which projected to these two follicles in neonatally nerve damage adult animals were almost completely intermixed (Fig. 5). Furthermore, injections of adjacent follicles in these animals invaribly produced a number of double labelled cells, a finding which suggested the possibility that a given ganglion cell might innervate more than one vibrissa follicle. This conclusion has been confirmed in our electrophysiological studies (Jacquin et al., 1987).

DISCUSSION

Most aspects of the reorganization we have observed after neonatal transection of the infraorbital nerve appear to be amplifications of phenomena that have been reported for adult animals after similar damage (see Aldskogius et al., 1985 for a review). One result that appears qualitatively different from those obtained after transections of sensory nerves in adults is the reorganization across branches of trigeminal peripheral projections. There are two possible sources of these multiply projecting fibers: axotomized (i.e. infraorbital) ganglion cells and ganglion cells which send their axons into other trigeminal branches at the time of

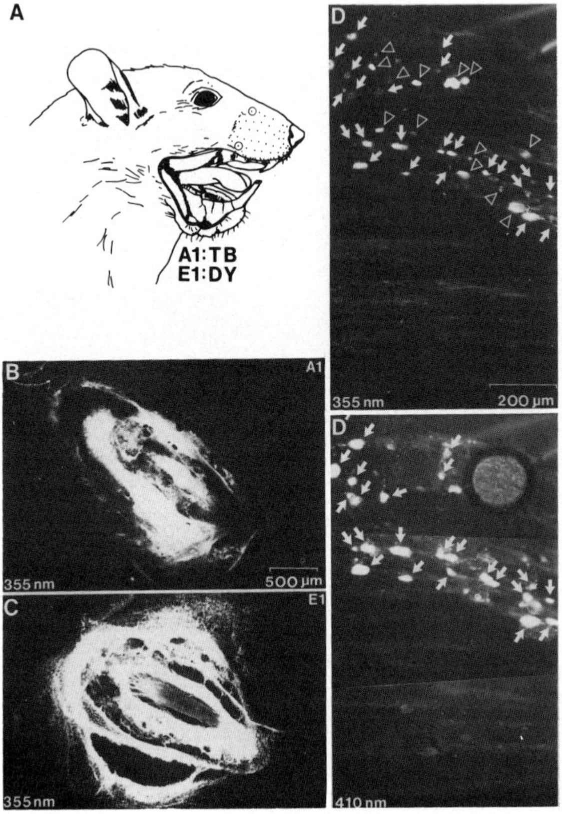

Figure 5. Data from a neonatally nerve damaged animal in which TB was injected into follicle A1 (A and B) and DY was injected into E1 (A and C). D and D' show the complete intermingling of TB (open arrowheads) and DY (solid arrows) labelled neurons. Compare with figure 1.

the lesion. With respect to the first possibility, a number of studies (eg. Greenman, 1913; Jenq and Coggeshall, 1984) have shown that nerve injury may result in supranormal numbers of fibers distal to the point of damage in the regenerate nerve. Other experiments have indicated that the branching which gives rise to at least some of these extra collaterals occurs proximally to the point of the lesion (Cajal, 1928; McQuarrie, 1985). It may be that the retrograde axonal degeneration which follows transection of the infraorbital nerve in neonatal rats extends to the ganglion. This would permit elaboration of axonal sprouts at a point that would allow access to different peripheral branches.

The development of multiple peripheral projections by undamaged ganglion cells, if it, in fact, occurs, would be more difficult to explain. Hulsebosch and Coggeshall (1983) have demonstrated that sprouting of undamaged dorsal root axons follows transection of adjacent roots in both neonatal and adult rats, but there is also evidence that such branching occurs for a smaller number of dorsal root ganglion cells in normal animals (Langford and Coggeshall, 1979). Our experiments have shown that only a very few trigeminal ganglion cells in normal neonates and none at all in adults have branched peripheral projections.

In summary, the data reviewed in this chapter show that neonatal transection of the infraorbital nerve in rats results in a substantial number of "errors" in the reinnervation of the periphery by regenerate axons. Our findings also suggest that some aspects of the central functional reorganization observed after neonatal nerve damage (eg. Killackey et al., 1978; Simons et al., 1984) may reflect abnormalities in these peripheral projections.

ACKNOWLEDGEMENT

Supported by grants from the National Institute of Dental Research and the National Science Foundation.

REFERENCES

Aldskogius H, Arvidsson J, Grant G (1985). The reaction of primary sensory neurons to peripheral nerve injury with particular emphasis on transganglionic changes. Brain Res Rev 10:27-46.

Arvidsson J (1982). Somatotopic organization of vibrissae afferents in the trigeminal sensory nuclei of the rat studied by transganglionic transport of HRP. J Comp Neurol 211:84-92.

Bates CA, Killackey HP (1985). The organization of the

neonatal rat's brainstem trigeminal complex and its role in the formation of central trigeminal patterns. J Comp Neurol 240:265-287.
Belford GR, Killackey HP (1979). The development of vibrissae representation in subcortical trigeminal centers of the neonatal rat. J Comp Neurol 188:63-74.
Belford GR, Killackey HP (1980). The sensitive period in the development of the trigeminal system of the neonatal rat. J Comp Neurol 193:335-350.
Chiaia NL, Hess PR, Rhoades RW (1986). Long-term consequences of neonatal transection of the infraorbital nerve in rat are not influenced by reestablishment of periphperal connections. Soc Neurosci Absts, in press.
Devor M, Schonfeld D, Zeltzer Z, Wall PD (1979) Two modes of cutaneous reinnervation following peripheral nerve injury. J Comp Neurol 185:211-220.
Durham D, Woolsey TA (1984). Effects of neonatal whisker lesions on mouse central trigeminal pathways. J Comp Neurol 223:424-447.
Erzurumlu RS, Killackey HP (1983). Development of order in the rat trigeminal system. J Comp Neurol 213:365-380.
Forbes DJ, Welt C (1981). Neurogenesis in the trigeminal ganglion of the albino rat. A quantitative autoradiographic study. J Comp Neurol 199:133-147.
Greenman MJ (1913). Studies on the peroneal nerve of the albino rat: number and sectional area of fibers: area relation of axis to sheath. J Comp Neurol 23:479-513.
Hulsebosch CE, Coggeshall RE (1983). Age related sprouting of dorsal root axons after sensory denervation. Brain Res 288:77-83.
Jackson PC, Diamond, J (1984). Temporal and spatial constraints on the collateral sprouting of low-threshold mechanosensory nerves in the skin of rats. J Comp Neurol 226:336-345.
Jacquin MF, Renehan WE, Klein BG, Mooney RD, Rhoades RW (1987) Functional consequences of neonatal infraorbital nerve section in rat trigeminal ganglion. J Neurosci, in press.
Jenq C-B, Coggeshall RE (1984). Effects of sciatic nerve regeneration on axonal populations in tributary nerves. Brain Res. 295:91-100.
Killackey HP, Ivy GO, Cunningham TJ (1978). Anomalous

organization of SmI somatotopic map consequent to vibrissae removal in the newborn rat. Brain Res 155: 136-140.

Klein, BG, Macdonald G, Szczepanik AM, Rhoades RW (1986). Topographic organization of peripheral trigeminal ganglionic projections in newborn rats. Dev Brain Res 27:257-262.

Klein BG, Renehan WE, Jacquin MF, Rhoades RW (1985). Effects of neonatal infraorbital nerve lesion upon the innervation of the vibrissae follicles in the rat. Anat. Rec. 211:99A.

Land PW, Lund RW (1979). Development of rat's uncrossed retinotectal pathway and its relation to plasticity studies. Science 205:698-700.

Langford LA, Coggeshall RE (1979). Branching of sensory axons in the dorsal root and evidence for the absence of dorsal root efferent fibers. J Comp Neurol 184:193-204.

Math M, Klein BG, Rhoades RW (1984). Topographic representation of vibrissae follicles in the trigeminal (V) ganglion of normal adult rats and adults subjected to neonatal transection of the infraorbital (IO) nerve. Soc Neurosci Absts 10:1156.

McQuarrie IG (1985). Effect of a conditioning lesion on axonal sprout formation at nodes of ranvier. J Comp Neurol 231:239-249.

Ramon y Cajal S (1928). "Degeneration and Regeneration of the Nervous System." London: Hafner, pp 172-166.

Renehan WE, Rhoades RW (1984) A quantitative electron microscopic analysis of the infraorbital nerve in the newborn rat. Brain Res 322:369-373.

Savy C, Margules S, Farkas-Bargeton E, Verley R (1981) A morphometric study of mouse trigeminal ganglion after unilateral destruction of vibrissae follicles at birth. Brain Res 217:265-277.

Simons DJ, Durham D, Woolsey TA (1984). Functional organization of mouse and rat SmI barrel cortex following vibrissal damage on different postnatal days. Somatosen Res 1:207-245.

Van der Loos H, Woolsey TA (1973) Somato-sensory cortex: structural alterations following early injury to sense organs. Science 179:395-398.

Waite PME, Cragg BG (1982) The peripheral and central changes resulting from cutting or crushing the afferent nerve supply to the whiskers. Proc R Soc Lond Biol 214:191-211.

Weddell G, Guttmann L, Gutmann E (1941). The local extension of nerve fibres into denervated area of skin. J Neurol Neurosurg Psychiatr 4:206-255.
Welt C (1982) Somatotopic organization of the rat trigeminal ganglion determined by horseradish peroxidase (HRP) mapping. Soc Neurosci Absts 8:1023.

Effects of Injury on Trigeminal and Spinal Somatosensory Systems, pages 61–68

ORIGIN AND MODULATION OF THE DERMATOTOPIC MAP

Bryce L. Munger and Terrell E. Jones

Department of Anatomy, The Milton S. Hershey Medical Center of The Pennsylvania State University, Hershey, Pennsylvania 17033

The concept that skin is trophically linked to the nervous system during embryonic development was clearly recognized by Cajal (1960), based on his studies of normal development. Cajal's perception of the phenomenon of trophic dependency is as follows (page 196, Cajal, 1960):

> "The cutaneous mucosal epithelia and their derivatives, the glands and hair follicles, exert a trophic and orienting action over the embryonic nerve fibers."

That statement was written almost 100 years ago and yet our understanding of the mechanism of communication between skin and nerves is far from complete as summarized in recent monographs such as those edited by Black (1984) or Sladek and Gash (1984). The present review will not deal directly with trophic infleunces, but rather concentrate on fundamental problems dealing with development of cutaneous innervation and the impact of selected neural lesions. As a result of our studies on these fundamental problems, we return to the concepts of Cajal and agree that a strong mutual trophic dependency exists between the skin and nervous system.

The skin and the afferent nervous system are trophically mutually interdependent. In order to justify this statement we will first show a relationship between the afferent nervous system and both hairy and glabrous skin. The nature of the sensory terminals in glabrous and hairy skin have been summarized in numerous reviews (Munger, 1971; Halata, 1975; Halata and Munger, 1983;

Munger and Halata, 1983; Iggo, 1974; Bannister, 1976). What is not generally appreciated is the complexity of the innervation of hairy skin as reviewed by Munger (1982). This complexity is the result of the simultaneous presence on single hairs of more than one identifiable sensory receptor in all species save the rabbit (Rice and Munger, 1986). Briefly, the sensorineural apparatus of typical guard (large) hairs in primates and most other mammals consists of an array or palisade of lanceolate terminals surrounded by a variable admixture of free nerve endings (FNE's) and Ruffini terminals (Munger, 1982; Halata and Munger, 1983). The sensory innervation of vellus, or down hairs, is variable. Some vellus hairs have typical lanceolate terminals and surrounding Ruffini and FNE terminals. However, the majority of vellus hairs lack a palisade of lanceolate terminals and have only FNE's and scattered isolated lanceolate terminals.

The sensory innervation of primate glabrous skin is similar in having a variety of sensory terminals associated with the papillary or sweat duct ridges. Halata and Munger (1983) noted that in each instance (glabrous and hairy skin) the sensory receptors are organized around the epidermal derivative, a conclusion stated earlier by Miller, Ralston, and Kasahara (1958). Meissner corpuscles and FNE's are present high in the dermal papillae and clusters of Merkel terminals are present between each duct of the sweat duct ridge as noted originally by Perez (1931) as intersudoriforal terminals. Ruffini and Pacinian corpuscles are present in the deeper dermis and FNE's can be found in all locations throughout the dermis. The physiological correlates of this innervation has been studied by Munger, Page, and Pubols (1979) in partially deafferented primate skin and Meissner corpuscles are the source of RA units and Merkel clusters the source of SA units as had been predicted from other studies (Munger, 1971, Iggo 1974, Halata, 1975).

The glabrous skin of animals other than primates has been shown to have neural - epithelial interactions although it has received less attention. Ide (1976) provided clear evidence that mouse digital toe pads contain Meissner corpuscles that are equivalent in every respect to those of primates. Papillary ridges have recently been described by Silverman, Munger and Halata (1986) in the glabrous skin of the rat rhinarium and this epidermis also contains Merkel cells at the base of the papillary ridges. The racoon has extremely large clusters of Merkel cells in the glabrous skin of their digits, but this animal lacks ridges - rather having cylindrical rete pegs (Munger, Pubols and Pubols, 1971; Munger and Pubols, 1972). In the glabrous skin of both the racoon digit and rat and racoon rhinarium the dermis contains only simple corpuscles (using the terminology of Halata and Munger, 1983) rather than Meissner corpuscles.

We have recently been able to confirm Cummins's statement (1964) that opossum glabrous palmar and plantar skin has a dermatoglyphic pattern resembling that of primates. The opossum (both Monodelphis domesticus and Didelphis virginiana) indeed has papillary ridges containing the ducts of sweat glands resembling primate glabrous digital skin. Meissner corpuscles are present at the apex of the dermal papillae and Merkel clusters can be identified at the base of the papillary ridges identical to those of primates. These findings suggest that the opossum, especially Monodelphis, will be an exciting model for experimental studies as its peripheral sensory system so closely resembles that of man. All of these examples clearly illustrate an anatomical or functional interrelationship between the afferent nervous system and epithelial derived structures.

In order to show a trophic interdependence between the afferent nervous system and the epithelial both components must be identified at very young ages. Dell and Munger (1986) and Jones and Munger (1986) in a study of primate and opossum glabrous skin development noted large Merkel cells lacking any sign of secretory granules over a large expanse of cytoplasm (English, Burgess and Norman, 1980). These studies provide examples of ultrastructurally identified profiles of growth cones. By being able to identify growth cones, peripheral neurites could be identified in much younger embryonic skin. Retrospectively, we can identify profiles of growth cones in micrographs from developing hairy skin in embryos considerably younger than those used by Bressler and Munger (1983).

Based on the presence of growth cones tightly abutting the epidermis in primate embryos prior to differentiation of papillary ridges, Dell and Munger (1986) suggested that afferent nerves might play an important role in the development of papillary ridges and thus the dermatoglyph. Since the afferent nerves are the basis for the spinal segmental innervation they further suggested that this early trophic interdependence would be the somatotopic basis of the dermatotopic map. The spacing of papillary ridges is constant, and once established remains fixed as noted by Hale (1952). However, the minutae or fine detail of a fingerprint is remarkably unique even between identical twins or between left and right hands (Cummins and Midlo, 1961). Only the distal digital pads of the fingers have distinctive prints and the ridges begin to form at the center of the distinctive pattern. A wave of differentiation spreads out circumferentially with the initiation and cessation of ridge formation giving rise to the distinctive pattern. The remainder of the glabrous digital skin is filled in with parallel ridges that lack a distinctive pattern. Proposing that the afferent nerves have a role in the distinctive pattern would suggest a logical link between abnormal finger prints and numerous congenital neurological disorders where abnormal finger prints are commonly observed (Schaumann and Alter, 1976 and see Discussion in Dell and Munger, 1986). These examples provide clear illustrations of a maturing or changing nervous system being correlated with a maturing or changing periphery.

We have recently been able to find other examples of successive waves of differentiation within the afferent nervous system in the mystacial pads of both rats (Munger and Rice, 1986) and opossum pups (Munger and Jones, 1986a). Rice (1985) had noted marked changes in the clarity of the cortical barrels in postnatal rat pups and these observations formed the basis of a developmental study of cutaneous innervation in rat mystacial skin (Munger and Rice, 1986). Cortical barrels representing the posterior mystacial pad begin to be visible in the rat by 4 days of age and are "remodeled" to their less prominent adult form between the third and fifth week postpartum. All vibrissae are differentiated by birth in the rat and they are all well innervated by most of their adult compliment of axons. A notable exception is the conus nerve and its associated lanceolate, FNE, and Ruffini terminals as identified by Renehan and Munger (1985). The conus innervation is not present at birth and develops over the first week of age that in no way correlates with the changes in cortical barrels. The pelage at birth has no distinctive terminals, rather, as described by Bressler and Munger (1983) in the monkey, the axons associated with differentiating hairs appear to be relatively undifferentiated FNE's. The lanceolate terminals that are distinctive in adult guard hairs begin to form by 2 weeks of age and relatively mature innervation can be identified on many guard hairs by 3 weeks of age. These changes in the innervation of the pelage precisely parallel the developmental changes of the barrel fields of SmI cortex and suggest that successive waves of differentiation within the afferent nervous system is probably a general phenomenon in neural development. Rubel (1984) has provided a similar argument for the normal sequence of development in the auditory system. The best studied system involving precise topological development is the visual system (Walsh and Polley, 1985; Fawcett and Cowan, 1985; Guillery, 1982) where this orderly progession of differentiation is clearly modulated by function (Schmidt, 1985).

On the basis of these considerations Munger and Jones (1986b) recently evaluated the sequence of differentiation within a spinal dermatome and have found an orderly progression from posterior to anterior. The spinal nerves are identifiable in an E13 day rat embryo and the first signs of cutaneous innervation can be identified by E13.5 but only in terminal branches of the posterior cutaneous nerves. The posterior cutaneous nerve in mammals is a branch of the dorsal ramus, and the lateral and anterior cutaneous nerves are terminal branches of the intercostal nerve that are branches of the ventral ramus. The lateral and anterior cutaneous nerves innervate the epidermis by E14.5-15. All of these cutaneous nerves are arrayed in a geometric pattern reminiscent of the geometric pattern seen in digital skin by Dell and Munger (1986). In each case the dermatotopic map is established in an orderly progression in space and time.

Finally, the trophically mutual interdependence of these systems can be shown by modulating one and causing a compensatory modulation of the other. Recently we have been able to experimentally verify the concept that afferent nerves have a role in cutaneous differentiation in both chicken embryos (Munger, Terry and Kirby, 1985) and opossum pups (Jones and Munger, 1986). If afferent nerves have a role in cutaneous differentiation, what would be the impact of deleting these nerves, specifically by deleting neural crest and thus dorsal root ganglia? We were most fortunate in having the collaboration of Dr. M. Kirby. Kirby and Bockman (1985) had been studying the impact of neural crest deletions on cardiac development. Much to our surprise we have found striking hyperplasia of the dorsal root ganglia and an expansion of the dermatotopic map following neural crest deletion (Munger, Terry and Kirby, 1985). In the area of deletion, feathers do not form confirming Mauger (1972). The skin and afferent nervous system are thus trophically mutually interdependent.

REFERENCES:

Bannister LH (1976) Sensory terminals of peripheral nerves. In Landon DN (ed): "The Peripheral Nerve," New York: Wiley, pp 396-343.

Black IB (1984) "Cell and Molecular Biology of Neuronal Development." New York: Plenum Press.

Bressler MF and Munger BL (1983) Embryonic maturation of sensory terminals of primate facial hairs. J Invest Dermatol 80:245-260.

Cajal SR (1960) "Studies on Vertebrate Neurogenesis." (translated by Guth L) Springfield, Illinois: Charles C. Thomas.

Cummins H (1964) Dermatoglyphics: a brief review. In: Montagna, W and Lobita WC Jr. (eds): "The Epidermis," New York: Academic Press, pp 375-386.

Cummins H and Midlo C (1961) "Finger Palms, Palms and Soles: An Introduction to Dermatoglyphics." New York: Dover Publications.

Dell DA and Munger BL (1986) The early embryogenesis of papillary (sweat duct) ridges in primate glabrous skin: the dermatotopic map of cutaneous mechanoreceptors and dermatoglyphics. J Comp Neurol 244:511-532.

English KB, Burgess PR and Norman DK. (1980) Development of rat merkel cells. J Comp Neurol 194:475-496.

Fawcett JW and Cowan WM (1985) On the formation of eye dominance stripes and patches in the doubly-innervated optic tectum of the chick. Dev Brain Res 17:149-163.

Guillery RW (1982) The optic chiasm of the vertebrate brain. Contri Sens Physiol 6:39-47.

Halata Z (1975) The mechanoreceptors of the mammalian skin ultrastructure and morphological classification. Adv Anat 50:1-77.

Halata Z and Munger BL (1983) The sensory innervation of primate facial skin. II. Vermilion border and mucosa of lip. Brain Res Rev 5:81-107.

Hale AR (1952) Morphogenesis of volar skin in the human fetus. Am J Anat 91:147-181.

Ide C (1976) The fine structure of the digital corpuscle of the mouse toe pad with special reference to nerve fibers. Anat Rec 147:329-356.

Iggo A (1974) Cutaneous receptors. In: Hubbard SJ (ed): "The Peripheral Nervous System," New York: Pergamon, pp 397-404.

Jones TE and Munger BL (1985) Early differentiation of the afferent nervous system in the glabrous snout skin of the opossum (Monodelphis domestica). Somatosensensory Res 3:169-184.

Jones TE and Munger BL (1986) Intraepidermal axonal invasion and epidermal hyperplasia secondary to partial neuralectomy in postnatal opossum pups. Anat Rec 214:62A.

Kirby MK and Stewart DE (1983) Neural crest origin of cardiac ganglion cells in the chick embryo: identification and extirpation. Develop Biol 97:433-443.

Mauger A (1972) A role du tube neural dans le development du plumage dorsal de l'embryo de poulet. William Roux Arch 170:244-266.

Miller MR, Ralston HJ III and Kasahara M (1958) The pattern of cutaneous innervation of the human hand. Am J Anat 102:183-217.

Munger BL (1971) Patterns of organization of peripheral sensory receptors. In: Loewenstein WR (ed): "Handbook of Sensory Physiology," New York: Springer-Verlag, pp 523-556.

Munger BL (1982) Multiple afferent innervation of primate facial hairs - Henry Head and Max von Frey revisited. Brain Res Rev 4:1-43.

Munger BL and Halata Z (1983) The sensory innervation of primate facial skin. I. Hairy skin. Brain Res Rev 5:45-80.

Munger BL and Jones TE (1986) Spatial and temporal gradients in the differentiation of sensory nerves and mystacial hairs in postnatal opossum (Monodelphis Domestica) and rat pups. Anat Rec 214:90A.

Munger BL, Page RB and Pubols BH (1979) Identification of specific mechanosensory receptors in glabrous skin of dorsal root ganglionectomized primates. Anat Rec 193:630-631 (abstract).
Munger BL and Pubols LM (1972) The sensorineural organization of the digital skin of the raccoon. Brain Behav Evol 5:367-392.
Munger BL, Pubols LM and Pubols BH (1971) The Merkel rete papilla - a slowly adapting sensory receptor in mammalian glabrous skin. Brain Res 29:47-61.
Munger BL and Rice FL (1986) Successive waves of differentiation of cutaneous afferents in rat mystacial skin. J Comp Neurol, in press.
Munger BL, Terry S and Kirby ML (1985) Hyperplasia of dorsal root ganglia and expansion of the dermatotopic map following neural crest deletion in chick embryos. Amer Assoc Anat, Toronto, Ontario, Canada, pp 134A.
Perez APR (1931) Contribution a las connaissance des terminaisons intersudorales. Travaux du Lab de Recher 27:339-343.
Renehan WE and Munger BL (1986) Degeneration and regeneration of peripheral nerve in the rat trigeminal system. I. Identification and characterization of the multiple afferent innervation of the mystacial vibrissae. J Comp Neurol 246:129-145.
Rice FL (1985) Gradual changes in the structure of the barrels during maturation of the primary somatosensory cortex in the rat. J Comp Neurol 236:496-503.
Rice FL and Munger BL (1986) A comparative light microscopic analysis of the sensory innervation of the mystacial pad in the hamster, mouse, rat, gerbil, rabbit, guinea pig and cat. II. The common fur between the vibrissae. Submitted.
Rubel EW (1984) Ontogeny of auditory system function. Am Rev Physiol 46:213-229.
Schaumann B and Alter M (1976) "Dermatoglyphics in Medical Disorders." New York: Springer-Verlag, 1976.
Schmidt JT (1985) Formation of retinotopic connections: selective stabilization by an activity dependent mechanisms. Cell Mol Neurobiol 5:65-84.
Silverman RT, Munger BL and Halata Z (1986) The sensory innervation of the rat thinarium. Anat Rec 214:210-225.
Sladek JR and Gash GM (1984) "Neural transplants: Development and Function." New York: Plenum Publishing.
Walsh C and Polley EH (1985) Topography of ganglion cell production in the cat's retina. J Neurosci 5:741-750.

Effects of Injury on Trigeminal and Spinal Somatosensory Systems, pages 69–76

IMPROVEMENTS IN PERIPHERAL NERVE REGENERATION WITH PERMEABLE TUBES AND PRELIMINARY DATA INDICATING THAT THE IMPROVEMENTS ARE ASSOCIATED WITH CELLS OF THE GENERAL CONNECTIVE TISSUE

Richard E. Coggeshall and Chung-Bii Jenq

Marine Biomedical Institute and Departments of Anatomy & Neurosciences and Physiology & Biophysics, University of Texas Medical Branch, Galveston, Texas 77550

INTRODUCTION

One of the important issues for a symposium on the effects of injury on somatosensory systems is mechanisms of regeneration following somatic nerve transection. In this regard attention is often focussed on the nerve stumps, particularly the distal stump, because the distal stump is thought to emit substances that attract regenerating axons (Ramon y Cajal, 1959; Politis et al., 1982) and it is also a major source of cells that migrate into the gap between the stumps to surround the regenerating axons and provide extracellular matrices through which they grow (Thomas, 1966). One way to obtain these substances and cells is to place the stumps of a transected nerve in an impermeable tube. This pools the factors from the stumps around the regenerating axons and separates this regenerating system from the rest of the organism. This is thus an important paradigm and the first question this paper deals with is whether or not this pool of substances and cells is optimal for nerve regeneration. Somewhat to our surprise, we found that when the tube was made permeable, thus destroying the pool and allowing influences from the body in general to contact the regenerating axons, regeneration was improved, at least in terms of axonal numbers and the length of the interstump gap regenerating axons can span. The next issue for the present study is what is the reason for this improvement and our preliminary data indicates that certain cells from the body in general vigorously support axon regeneration after peripheral nerve transection.

MATERIALS AND METHODS

The experiments are done on adult Sprague-Dawley rats of either sex. Details of anesthesia, perfusion, fixation, embedding and examination for light and electron microscopy have been published in the articles cited from this laboratory. Each animal was subjected to 1 of the following procedures, 1) 8mm of sciatic nerve are removed in the thigh and the stumps are placed in a regular impermeable silicone tube with either an 8mm or 16mm gap maintained between the stumps (the impermeable tube), 2) 8mm of sciatic nerve are removed in the thigh and the stumps are placed in a silicone tube made completely permeable by drilling holes in its sides with either an 8 or a 16mm gap between the stumps (the permeable tube), 3) the sciatic nerve is transected, the distal stump turned aside, and the proximal stump inserted into a regular silicone tube 6mm long sealed at its distal end (the sealed tube), 4) the sciatic nerve is transected, the distal stump extensively removed, and the proximal stump inserted 2mm into a regular silicone tube 8mm long the distal end of which is covered by a nucleopore filter with a pore size of 1.2 μ (the small pore tube) and 5) the sciatic nerve is transected, the distal stump extensively removed, and the proximal stump inserted into a regular silicone tube the distal end of which is covered by a nucleopore filter of 5 μ size (the large pore tube).

RESULTS

Impermeable Tubes

Numbers of axons that regenerate across an 8mm gap in this paradigm have been published (Jenq and Coggeshall, 1985), but the actual numbers are not particularly important for the present argument. The major point is that both myelinated and unmyelinated axon numbers are significantly decreased in the gap after 8 weeks of regeneration although they have returned to normal after 9 months. By contrast, there is usually no regeneration of any kind across a 16mm gap, except in one instance where we found a tiny strand with 232 axons bridging the gap. These results are consistent with previous observations showing that transected rodent sciatic nerve axons can cross gaps of up to 10mm but no more if the stumps are placed in an impermeable tube (Lundborg et al., 1982; Seckel et al., 1984; Henry et al., 1985).

Permeable Tubes

When the silicone tube into which the nerve stumps are placed is made permeable by cutting macroscopic holes in its walls, the numbers of both myelinated and unmyelinated axons are closer to normal in the 8mm gap paradigm after 8 weeks of regeneration than after similar regeneration in a permeable tube (Jenq and Coggeshall, 1985). Of even more interest, however, is the fact that sizeable numbers of axons regenerate across the 16mm gap after 6 weeks of regeneration in this paradigm (preliminary data). The numbers of axons in the distal stumps of the 16mm permeable tube animals are approximately 3200 (± 1600 S.D.). The differences between the permeable and impermeable tube regeneration, in terms either of numbers of regenerated nerves or of numbers of regenerated axons, are statistically significant. Furthermore the nerve to the medial gastrocnemius muscle in 3 of the animals with successful 16mm regeneration contained an average of 37 axons. This indicates that some axons crossed the gap, passed into the distal stump and then into a tributary nerve, a distance approximately 31mm from the start of the regeneration at the distal end of the proximal stump, 6 weeks after nerve transection.

On the basis of the above data, we made the working hypothesis that cells from the general connective tissue provide something not available from the nerve stumps that facilitates regeneration. Three sets of data support this conclusion (see below). Because the work is underway, however, all we have at present are the relatively simple observations as to whether a nerve regenerated in a particular type of tube or not. Cytologic descriptions and axon numbers will be available in the future.

Blind Tubes

Five animals had the proximal stump of a transected sciatic nerve inserted into the proximal end of a silicone tube whose distal end was sealed. There was no growth in the tube in 4 animals and 1 animal had a tiny filament passing from the proximal stump down the middle of the tube. These results will be taken to imply that there is essentially no regeneration when proximal stumps are placed into blind but otherwise untreated silicone tubes.

Small Pore Tubes

Six animals had the proximal stump of a transected sciatic nerve inserted into the proximal end of a silicone tube whose distal end was covered by a nucleopore filter with a pore size of 1.2 μ. In 3 of these animals there was no regeneration. In the other 3 there was a small regenerated nerve that passed from the end of the proximal stump, as illustrated in the upper regenerate in Figure 1. Electron microscopic examination of the filter revealed that cell processes did not penetrate the 1.2 μ pores.

Large Pore Tubes

Six animals had the proximal stump of a transected sciatic nerve inserted into the proximal end of a silicone tube whose distal end was covered by a nucleopore filter with a pore size of 5 μ. In all of these animals, a large nerve cable regenerated to the filter, as illustrated in the lower regenerate in Figure 1. Electron microscopic examination of the filter revealed that cells passed through the 5 μ pores of the filters.

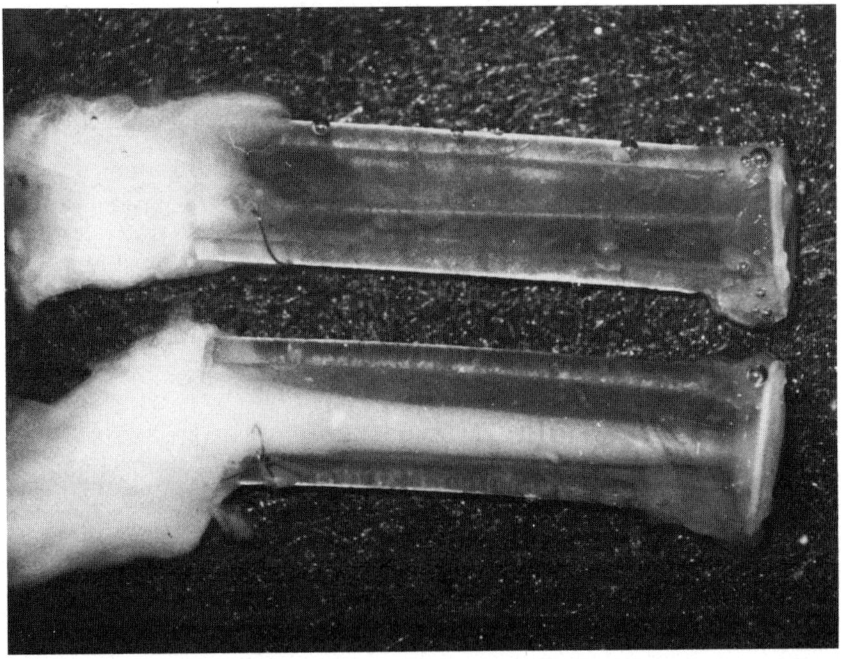

DISCUSSION

The ultimate goal of the research described in this paper and in much recent work from other laboratories is to obtain an understanding in cellular and molecular terms of the mechanisms of peripheral nerve regeneration. As indicated in the introduction, in the particular case of a transected nerve, attention has usually focussed on the nerve stumps, the proximal stump because it contains the regenerating axons and the distal stump because it seems to emit substances that attract regenerating axons and is a major source of cells that migrate between the stumps to surround the axons and provide them with extracellular matrices (Ramon y Cajal, 1958; Thomas, 1966). To study these processes in the animal, it is important to keep the system as simple as possible, and one way to do this is to keep factors from the stumps separate from factors from the body in general. To do this, Longo and associates (Longo et al., 1983a & b, 1984) modified a procedure previously used to guide axons from the proximal to the distal stump, namely placement of a transected nerve in an impermeable tube. When this was done, an important observation was that there was a limit to the gap the regenerating axons could span. In the case of rodent sciatic nerve, the gap was approximately 10mm (Lundborg et al., 1982; Seckel et al., 1984; Henry et al., 1985). In addition, axonal numbers in the gap had not returned to normal after 8 weeks of regeneration.

Because of the importance of the silicone tube paradigm in peripheral nerve regeneration research, we felt it desireable to test whether the pool of cells and soluble factors maintained around the regrowing axons was optimal for regeneration. Accordingly we made the tubes completely permeable by drilling holes in their sides. When this was done, axon numbers were closer to normal (Jenq and Coggeshall, 1985) and the axons could span considerably longer gaps than if an impermeable tube was used (preliminary data). Since it is a reasonable hypothesis that regeneration is better

---

Figure 1. These are 2 silicone tubes which have had the proximal stump of a transected sciatic nerve inserted into one end (the left in this picture) and a nucleopore filter seals the other end. The upper tube has a filter of pore size 1.2 μ and the lower a filter size of 5.0 μ. Note the much greater size of the regenerate in the lower regenerate.

when axonal numbers are closer to normal and when axons can span longer gaps, we feel that it is permissible to conclude that making an impermeable tube permeable improves peripheral nerve regeneration, at least for the parameters we measured.

The next question concerns the mechanisms which lead to more normal axon numbers and greater length of gap the axons span when a permeable tube is used. It seemed to us that there were 2 possibilities, 1) that pooling of material around the stumps is deleterious, perhaps for as simple a reason as a buildup of metabolites or a lack of oxygen or 2) that there was something not in the nerve stumps, or at least not enough of something in the nerve stumps for optimal regeneration. Thus we designed the experiments with the proximal stump alone to begin to get some preliminary data on these questions (see results). We emphasize that these findings are preliminary, but what we can infer at present is that when a proximal stump is placed in a blind but otherwise unmanipulated silicone tube there is no significant regeneration, when the proximal stump is placed in a similar tube but the distal end is opened enough to allow fluid to pass but not cells (the small pore tubes), regeneration is poor, but when the regeneration is into a similar tube but the distal end is open enough for cells and fluid to penetrate (the large pore tubes), regeneration is very good. This allows us to conclude tentatively that cells from the body in general, as distinct from cells from the nerve stumps, have some role, presumably an important role, in nerve regeneration. Further work to confirm the above observations, to get axon numbers and an accurate cytologic description of each of the regenerated nerves, to identify into what these cells are doing are underway.

In summary, placing nerve stumps in an impermeable tube was first used as a general procedure for guiding regenerating axons from the proximal to the distal stump of a transected nerve. For various technical reasons, this procedure is not regarded as the equal of an autologous transplant for long gap repair of human nerve transection (Sunderland, 1976), but if the difficulties can be overcome, the use of a tube might alleviate the necessity of taking another nerve from the patient for a transplant. The silicone tube paradigm is also useful in basic nerve regeneration research because it pools factors from the stumps around the regenerating axons and isolates them from the rest of the organism. Most previous attention has focussed on the factors from the stumps, as compared to the factors from the body in general, but finding that regeneration is superior with a permeable tube suggests that attention should also be devoted to the general body factors. The present report also discusses evidence indicating that the general factors that improve regeneration are associated with the entry of cells into the tube. Thus the silicone tube paradigm offers a useful preparation for those whose goal it is to understand the cellular and molecular bases of nerve regeneration in the living animal.

CONCLUSIONS

1. When stumps of transected rodent nerves are placed in impermeable tubes, there is a limit to the length of the interstump gap the axons can cross and axon numbers are less than normal in the regenerate 8 weeks after transection.
2. When the tube is made permeable, the axons can span a longer gap and axon numbers are closer to normal 8 weeks after transection.
3. Thus certain aspects of regeneration are improved when a previously impermeable tube is made permeable.
4. This suggested that certain factors from the body in general, as distinct from factors in the stumps, might also be important for peripheral nerve regeneration.
5. Preliminary evidence indicates that the important factors from the body in general are cells as opposed to soluble compounds.
6. Further work to confirm these findings, to identify the cells and to specify their role in nerve regeneration is underway.

REFERENCES

Henry EN, Chiu T-H, Nyilas E, Brushart TM, Dikkes P, Sidman RL (1985). Nerve regeneration through polyester biodegradeable tubes. Exp Neurol 90:652-676.

Jenq CB, Coggeshall RE (1985). Nerve regeneration through holey silicone tubes. Brain Res 361:233-241.

Longo FM, Manthorpe M, Skaper SD, Lundborg G, Varon S (1983) Neuronotrophic activities accumulate _in vivo_ within silicone nerve regeneration chambers. Brain Res 261: 109-117.

Longo FM, Skaper SD, Manthorpe M, Williams LR, Lundborg G,

Varon S (1983). Temporal changes of neuronotrophic activities accumulating in vivo within nerve regeneration chambers. Exp Neurol 81:756-769.

Longo FM, Hayman EG, Davis GE, Ruoslahti E, Engvall E, Manthorpe M, Varon S (1984). Neurite-promoting factors and extracellular matrix components accumulating in vivo within nerve regeneration chambers. Brain Res 309:105-117.

Lundborg G, Dahlin LB, Danielsen N, Gelberman RH, Longo FM, Powell HC, Varon S (1982). Nerve regeneration in silicone chambers: influence of gap length and of distal stump components. Exp Neurol 76:361-375.

Politis MJ, Ederle K, Spencer PS (1982). Tropism in nerve regeneration in vivo. Attraction of regenerating axons by diffusible factors from cells in distal nerve stumps of transected peripheral nerves. Brain Res 253:1-12.

Ramon y Cajal S (1959) "Degeneration and Regeneration of the Nervous System." New York, Hafner Publishing Co.

Seckel BR, Chiu T-H, Nyilas D, Sidman RL (1984). Nerve regeneration through synthetic biodegradeable nerve guides: Regulation by the target organ. Plas Recon Surg 74:173-181.

Sunderland S (1978). "Nerves and Nerve Injury." Edinburgh, Churchill Livingston.

Thomas PK (1966). The cellular response to nerve injury. I. The cellular outgrowth from the distal stump of the transected nerve. J Anat 100:287-303.

ACKNOWLEDGEMENTS

This research is supported by NIH grants NS10161, 17039, 11255, 07185 and the Texas Neurofibromatosis Foundation.

Effects of Injury on Trigeminal and Spinal Somatosensory Systems, pages 77–83

HAS THE AMOUNT OF SPONTANEOUS ELECTRICAL ACTIVITY IN EXPERIMENTAL NEUROMAS BEEN OVERESTIMATED?

Kim J. Burchiel and Lisa C. Russell
Dept. of Neurological Surgery
University of Washington
Veteran's Administration Hospital
Seattle, Washington 98108

INTRODUCTION

Abnormal sensations which occasionally develop after peripheral nerve injury may be related to spontaneous discharges which appear to originate in neuromas (Burchiel, 1984a, 1984b; Burchiel and Russell, 1985a, 1985b, 1985c; Govrin-Lippmann and Devor, 1978; Scadding, 1981; Wall and Gutnick, 1974a, 1974b). Previous investigations indicated that a profusion of spontaneous activity was found in experimental neuromas, and it has been proposed that this activity may contribute to clinical symptoms such as mechanosensitive and spontaneous pains. Although mechanosensitivity of neuromas and partial nerve injuries is well-known (Tinel's sign), the clinical correlate of ongoing spontaneous activity, commonly recorded in experimental neuromas, has been problematic, since the vast majority of human neuromas are described as nonpainful.

We and others (Devor, 1983) have previously reported that potassium channel-blocking agents can markedly increase the incidence of spontaneously active fibers recorded in an experimental neuroma. Furthermore, Smith and Schauf (1981) have demonstrated that an agent commonly used for muscular paralysis in animal experiments, gallamine, has potent potassium channel-blocking properties. When gallamine is used during acute microfilament recording from neuromas it can increase the apparent level of spontaneous activity in a given axon (Burchiel and Russell, 1985b, Devor, 1983).

We hypothesized that the results of previous studies of experimental neuromas may have, in many cases, been confounded by the use of gallamine, resulting in an overestimation of the incidence of spontaneous activity. We conducted the present series of experiments to investigate this possibility. We have also refined our recording protocol to better quantitate both the velocity and direction of propagated action potentials (APs) as recorded by the microfilament technique.

METHODS

Forty-two adult male Sprague-Dawley rats were used in these experiments. At the time of the initial surgeries, all rats were anesthetized with pentobarbital (60 mg/Kg IP intial dose and 10 mg IV every 20-30 minutes thereafter) and the left saphenous nerve was exposed along the medial hindlimb at the level of the distal femur. A 3-5 mm section of the nerve was isolated then ligated with 6-0 polypropylene suture and divided distal to the suture.

From 6-28 days after saphenous nerve section, rats were anesthetized as above, and acute recording was performed in the nerve using a modification of the microfilament technique. This technique involved recording of propagated APs at two points along the nerve: At the microfilament and an averaged AP obtained from the whole nerve trunk some distance away.

Microfilament recordings were performed in control animals and those with saphenous neuromas both before and after the administration of gallamine (20 mg IV initially and 10 mg every half hour thereafter).

RESULTS

In 6 rats, no prior saphenous neurotomy was performed and recordings of spontaneous activity in an isolated saphenous segment were made. Spontaneous activity in these nerves was rare and was not significantly affected by the administration of gallamine.

An additional 36 rats with saphenous neurotomies made from 6-28 days prior to acute microfilament recording were studied. To summarize our results, in our preparation and in animals not treated with gallamine, spontaneous activity originating in the neuroma was rare. In addition, many spontaneous discharges which might have been previously confused with neuroma activity actually originated in along adjacent small arteries, within the fascia surrounding the nerve, or in the hairy skin and subcutaneous tissue of the medial hindlimb. Although uncommon, it was surprising to find apparently intact cutaneous receptive fields for saphenous microfilaments, despite the appearance of complete nerve transection distally by inspection under the dissecting microscope.

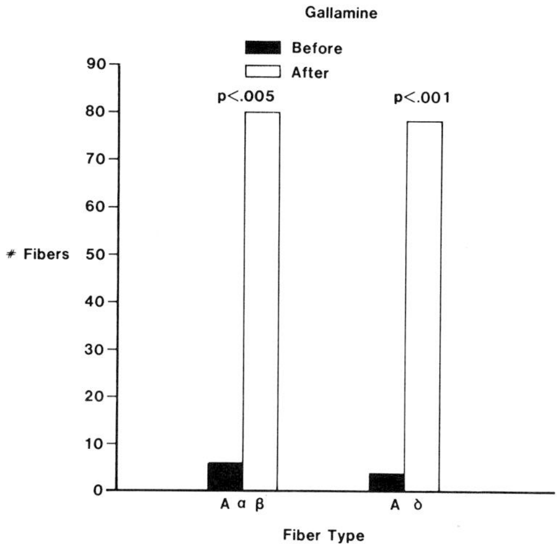

Figure 1. Axons exhibiting spontaneous discharges from 6-28 day rat neuromas before and after gallamine. Gallamine produced significantly more A-alpha/beta and A-delta spontaneous activity. No on-going C-fiber activity originating in the neuroma was recorded before or after gallamine.

The total number of microfilaments recorded showing spontaneous activity after gallamine treatment in all animals with neuromas increased by a factor of 12.75 in comparison to recordings made in those same animals before the administration of gallamine (Figure 1). No spontaneous C-fiber activity originating in the neuroma was recorded either before or after gallamine administration (Figure 2).

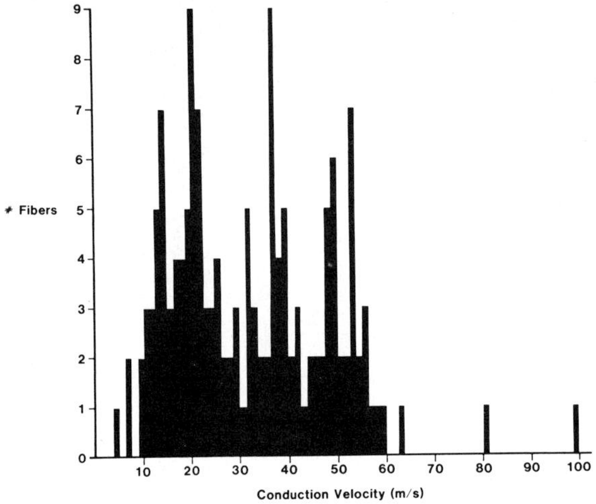

Figure 2. Conduction velocity spectrum of spontaneously active axons from 6-28 day saphenous neuromas after gallamine treatment. Most fibers fell within the A-beta and A-delta range.

DISCUSSION

Previous reports have speculated that ectopic discharge may emanate from regenerating primary afferents in neuromas and thus may be responsible for the genesis of painful paresthesias which can develop after nerve injury (Burchiel, 1984a, 1984b; Burchiel and Russell, 1985a, 1985b, 1985c; Devor and Govrin-Lippmann, 1983; Govrin-Lippmann and Devor, 1978; Scadding, 1981; Wall and Gutnick, 1974a, 1974b). Large numbers of spontaneously active fibers recorded in experimental neuromas have been defined within the A-alpha/beta and A-delta ranges (Burchiel, 1984a, 1984b; Burchiel and Russell, 1985a, 1985b, 1985c; Meyer et al., 1985; Wall and Gutnick, 1974a, 1974b) yet information on spontaneous activity in neuroma C-fibers is incomplete (Devor and Raber, 1983). Our data from a purely sensory nerve depicts a neuroma as a structure which only rarely produces spontaneous impulses in myelinated fibers and never in unmyelinated axons.

The use of gallamine, a potent potassium channel-blocking agent, in previous studies may have resulted in the overestimation of spontaneous activity in experimental neuromas. Furthermore, C-fiber recordings presumably originating in the neuroma, may have been from intact surrounding receptive fields. This, combined with less precise measures for determination of conduction velocity in unmyelinated axons, may have resulted in the erroneous conclusion that neuromas contained C-fibers that were spontaneously active. We have not been able to demonstrate that neuromas produce C- fiber discharges, despite the use of a technique that can discriminate propagated C-fiber activity produced by simulation of intact receptive fields.

Lastly, these results are concordant with the clinical characteristics of neuromas: While the majority of neuromas are mechanosensitive, very few produce a clinical pain syndrome. Our results indicate that neuromas are, for the most part, electrically silent unless stimulated by either perturbing the ionic flux of the axon membrane or by mechanical stimulation.

CONCLUSIONS

(1) Neuromas exhibit only rare spontaneous discharges unless exposed to potassium channel-blocking agents.

(2) All C-fiber activity recorded in saphenous nerve with a distal neuroma is derived from vascular, fascial and other receptive fields rather than the neuroma.

(3) These data are consistent with known clinical phenomena in that neuromas are not usually spontaneously painful.

REFERENCES

Burchiel KJ (1984a). Effects of electrical and mechanical stimulation on two foci of spontaneous activity which develop in primary afferent neurons after peripheral axotomy. Pain 18:249-265.

Burchiel KJ (1984b). Spontaneous impulse generation in normal and denervated dorsal root ganglia: Sensitivity to alpha-adrenergic stimulation and anoxia. Exp Neurol 85:257-272.

Burchiel KJ, Russell LC (1985a). Spontaneous activity of ventral root axons following peripheral nerve injury. J Neurosurg 62:408-413.

Burchiel KJ, Russell LC (1985b). Effect of potassium channel-blocking agents on spontaneous discharges from neuromas in rats. J Neurosurg 63:246-249.

Burchiel KJ, Russell LC (1985c). Glycerol neurolysis: neurophysiological effects of topical glycerol application on rat saphenous nerve. J Neurosurg 63:784-788.

Burchiel KJ, Russell LC (1986). A method for determination of conduction velocities in myelinated and unmyelinated single axons. Exp Neurol submitted.

Devor M (1983). Potassium channels moderate ectopic excitability of nerve-end neuromas in rats. Neurosci Lett 40:181-186.

Devor M, Govrin-Lippmann R (1983). Axoplasmic transport block reduces ectopic impulse generation in injured peripheral nerves. Pain 16:73-85.

Devor M, Raber P (1983). Autotomy after nerve injury and its relation to spontaneous discharge originating in nerve-end neuromas. Behav Neural Biol 37:276-283.

Govrin-Lippmann R, Devor M (1978). Ongoing activity in severed nerves: Source and variation with time. Brain Res 159:406-410.

Meyer RA, Raja SN, Campbell JN, Mackinnon SE, Dellon AL (1985). Neural activity originating from a neuroma in the baboon. Brain Res 325:255-260.

Scadding JW (1981). The development of on-going activity, mechanosensitivity and adrenaline sensitivity in severed peripheral nerve axons. Exp Neurol 73:345-364.

Smith KJ, Schauf CL (1981). Effects of gallamine triethiodide on membrane and currents in amphibian and mammalian peripheral nerve. J Pharmacol Exp Ther 217: 719-726.

Wall PD, Gutnick M (1974a). Properties of afferent nerve impulses originating from a neuroma. Nature 248: 740-743.

Wall PD, Gutnick M (1974b). Ongoing activity in peripheral nerves. The physiology and pharmacology of impulses originating from a neuroma. Exp Neurol 43: 580-593.

Effects of Injury on Trigeminal and Spinal Somatosensory Systems, pages 85–92

CHANGES IN PRIMARY AFFERENT NEURONS FOLLOWING LESIONS OF THEIR AXONS

Helmut Blumberg and Wilfrid Jänig

Universität Kiel, Physiologisches Institut, Olshausenstr. 40, 2300 Kiel, FRG (W.J.)
Neurologische Klinik, Universität Freiburg, Hansastr. 9, 7800 Freiburg, FRG (H.B.)

INTRODUCTION

Peripheral nerve lesions are followed by reactions of the primary afferent neurons which may be considered as an attempt of the neurons to repair the interruption between axon and target organ (see Lieberman, 1974; Jänig, 1985). These neurobiological changes entail many clinical phenomena (including pain) in patients who have accidentally undergone such nerve lesions. It is difficult to relate the clinical (sensory, skeleto-motor, autonomic and other) phenomena which are observed in patients to individual pathobiological processes which can be measured under controlled experimental conditions in animals. The following article summarizes some of the neurophysiological changes which occur in primary afferent cutaneous axons when the peripheral nerve trunk is transected and regeneration of its axons is prevented. Most data discussed were obtained on afferent fibers that ended in neuromas of the superficial peroneal nerve of the cat (see Blumberg and Jänig, 1982a, 1982b, 1984).

RESULTS

1) Morphological changes

Neurons projecting in a skin nerve undergo considerable changes when their peripheral axons are transected and regeneration is prevented. The axon central to the lesion generates multiple sprouts which mostly originate close to the lesion, but possibly also in the nerve proximal to the lesion. Axons and cell bodies shrink. These changes occur in neurons with myelinated axons as well as those with unmyelinated ones and are reflected in a decrease of the conduction velocity of these axons (Cragg and Thomas, 1961; Davis et al, 1978, Blumberg and Jänig, 1982a). The neurons with unmyelinated axons seem to be more affected than the neurons with myelinated ones: many of the former may finally die (Jänig and McLachlan, 1984; Aldskogius et al, 1985; Arvidson et al, 1986). The time course and degree of shrinkage and cell death varies according to the distance of the lesion from the cell body. Both phenomena may also occur in the postganglionic sympathetic neurons which project in the lesioned peripheral nerve (Jänig and McLachlan, 1984). Experimental results obtained so far on cats and rats are somewhat controversial concerning the latter point (see Peyronnard et al, 1986). It has, however, been shown in cats that many postganglionic sympathetic neurons projecting in a skin nerve which was cut and ligated some 4 to 33 weeks before cannot any longer be activated by electrical stimulation of the preganglionic axons in the sympathetic chain; this is probably due to failure and inefficiency of synaptic transmission in sympathetic ganglia after depriving the postganglionic neurons of their target organs (see Blumberg and Jänig, 1982a).

2) Ongoing activity

Lesioned primary afferents which end in a neuroma may develop ongoing activity. This activity originates in the neuroma: cutting the nerve proximal to the recording electrode does not affect rate and pattern of ongoing activity. There are considerable variations between cats in the frequency of afferent fibers with ongoing activity: in the first 4-7 weeks only few fibers discharge spontaneously (0 - 10%), thereafter the percentage increases (about 3 to 40%). The rate of ongoing activity is mostly below 1 Hz, some fibers discharge at rates above 1 Hz and few at higher rates of 4 to maximally 15 Hz. The high dischage rates were nearly almost only found in myelinated fibers and in young neuromas (below 27 days). Ongoing activity in unmyelinated fibers had mostly rates of less than 1 Hz, was irregular and exhibited frequently considerable spontaneous fluctuations which were not correlated to any changes occurring in the animal or in the environment of the neuroma. Myelinated fibers tended to discharge more regularly and sometimes in bursts. Generally only very few myelinated fibers from cat neuromas discharged spontaneously.

The results obtained on afferent fibers from neuromas of cutaneous nerves of the cat are quantitatively different to those obtained on afferent fibers of neuromas of the sciatic nerve of mice and certain strains of rats (see Govrin--Lippmann and Devor, 1978; Devor and Bernstein, 1982; Scadding, 1981). First, in rats and mice the rate of ongoing activity is very high and may reach values of more than 50 Hz (means about 23 to 25 Hz). Second, the frequency of fibers with ongoing activity from neuromas of the sciatic nerve in rodents increases to about 20 to 30% in the second to third week after the nerve lesion and drops thereafter to values of 5% or less. However, it should be kept in mind that almost all fibers investigated in these experiments were myelinated, whereas in the cat 70% of the analyzed afferents or more conducted at less than 2 m/s (Blumberg and Jänig, 1984). Recently it was reported that unmyelinated fibers from rat neuromas also discharge spontaneously at very low rates, and that this ongoing discharge is also seen in neuroma nerves which are older than 3-4 weeks (Devor and Govrin-Lippmann, 1985).

3) Mechanosensitivity

Many fibers from a neuroma can be activated by mechanical stimulation of the neuroma (Scadding, 1981; Blumberg and Jänig, 1984). Fibers with ongoing activity are also mechanosensitive, but so are many silent fibers. The frequency of afferent units being mechanosensitive may reach 50% or more and varies considerably between animals. The percentage of mechanosensitive afferent units from old neuromas seem to be higher in cats than in mice. The mechanosensitivity was restricted to the neuroma. No afferent units were found which responded to mechanical stimulation of the neuroma nerve.

The mechanical thresholds to activate the fibers vary from very low to high. This is probably due to the location of the mechanosensitive endings in the neuroma. The afferent units have often well-defined "receptive fields" on the neuroma surface. Some afferent units exhibit afterdischarges upon mechanical stimulation of the neuroma. This afterdischarge lasted for about 1 to 5 min after removing the stimulus of about 10 s length. The afterdischarges were particularly observed after strong mechanical stimuli. The afferent discharges during and after the mechanical stimuli were accompanied by increases of the blood pressure.

4) Chemosensitivity

It is of considerable interest whether the afferent fibers which end in neuromas are excited by stimulation of the sympathetic supply to the neuromas and by adrenaline and noradrenaline injected i.v. or i.a.. In the cat the effects of repetitive electrical stimulation of the sympathetic preganglionic axons in the sympathetic chain (20 to 25 Hz for 2 to 10 s, maximal strength for all fibers) which synapse with postganglionic neurons projecting to the neuroma were very subtle. This may have been partly due to degeneration of postganglionic neurons and due to impaired impulse transmission in sympathetic ganglia following the peripheral nerve lesion (see Blumberg and Jänig, 1984; Jänig and McLachlan, 1984). However, adrenaline and noradrenaline injected in doses of up to 20 µg i.v. were also relatively ineffective. Responses to mechanical stimuli applied to the neuroma were not enhanced by adrenaline injected i.v. or by electrical stimulation of the lumbar sympathetic chain. The weak effects produced by the relatively high doses of catecholamines injected i.v. may have been due to a too low concentration of the catecholamines in the neuroma and it is possible that under favorable conditions noradrenaline released from varicosities reach very high local concentrations.

Data obtained on afferent units from neuromas in rodents (particularly Sabra albino rats; see Devor and Jänig, 1981; Korenman and Devor, 1981) differ quantitatively from those obtained in cats. Many fibers with ongoing activity from sciatic nerve neuromas were excited by systemically applied adrenaline and noradrenaline and upon electrical stimulation of the sympathetic supply to the neuroma. These effects could be blocked by α-adrenergic antagonists.

As interesting as these results are, it must be kept in mind that the sympathetic supply had to be stimulated at 10 Hz or more for 1 to 10 s in order to see the effects. Discharge frequencies of 10 Hz or more are only observed in sympathetic neurons under extreme conditions, if at all (Jänig, 1985b).

These somewhat disappointing results concerning the postganglionic adrenergic effects on discharges of neuroma fibers does not mean that the chemical postganglionic-afferent link does not exist. The experiments show , first, that quantitatively large responses are rare (and this might be expected from the clinical experience), second, that there are possibly species and genetic differences (see Devor, 1983) and, third, that other types of experimental nerve lesions have to be designed which increase the likelihood that this chemical coupling between postganglionic noradrenergic axons and afferent axons develops.

5) Ephaptic transmission

Fibers which are isolated from a neuroma nerve and cut centrally, thus leaving the connection to the neuroma intact, may be excited by stimulation of other fibers in the same nerve. Blocking the conduction in the nerve just proximal to the neuroma by cooling normally abolishes this response, arguing that the transmission of impulses occurs in the neuroma. The responses normally follow high frequency stimulation and have constant latencies and thresholds. The stimulated and recorded fibers are myelinated and unmyelinated. In the first 30 days after the nerve cut the event is rare though not absent, later it is more common attaining up to 15 - 25% of all tested axons. Postganglionic axons are probably not involved. Similar results have been obtained on lesioned cutaneous nerves in the cat (Blumberg and Jänig 1982b; Lisney and Power, 1982a,b) and on the lesioned sciatic nerve in the rat (Seltzer and Devor, 1979).

The phenomenon may be explained in either of two ways: first, ephaptic transmission ("cross talk") between fibers in the neuroma or, second, retrograde sprouting of fibers in the nerve over long distances. We favor the first possibility since the phenomenon was already occasionally observed at short time intervals of 6 and 13 days following cutting and ligating the skin nerve. Retrograde sprouting would have to occur in these experiments at speeds of 6 to 12 mm/day over distances of 60 to 75 mm (Blumberg and Jänig, 1982b). Furthermore ephaptic transmission may occur via close appositions between nerve fibers without intervening isolating tissue such as Schwann cell cytoplasm. These appositions have been described to occur quite frequently in neuromas (Bernstein and Pagnanelli, 1982; Devor and Bernstein, 1982;

Jänig, 1985a).

Some afferent units in neuroma nerves which can be excited (probably ephaptically) by stimulation of other fibers exhibit also ongoing activity and can be activated by mechanical stimulation of the neuroma (Blumberg and Jänig, 1984). This means that the ephaptically excited units generate the ongoing activity and are mechanosensitive or that the afferent units are ephaptically excited by other units which exhibit ongoing activity and mechanosensitivity.

There are also indications from neurophysiological experiments on cats that fibers may either sprout or be coupled ephaptically in the neuroma nerve at considerable distances proximal to the neuroma. It has been shown that some fibers which are cut distally can be activated by electrical stimulation of the neuroma nerve distal to the recording site and sometimes even by mechanical stimulation of the neuroma. The responses elicited electrically have constant latencies and thresholds and follow short trains of electrical stimuli at 10 to 50 Hz. These responses can only very rarely be observed (less than 1%) in normal skin nerves (Blumberg and Jänig, unpublished observations). Close appositions between unmyelinated fibers have been observed in neuroma nerves (Vahle-Hinz, unpublished observation).

Generally it can be concluded that ephaptic transmission between fibers in the neuroma and in the neuroma nerve can lead to impulse multiplication. Small excitations produced by trivial events may in this way lead to large barrages of impulses to the spinal cord.

SUMMARY

When the peripheral axons of primary afferent neurons are cut and regeneration of their axons to the target organs is prevented, many functional changes may occur in the afferent neurons. 1) The neurons shrink and may eventually die. The latter may particularly apply to neurons with unmyelinated axons. 2) The axons sprout and form together with the proliferated Schwann cells a neuroma. 3) The sprouts of many myelinated and unmyelinated fibers in the neuroma develop ongoing activity, mechanosensitivity and chemosensitivity, thus they are excited by mechanical stimulation of the neuroma and by chemical agents (such as e.g. noradrenaline). 4)

In the neuroma sprouts may be electrically coupled via close appositions of axon profiles, leading to ephaptic transmission ("cross talk") between fibers. This pathophysiological mechanism may lead to multiplication of afferent impulses. 5) Also in the neuroma nerve fibers may be ephaptically coupled and sprout.

REFERENCES

ALDSKOGIUS H, ARVIDSON J, GRANT G (1985). The reaction of primary sensory neurons to peripheral nerve injury with particular emphasis on transganglionic changes. Brain Res Reviews 10: 27-46.

ARVIDSON J, YGGE J, GRANT, G (1986). Cell loss in lumbar dorsal root ganglia and transganglionic degeneration after sciatic nerve resection in the rat. Brain Res 373: 15-21.

BERNSTEIN JJ, PAGNANELLI D (1982). Long-term axonal apposition in rat sciatic nerve neuroma. J Neurosurg 57: 682-684.

BLUMBERG H, JÄNIG W (1982a). Changes in unmyelinated fibers including sympathetic postganglionic fibers of a skin nerve after peripheral neuroma formation. J Auton Nerv Syst 6: 173-183.

BLUMBERG H, JÄNIG W (1982b). Activation of fibers via experimentally produced stump neuromas of skin nerves: ephaptic transmission or retrograde sprouting? Exp Neurol 76: 468-482.

BLUMBERG H, JÄNIG W (1984). Discharge pattern of afferent fibers from a neuroma. Pain 20: 335-353.

CRAGG GB, THOMAS PK (1961). Changes in conduction velocity and fibre size proximal to peripheral nerve lesions. J Physiol (Lond) 157: 315-327.

DAVIS LA, GORDON T, HOFFER JA, JHAMANDAS J, STEIN RB (1979). Compound action potentials recorded from mammalian peripheral nerves following ligation and resuturing. J Physiol (Lond) 285: 543-559.

DEVOR M (1983). Nerve pathophysiology and mechanisms of pain in causalgia. J Auton Nerv Syst 7: 371-384.

DEVOR M, BERNSTEIN JJ (1982). Abnormal impulse generation in neuromas: electrophysiology and ultrastructure. In WJ Culp, J Ochoa (eds), Abnormal Nerves and Muscles as Impulse Generators, Oxford University Press, London, pp 363-380.

DEVOR M, GOVRIN-LIPPMANN R (1985). Spontaneous neural discharge in neuroma C-fibers in rat sciatic nerve.

Neurosci Lett Suppl 22: S32.
DEVOR M, JÄNIG W (1981). Activation of myelinated afferents ending in a neuroma by stimulation of the sympathetic supply in the rat. Neurosci Lett 24: 43-47.
GOVRIN-LIPPMANN R, DEVOR M (1978). Ongoing activity in severed nerves: source and variation with time. Brain Res 159: 406-410.
JÄNIG W (1985a). Causalgia and reflex sympathetic dystrophy: in which way is the sympathetic nervous system involved? Trends in Neurosci 8: 471-477.
JÄNIG W (1985b). Organization of the lumbar sympathetic outflow to skeletal muscle and skin of the cat hindlimb and tail. Rev Physiol Biochem Pharmacol 102: 119-213.
JÄNIG W, MCLACHLAN EM (1985). On the fate of symapthetic and sensory neurons projecting into a neuroma of the superficial peroneal nerve in the cat. J Comp Neurol 225: 302-311.
KORENMAN EMD, DEVOR M (1981). Ectopic adrenergic sensitivity in damaged peripheral nerve axons in the rat. Exp Neurol 72: 63-81.
LIEBERMAN AR (1974). Some factors affecting retrograde neuronal responses to axonal lesions. In R Bellairs, EG Gray (eds), Esays on the Nervous System. A Festschrift for Prof JZ Young. Clarendon Press, Oxford, pp 71-105.
LISNEY SJW, POVER CM (1982a). Coupling between fibres in sensory nerve neuromas in cats. J Physiol (Lond) 327: 6-7P.
Lisney SJW, POVER CM (1982b) Coupling between regenerated sensory nerve fibres in the cat. J Physiol (Lond) 334: 71-72P.
PEYRONNARD JM, CHARRON L, LAVOIE J, MESSIER JP (1986). Differences in horseradish peroxidase labeling of sensory, motor and sympathetic neurons following chronic axotomy of the rat sural nerve. Brain Res 364: 137-150.
SCADDING JW (1981). Development of ongoing activity, mechanosensitivity, and adrenaline sensitivity in severed peripheral nerve axons. Exp Neurol 73: 345-364.
SELTZER Z, DEVOR M (1979). Ephaptic transmission in chronically damaged peripheral nerves. Neurology (Mineap) 29: 1061-1064.

Effects of Injury on Trigeminal and Spinal Somatosensory Systems, pages 93–106

RESPONSE CHARACTERISTICS OF FIBERS IN REGENERATING AND REGENERATED CUTANEOUS NERVES IN CAT AND RAT

Manfred Zimmermann, Gabriele-Monika Koschorke and Karl Sanders
Department of Physiology, University of Heidelberg, Heidelberg, FRG

INTRODUCTION

A patient with a regenerating or regenerated somatosensory nerve may complain about various abnormal sensations: anesthesia, dysesthesia, paresthesia, hyperesthesia, pain and causalgia (Sunderland, 1978). What are the neurobiological mechanisms behind these clinical phenomena? The state of anesthesia has a rather simple explanation: absence of sensory nerve endings in the denervated territory. The other abnormal sensory phenomena, including pain, have been assumed to be due to some form of hyperexcitability of the regenerative sensory nerve sprouts or the regenerated sensory fibers.

I would like to give an outline of our recent work in this field. We have performed two kinds of experiments in cutaneous nerves of cats and rats:

- Neuroma were produced to investigate the responsiveness of the nerve sprouts to endogenous chemical substances.
- Fiber regrowth was induced by nerve crush to assess the functional restitution of cutaneous mechanoreceptors and nociceptors after reinnervation of the skin.

CHEMOSENSITIVITY OF NERVE SPROUTS IN A NEUROMA

Several laboratories have contributed to the analysis of impulse generation in the neuroma, using electrophysiological recording from the fibers of the neuroma nerve (Wall and Gutnick, 1974; Korenman and Devor, 1981; Scadding, 1981; Blumberg and Jänig, 1984; Burchiel, 1984). Sprouts of the regenerating fibers show discharges in response to mechanical stimulation, to administration of adrenaline, and to activation of the sympathetic trunk. Ongoing activity was also observed. Here, we report on the modulation of excitability of neuroma sprouts by bradykinin, substance P, adrenaline, and noradrenaline.

Methods. To produce a neuroma, the sural nerve was transected and ligated unilaterally in cats under anesthesia with pentobarbital sodium (35 or 40 mg/kg intraperitoneally). Postoperatively no signs of pain or discomfort could be observed: in particular, scratching or self-mutilation of the denervated nerve territory did not occur. Weeks afterwards, the animals were again anesthetized. The perineurial sheath around the neuroma was opened and the neuroma was put into a small perspex chamber for superfusion with various solutions. A filament was separated from a desheathed proximal section of the nerve for recording of unit action potentials in A- and C-fibers, as could be identified by electrical nerve stimulation close to the neuroma (Fig. 1A). Multi-fiber discharges were plotted as histograms (Fig. 1B to E).

Results. Within 3 weeks following nerve transection a neuroma had developed on the nerve stump. In most filaments ongoing activity was seen, usually arising in one or two single C-fibers, at discharge rates below 1 imp/s (Fig. 1B). No ongoing activity was seen in A-fibers. Responses could be elicited in A- and C-fibers by mild mechanical probing of the neuroma. We did not quantify these responses as they have been extensively studied by others (Scadding, 1981; Devor and Bernstein, 1982; Blumberg and Jänig, 1984).

Discharges were elicited for about 60 s in C-fibers when the neuroma was superfused with bradykinin (Fig. 1C) starting after latencies between 15 and 125 s. The maximum discharge rate or the total number of impulses increased dose-dependently. Thresholds of discharges were between 1 and 10 µg/ml of bradykinin. In part of the filaments, repeated periods of discharges appeared during a continuous irrigation with bradykinin. After exposure to bradykinin for about 5 min the responding fibers showed prolonged desensitization to a subsequent administration of the same substance, which could last for more than 15 min.

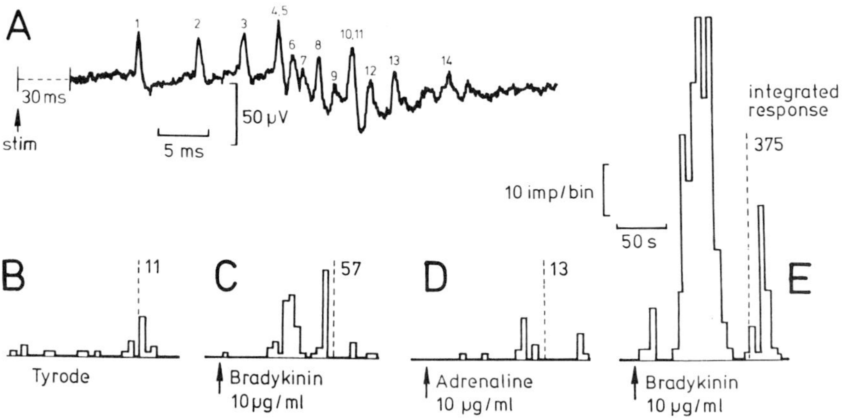

Figure 1. Discharges of neuroma C-fibers evoked and sensitized by chemical substances. (A) Recording from a filament of a cat's sural nerve, after electrical stimulation 40 mm distally. C-fiber action potentials are labelled 1 to 14. (B to E) Histograms of C-fiber discharges recorded from a filament during superfusion of the neuroma with Tyrode solution (B), with a solution containing bradykinin (C) or adrenaline (D) and then again bradykinin (E). Superfusions lasted 5 min, starts were indicated by arrows. The numbers at the vertical broken lines indicate the integrated responses from the start of superfusion. The time separation between (C) and (D) was 10 min. Bradykinin superfusion in (E) was started immediately at the end of the 5 min superfusion with adrenaline in (D).

The fibers activated by bradykinin were almost exclusively C-fibers. We found that 26% of the C-fibers contained in the recorded filaments responded to bradykinin. No responses occurred in A-beta-fibers, and of 50 A-delta-fibers tested only 2 responded to bradykinin.

Responses to bradykinin were facilitated by a preceding superfusion with a solution containing adrenaline or noradrenaline, at concentrations of 10 or 100 µg/ml (Fig. 1D,E). However, when given alone these catecholamines produced responses only in rare cases, in contrast to the occurrence of responses to adrenaline and noradrenaline in rat neuroma (Korenman and Devor, 1981; Welk and Zimmermann, to be published). We have seen this enhancement of discharges by a catecholamine in the majority of filaments tested. The facilitated responses were greater by up to 10 times the original response, average facilitation of all fibers tested was to about 5 times the control responses.

When superfusion with substance P at concentrations of 1 to 100 µg/ml preceded bradykinin, responses to bradykinin were reversibly suppressed for periods of about 15 min (Fig. 2). Spontaneous activity and discharges evoked in C-fibers by heating the neuroma to 50°C were also suppressed by preceding superfusion with substance P.

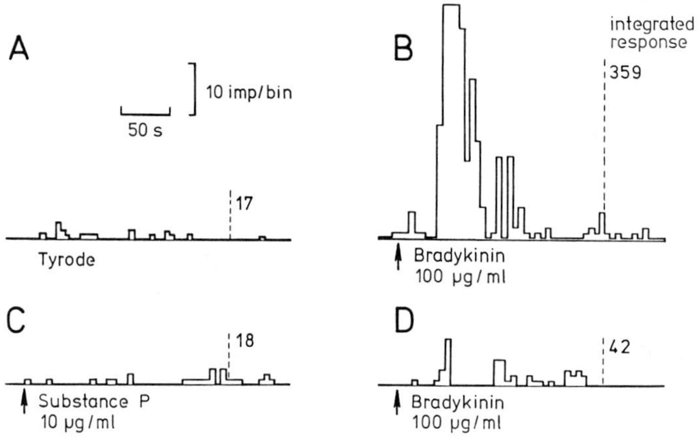

Figure 2. Suppression of the bradykinin response in neuroma C-fibers by substance P. Histograms of C-fiber discharges recorded from a sural multi-unit filament (cat) during superfusion of the neuroma with Tyrode solution (A) or solutions containing bradykinin (B), substance P (C), and then again bradykinin (D). Superfusions lasted 5 min. Time separation between (B) and (C) was 10 min, whereas the second bradykinin superfusion (D) was started 30 min after the end of the superfusion with substance P (C). The numbers at the vertical broken lines indicate the integrated responses during periods from the starts of superfusions, labelled by arrows.

Discussion. It is likely that the excitatory actions reported here are mediated by biochemical receptors for bradykinin, as fibers in normal or acutely damaged nerve do not respond (Zimmermann and Sanders, 1982). Bradykinin excites sensory receptors in skin, muscle, joints and viscera (e.g., Kanaka et al. 1985) and these excitations have been associated with pain produced by bradykinin in humans (Keele and Armstrong, 1964). Therefore, it is conceivable that our results are related to pain originating from a neuroma in patients when algesic substances are present.

Responsiveness to bradykinin was enhanced by preceding superfusion with adrenaline or noradrenaline. Thus, an interaction between a catecholamine and bradykinin seems to occur at the sprouts. This is reminiscent of the interaction between prostaglandin E2 or 5-hydroxytryptamine and bradykinin at nociceptors of skeletal muscle (Mense, 1981). We hypothesize here that facilitatory interactions of two or more neuroactive substances may be a mechanism by which nociceptive nerve endings or nerve sprouts are sensitized during disease processes involving the release of endogenous substances, e.g., inflammatory processes.

The facilitations produced by adrenaline and noradrenaline might be inherent to the pathophysiology by which pain due to nerve lesions is enhanced in states of sympathetic activation (Nathan, 1983): as regenerating sympathetic efferent (postganglionic) fibers are contained in the neuroma, the catecholamines released during sympathetic activation could have the same facilitatory effect as irrigation of the neuroma with exogenous adrenaline or noradrenaline. Interestingly, excitatory effects of sympathetic trunk stimulation have been observed in neuroma of the rat (Devor and Jänig, 1981).

Suppression by substance P of discharges evoked from the neuroma by bradykinin or heating is an unexpected effect, as substance P was considered a pain-producing substance previously (Keele and Armstrong, 1964). As we know that substance P is released from neuroma sprouts (Koschorke et al., 1985), suppression of afferent activity in neuroma sprouts might be meaningful as a negative feedback process decreasing the sensitivity of nerve sprouts to excitatory factors. This would fit the role of substance P in neurogenic inflammation (Chahl et al., 1984), thought to counteract the traumatic events eliciting substance P release.

REDEVELOPMENT OF CUTANEOUS NOCICEPTORS

Patients with an injured cutaneous nerve complain about pain and hyperpathia persisting even when the nerve has grown back to the original skin territory. From this clinical evidence it is conceivable that nociceptors exist in the skin after nerve regeneration. We have studied regenerated nociceptors in cats after experimental crush lesions of the plantar nerves.

Methods. The lateral and medial plantar nerves were exposed unilaterally in anesthetized cats (halothane and N_2O). Both nerves were squeezed repeatedly with watchmaker forceps over a section of 5 mm, which is sufficient to interrupt all the axons irreversibly. Between 1 and 92 days later cats were reanesthetized, fine nerve strands were dissected from the nerves at sites proximal to the previous crush, and investigated for impulse discharges in single C-fibers. When C-fibers could be identified by electrical stimulation of the nerves distally to the previous crush, they were tested systematically for responses to adequate mechanical and thermal stimulation of the foot skin.

Results. At regeneration periods longer than 22 days an increasing proportion of C-fibers could be excited by natural skin stimulation. As the nerve crush was 20 to 40 mm from the large foot pad, this time delay probably reflects growth of the fibers to the original territory. We could discern redeveloped C-fibers with low threshold mechanoreceptors, mechanosensitive nociceptors and heat sensitive nociceptors occurring in normal skin (Zimmermann 1975).

We tested systematically the responsiveness of C-fibers to noxious heat, as heat sensitive nociceptors in the cat's hind foot have well defined characteristics (Beck et al., 1974). Radiant heat to the skin 10 s in duration was used. The skin temperature was controlled by feedback from a thermocouple in contact with the skin. In a regenerated C-heat nociceptor the number of impulses per heat stimulus increased linearly with the skin temperature, much the same as in nociceptors from normal plantar nerves (Beck et al., 1974). Thus, after nerve crush C-fiber endings redevelop encoding the intensity of the thermal stimulus. However, the thermal thresholds of regenerated C-nociceptors tend to be lower than in normal nerves (see below).

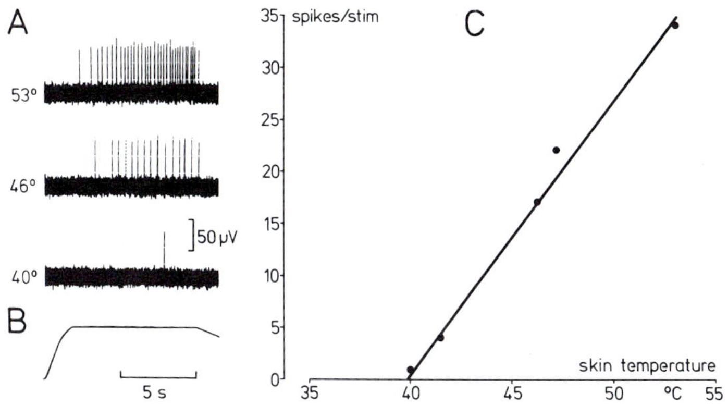

Figure 3. Redevelopment of heat nociceptors after nerve regeneration in the cat. (A) Time course of occurrence of redeveloped heat nociceptors with C-fibers after crush of the plantar nerves. The ordinate plots the percentage of heat nociceptors relative to the number of C-fibers identified by electrical nerve stimulation, absolute numbers are indicated at each point. The control value is from experiments performed under identical conditions of thermal stimulation in the absence of nerve lesions (Beck et al., 1974). (B) The continuous curve plots the cumulative probability (ordinate) of temperature thresholds (abscissa) for a population of 13 regenerated C-heat nociceptors. The broken line shows the cumulative probability function of 40 heat nociceptors from normal nerves (from Dickhaus et al., 1976).

At day 28 after nerve crush the first heat nociceptor appeared, at day 42 and later about 16% of the plantar C-fibers could be activated by skin heating (Fig. 3A). This proportion is the same as in control experiments (Beck et al., 1974).

The thresholds of 13 regenerated fibres to heating the skin of the receptive field ranged from 32° to 46°C, the median value was 38.7°C (Fig. 3B). The corresponding distribution of thresholds in a control sample of 40 C-heat nociceptors had its median at 42.4°C (Fig. 3B, broken line). Thus, the threshold distribution of regenerated C-heat nociceptors is significantly shifted to lower temperatures by about 3.7°C relative to the thresholds in normal nerves.

Discussion. The proportion of C-fibers responding to radiant heat at a regeneration time of 42 days and longer is the same as in normal nerve: 16%. This suggests that virtually all the afferent C-fibers have regenerated within less than 90 days after the nerve crush. The decrease in threshold of the heat response in the C-nociceptors might provide a neurophysiological basis for the hyperpathia observed in man during nerve regeneration (Sunderland, 1978). Hyperpathia to thermal skin stimuli has been described also by Sir Henry Head in the nerve lesion experiments done on himself; during skin nerve regeneration his heat pain threshold was at 38°C, which is well below the normal threshold values around 45°C.

FUNCTIONAL RESTITUTION OF CUTANEOUS MECHANORECEPTORS AFTER NERVE REGENERATION

The characteristics of sensitive cutaneous mechanoreceptors after nerve regeneration have been investigated in animals (Burgess and Horch, 1973; Dykes and Terzis, 1979; Terzis and Dykes, 1980; Terzis, this volume; Sanders and Zimmermann, 1986) and in man (Hallin et al. 1981; Mackel et al. 1983). After several months part of the regenerated A-beta-fibers revealed of mechanosensitivity which virtually could not be distinguished from normal types of specific cutaneous mechanoreceptors. Usually, these are classified as SA- (slowly adapting), RA- (rapidly adapting) and PC- (Pacinian-like) receptors, having distinct encoding characteristics (Jänig et al., 1968; Zimmermann, 1978). Here, we report the time course of the transition from mechanosensitive sprouts of regenerating fibers to functionally defined mechanoreceptors in rats (Sanders and Zimmermann, 1986).

Methods. Nerve lesions were performed by repeatedly crushing the plantar nerves of ether anesthetized rats at sites 10 mm proximal to the heel, resulting in fiber discontinuity and proximal regeneration of fibers. From 1 to 24 weeks afterwards, animals were anesthetized with thiobutabarbital (Inactin, Byk Gulden, 100 mg/kg i.p.). Single A-fiber action potentials were recorded from nerve strands at sites proximal to the previous lesion. All fibers encountered were tested for a receptive field with mechanical stimuli, and electronically controlled skin displacements were applied to quantitatively assess the encoding characteristics of the mechanosensitive fiber endings.

Results. Mechanosensitivity of sprouts was observed in the nerve trunk a few days after the nerve crush already, which probably is similar as in neuroma sprouts (see above). On the average, 20% of A-fibers responded to mechanical probing. The site of mechanosensitivity proceeded distally with increasing time after the lesion. These responses did not show the distinctive characteristics of sensitive mechanoreceptors, i.e. SA-, RA- or PC-receptors: one or a few action potentials only were usually elicited at any stimulus strength, and mechanical thresholds were rather high compared to those of the specific mechanoreceptors. A considerable proportion of the regenerating A-beta fibers showed erratic behaviour which never has been observed in the low threshold cutaneous mechanoreceptors, e.g., large variations in excitability to successive stimuli, afterdischarges outlasting a mechanical stimulus, excitation by heating the skin to noxious temperatures.

Such unspecifically mechanosensitive nerve endings were still observed when the regenerating nerve had reached the foot skin (Fig. 4A). We used the term HT-units (high threshold). Within the following weeks receptive fields shifted to distal sites, and increasing numbers of specific SA- and RA-receptors were observed (Fig. 4B,C), whereas the number of HT-units decreased. At 24 weeks after the nerve lesions the frequency of occurrence and spatial distribution of SA- and RA-receptors could not be distinguished from the situation in control animals.

The capacity of units to encode the intensity of the stimulus was studied in SA-receptors (Fig. 4D). Mean stimulus-response functions were calculated for the samples of SA-receptors found at various periods after nerve crush. The sensitivity of the SA-receptors, expressed as the mean discharge frequency, and the capacity of intensity coding, expressed as the slope of the stimulus-response function, both gradually improved with time of regeneration. At 24 weeks after the nerve lesions these properties of SA-receptors could not be discerned from a control sample. Corresponding findings were obtained for regenerating RA-receptors: here, the discharge frequency was plotted versus the velocity of skin indentation to quantify the coding capacity (Sanders and Zimmermann 1986).

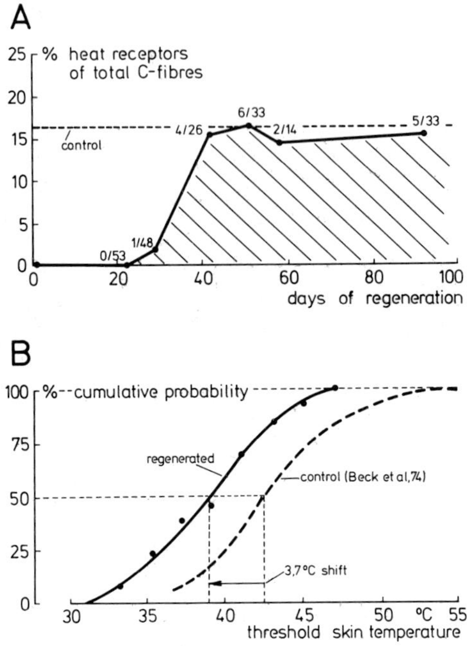

Figure 4. Functional maturation of slowly adapting (SA-) mechanoreceptors in the hind foot of the rat after crush lesions of the plantar nerves. (A) The triangles show the sites of responses to mechanical stimuli of single A-beta-fibers recorded from nerve filaments 1 w (week) after the crush. Responses were classified as high threshold or HT-units. (B) Sites of responses to mechanical stimulation of regenerating fibers 2 w after the nerve crush. Triangles denote HT-units as in (A), circles denote SA-receptors. (C) As in (A) and (B), 24 weeks after nerve crush. (D) Mean stimulus-response functions of redeveloped SA-receptors measured between 2 w and 24 w after nerve crush. The stimulus was a skin indentation to the receptive field of the unit. The numbers of units used for the mean curves are given in parentheses (from Sanders and Zimmermann, 1986).

The only parameters that still had not reached control values after 24 weeks of regeneration were the conduction velocities of the afferent axons which were considerably lower than normal, and the time course of discharge rate in SA-receptors during prolonged skin indentations, which showed a faster decline than in control receptors (Sanders and Zimmermann, 1986).

Discussion. In the rat, HT-units represented the first sign of mechanosensitivity in the foot skin 1 week after crush lesions of the plantar nerves near the heel. The HT-responses presumably originated in the sprouts of fibers still growing out. It is conceivable that most HT-units found after nerve crush represent an intermediate and immature state of fiber endings before or during redevelopment of specific mechanoreceptors.

Newly regenerated RA- and SA-receptors in the rat were less sensitive than in normal skin, as stimulus-response functions were generally attenuated. Within 24 weeks the receptors had gradually regained their normal characteristics. An initially lower excitability has also been reported during ontogenetic development (Ferrington and Rowe, 1980). Maturation of the nerve ending-receptor complex might be a common mechanism to explain both cases of functional development. It is conceivable that receptor excitations originating in individual end organs summate at branching sites of the parent axon. Thus, the increase in excitability of RA- and SA-receptors after regeneration may be due to an increasing number of axon-end organ connections.

Nerve crush caused a slowing of conduction in the nerve fibers proximal to the lesion. This decrease in conduction velocity was most pronounced immediately after the crush, and persisted beyond our observation time of 24 weeks. Factors involved in this change might be transient retrograde degeneration, decrease in axonal volume due to changes in axonal flow and biochemical sequaelae of trauma which are signalled by chromatolysis. While our observation of early decreases in velocity are unprecedented, the long-lasting slowing in conduction is in agreement with previous reports (Cragg and Thomas, 1961; Dykes and Terzis, 1979).

SUMMARY AND CONCLUSION

In conclusion, abnormal sensory responsiveness was observed in various stages of regenerating somatosensory nerve fibers. As long as the nerve sprouts have not reached the skin territory, responses to mechanical stimuli are unspecific in the sense that they are not related in a clearcut way to stimulus parameters. When regenerative sprouts are confined in a neuroma, the C-fibers show chemosensitivity to endogenous substances. Responsiveness to bradykinin was facilitated by adrenaline or noradrenaline, and suppressed by substance P. These modulations indicate complex biochemical interactions at the nerve fiber sprouts. When the regenerative nerve sprouts reach the skin, specific mechanoreceptors and nociceptors redevelop. The tactile mechanoreceptors reveal functional maturation within 24 weeks. Regenerated thermal nociceptors show considerable hypersensitivity which might account for the hyperpathia observed after cutaneous nerve regeneration in patients.

Acknowledgements. The authors are grateful to Frau Hannelore Ehlers for typing and editing the manuscript and Frau Almuth Manisali for the graphics. This work is being supported by the Deutsche Forschungsgemeinschaft (Grants Zi 110).

REFERENCES

Beck PW, Handwerker HO, Zimmermann M (1974). Nervous outflow from the cat's foot during noxious radiant heat stimulation. Brain Res 67: 373-386.

Blumberg H, Jänig W (1984): Discharge pattern of afferent fibers from a neuroma. Pain 20: 335-353.

Burchiel KJ (1984). Spontaneous impulse generation in normal and denervated dorsal root ganglia: sensitivity to alpha-adrenergic stimulation and hypoxia. Exp Neurol 85: 257-272.

Burgess PR, Horch KW (1973). Specific regeneration of cutaneous fibres in the cat. J Neurophysiol 36: 101-114.

Chahl LA, Szolcsanyi J, Lembeck F (eds) (1984). "Antidromic Vasodilatation and Neurogenic Inflammation." Budapest: Akademiai Kiado.

Cragg BG, Thomas PK (1961). Changes in conduction velocity and fibre size proximal to peripheral nerve lesions. J Physiol (Lond) 157: 315-327.

Devor M, Bernstein JJ (1982) Abnormal impulse generation in neuromas: electrophysiology and ultrastructure. In Culp WJ, Ochoa J (eds): "Abnormal Nerves and Muscles as Impulse Generators," New York, Oxford: Oxford University Press, pp 363-380.

Devor M, Jänig W (1981). Activation of myelinated afferents ending in a neuroma by stimulation of the sympathetic supply in the rat. Neurosci Lett 24: 43-47.

Dickhaus H, Zimmermann M, Zotterman Y (1976). The development in regenerating cutaneous nerves of C-fibre receptors responding to noxious heating of the skin. In Zotterman Y (ed): "Sensory functions of the skin in primates," Oxford: Pergamon Press, pp 415-425.
Dykes RW, Terzis JK (1979). Reinnervation of glabrous skin in baboons: properties of cutaneous mechanoreceptors subsequent to nerve crush. J Neurophysiol 42: 1461-1478.
Ferrington DG, Rowe MJ (1980). Functional capacities of tactile afferent fibers in neonatal kittens. J Physiol (Lond) 307: 335-353.
Hallin RG, Wiesenfeld Z, Lindblom U (1981). Neurophysiological studies on patients with sutured median nerves: faulty sensory localization after nerve regeneration and its physiological correlates. Exp Neurol 73: 90-106.
Jänig W, Schmidt RF, Zimmermann M (1968). Single unit responses and the total afferent outflow from the cat's foot pad upon mechanical stimulation. Exp Brain Res 6: 100-115.
Kanaka R, Schaible H-G, Schmidt RF (1985). Activation of fine articular afferent units by bradykinin. Brain Res 327: 81-90.
Keele CA, Armstrong D (1964). "Substances Producing Pain and Itch." London: Edward Arnold.
Korenman EMD, Devor M (1981). Ectopic adrenergic sensitivity in damaged peripheral nerve axons in the rat. Exp Neurol 72: 63-81.
Koschorke GM, Helme RD, Zimmermann M (1985). Substance P suppresses the response to bradykinin and to heat of nonmyelinated fibers in experimental neuroma of the cat's sural nerve. Soc Neurosci Abstr 11: 118.
Mackel R, Kunesch E, Waldhör F, Struppler A (1983). Reinnervation of mechanoreceptors in the human glabrous skin following peripheral nerve repair. Brain Res 268: 49-65.
Mense S (1981). Sensitization of group IV muscle receptors to bradykinin by 5-hydroxytryptamine and prostaglandin E2. Brain Res 225: 95-105.
Nathan PW (1983) Pain and the sympathetic nervous system. In Yokota T, Dubner R (eds): "Current topics in pain research and therapy," Amsterdam, Oxford, Princeton: Excerpta Medica, pp 241-247.
Sanders KH, Zimmermann M (1986). Mechanoreceptors in rat glabrous skin: Redevelopment of function after nerve crush. J Neurophysiol 55: 644-659.

Scadding JW (1981). Development of ongoing activity, mechanosensitivity, and adrenaline sensitivity in severed peripheral nerve axons. Exp Neurol 73: 345-364.

Sunderland S (1978). "Nerves and Nerve Injuries, 2nd ed." Edinburgh, London: Churchill Livingstone.

Terzis JK, Dykes RW (1980). Reinnervation of glabrous skin in baboons: properties of cutaneous mechanoreceptors subsequent to nerve transection. J Neurophysiol 44: 1214-1225.

Wall PD, Gutnick M (1974). Properties of afferent nerve impulses originating from a neuroma. Nature 248: 740-743.

Zimmermann M (1975). Cutaneous C fibers: peripheral properties and central connections. In Kornhuber HH (ed): "The Somatosensory System," Stuttgart: Thieme, pp 45-53.

Zimmermann M (1978). Mechanoreceptors of the glabrous skin and tactile acuity. In Porter R (ed): "Studies in Neurophysiology presented to A.K. McIntyre," Cambridge: University Press, pp 267-289.

Zimmermann M, Sanders KH (1982). Responses of nerve axons and receptor endings to heat, ischemia, and algesic substances. Abnormal excitability of regenerating nerve endings. In Culp WJ, Ochoa J (eds): "Abnormal nerves and muscles as impulse generators," New York, Oxford: Oxford University Press, pp 513-532.

Effects of Injury on Trigeminal and Spinal Somatosensory Systems, pages 107–114

STUDIES ON UNMYELINATED FIBRE REGENERATION IN RAT PERIPHERAL NERVE

S.J.W.Lisney

Department of Physiology, The Medical School, University Walk, Bristol BS8 1TD, U.K.

Peripheral nerves in the limbs, whether they are articular, cutaneous, or muscle nerves, contain several times more unmyelinated fibres than they do myelinated ones. These unmyelinated fibres are either afferents or postganglionic sympathetic fibres. In cat cutaneous nerves there are about three times as many unmyelinated afferents as there are postganglionic sympathetic fibres; the relative proportions in the other types of peripheral nerve have not been determined. Of the unmyelinated sensory fibres, experiments on mammalian cutaneous nerves have shown that here most are associated with polymodal nociceptors; whether or not this is also true for articular and muscle nerves is not yet clear.

Much work has been carried out into various aspects of the regeneration of injured myelinated fibres in cutaneous and muscle nerves. Information has been obtained to show what proportion of fibres can be expected to regenerate across the injury site and resupply the skin after different types of injury. A number of pathophysiological properties of regenerated myelinated fibres have also been described. Paradoxically, relatively little is known about the regeneration of damaged unmyelinated fibres in peripheral nerves, despite the fact that they easily outnumber the myelinated ones.

Here I shall describe some simple electrophysiological and anatomical experiments that I have been doing to try and get some idea of how these fibres respond to injury and how their regeneration compares with that of myelinated fibres.

MATERIALS AND METHODS

All the experiments were carried out on the saphenous nerves of male, Wistar rats which were within a few days of being 3 months old at the time of nerve injury. The nerve injuries, a simple transection at knee level in each case, were made during a brief operation under sodium pentobarbitone anaesthesia. After a recovery period of between 1 and 26 weeks a final, acute experiment was performed; again the anaesthetic was sodium pentobarbitone.

In some experiments electrophysiological recordings were made from fine strands dissected from the exposed nerve high in the groin. Strands which were found to show 1-7 clearly distinguishable action potentials with conduction velocities in the C-fibre range following electrical stimulation of the nerve proximal to the injury site were selected for study. Electrical stimulation distal to the injury site showed which of the fibres in each strand had managed to grow into the distal stump; collision procedures were used to confirm the identity of action potentials recorded with stimulation at the two sites. Latencies and conduction distances were measured so that conduction velocities could be calculated.

In other experiments the extent of reinnervation of the skin by polymodal nociceptor afferents was assessed. Kenins (1981) has shown that antidromic activation of polymodal nociceptor afferents results in changes in the properties of blood vessels adjacent to the sensory endings associated with the stimulated afferents; arterioles become dilated and capillary permeability is increased. If Evan's Blue dye is injected into the circulation before the stimulation it has time to attach to plasma proteins. Then when nerve stimulation is carried out and capillary permeability increases, the plasma protein/Evan's Blue complex leaks out into the extravascular space and the immediately adjacent area becomes blue. Brenan (1982,1984) has demonstrated that this technique can be used in rats to map the distribution of polymodal nociceptors with afferents in particular cutaneous nerves. Thus at various times after nerve injury both saphenous nerves, one normal and the other regenerated, were prepared for electrical stimulation. After Evan's Blue administration both nerves were stimulated simultaneously with the same stimulus strength. The areas of skin that turned blue were drawn onto scale figurines of the legs and then measured by simple planimetry. Reinnervation of skin by polymodal nociceptor afferents in the regenerated nerve was expressed in terms of the area that went blue in that leg compared with the area that went blue in the normal, control leg.

A third set of experiments provided histological material for nerve fibre counting. Six months after transection of one saphenous nerve animals were perfused with buffered gluteraldehyde/formaldehyde. Small pieces of nerve from proximal and distal to the injury site and from equivalent positions of the contralateral, normal nerve were then removed. These were post-fixed in osmium tetroxide, embedded in Epon resin and finally sectioned ready for examination in a Philips 300 electronmicroscope. The total number of myelinated fibre profiles in each sample of nerve was counted from a low-power montage. The total number of unmyelinated fibres in each sample was then estimated by multiplying the number of myelinated fibres it contained by the ratio of myelinated:unmyelinated fibres for that sample, as determined from high-power examination of just a part (average of 58%) of the entire nerve area.

RESULTS

Regeneration across the Injury Site

About 10% of the unmyelinated fibres that had survived in the proximal stump had grown into the distal stump by 1 week after the injury. By 2 weeks this proportion had risen to 40% and by 8-12 weeks it had reached 75%. At 26 weeks about 85% of the unmyelinated fibres in the proximal stump had regenerated into the distal part of the nerve. As the time allowed for regeneration was increased the variability in results between animals became less. Similar experiments on the regeneration of myelinated fibres in the same nerve have given virtually the same results.

Conduction Velocity Changes

Conduction velocities proximal to the injury site were calculated for all the fibres studied in the experiments mentioned above. It was not possible to get an estimate of conduction velocity in the distal stump alone because there was not enough room on the nerve for the extra set of electrodes that would have been needed. It was possible, however, to get a measure of conduction velocity in a portion of nerve that included a small part of the proximal stump, the neuroma, and the first part of the distal stump. The mean conduction velocity of unmyelinated fibres in the proximal portions of normal nerves was 0.88 $m.s^{-1}$, S.D. ±0.19, n=200. Similar numbers of fibres were studied in each of the groups of experimental rats (1,2,4,8,12,19,and 26 weeks after injury) but in no case was the mean value or the distribution significantly different from that of the controls. Conduction velocity in the proximal and distal portions of fibres in normal saphenous nerves were uniform but in regenerated nerves the distal conduction velocities tended to be slower. This was true at all recovery times.

Reinnervation of Skin by Polymodal Nociceptors

Twelve weeks after nerve injury something like 75% of unmyelinated fibres from the proximal stump had regenerated into the distal stump. By this time, however, it seemed that there was only about 20% reinnervation of the leg by polymodal nociceptors. At 26 weeks there was about 50% reinnervation of the leg: this is comparable with the proportion of low threshold, myelinated mechanoreceptor afferents that manage to reestablish functional endings in the skin following the same sort of injury to the same nerve.

Fibre Numbers in Regenerated Nerves

So far, fibre counts have been completed on the material from 3 animals. Although the numbers given here are the averages of these counts, the trends they show are a reflection of the changes that had occurred in each animal. The average numbers of myelinated and unmyelinated fibres in the proximal portions of the normal saphenous nerves were 1082 and 4460 respectively. In the distal stumps the corresponding figures were 1012 and 3475; this fall in fibre numbers is presumably because small branches leave the main nerve trunk as it courses distally. In the proximal stumps of the regenerated nerves the average numbers were 1062 myelinated fibres and 2151 unmyelinated ones. The difference in the number of myelinated fibres in the proximal portions of normal and regenerated nerves is negligible but there was about a 50% reduction in the number of unmyelinated ones. In the distal stumps of the regenerated nerves the average number of myelinated fibres had increased to 1671; this sort of result has been reported before (Horch & Lisney,1981) and comes about because many regenerated myelinated fibres support more than one process in the distal stump. The number of unmyelinated fibres found in the distal stump also increased but only very slightly to an average figure of 2227; this increase is insignificant.

DISCUSSION

The most important observation from these experiments is that there is a very significant loss of unmyelinated fibres from regenerated rat cutaneous nerves. As far as I am aware, no other directly comparable experiment has been performed against which this finding can be judged. Jenq & Coggeshall (1984,1985) have carried out several sets of experiments involving fibre counts of regenerated rat peripheral nerves and although none of the paradigms they used is similar to that adopted here, their general conclusion that there is a loss of unmyelinated fibres from regenerated rat cutaneous nerves fits with the present results. Janig & McLachlan (1984) have reported a loss of unmyelinated fibres from a cat cutaneous nerve following section, ligation, and neuroma formation, but again this situation is not directly comparable with the present one where the cut nerve was allowed to regenerate.

The present experiments do not show whether or not one of the subgroups of unmyelinated fibres is affected more than the others. All that can be said in this respect is that in regenerated cat sural nerves the relative proportions of unmyelinated afferents and postganglionic sympathetic fibres are the same as in normal sural nerves (Lisney,1986).

Another question that needs to be answered is does the fall in unmyelinated fibre numbers in the regenerated nerves indicate that neurones have died. An equally good explanation of the results would be that some unmyelinated axons in the proximal stump died back several millimetres from the injury site, and so were absent from the sample taken for histology, but that the remaining parts of these neurones were still alive. Several groups have reported evidence for loss of neurones after peripheral nerve injury (e.g. Devor et al.,1985; Arvidsson et al.,1986; for a recent review see Aldskogius et al.,1985), but in most instances the nerve injury was such that regeneration back into the distal stump was not possible. The events that take place in a neurone which is damaged but which cannot regenerate may be quite different from those that occur in a one which is damaged but which then regenerates and reforms a peripheral ending.

There is very little other work with which the results described here can be compared. Shea and Perl (1985) have described the electrophysiological properties of regenerated unmyelinated afferents supplying the skin of the rabbit's ear but I know of no other similar studies. They found that 5-8 months after nerve injury and repair about 75-80% of the unmyelinated fibres from which they made recordings could be excited by stimulation distal to the injury site; this is very similar to my own result. Generally speaking there were no differences in the properties of the different types of afferent after regeneration except for some small changes in the thresholds for activation of some polymodal nociceptors by some forms of stimulation.

So that some sort of comparison could be made with the regeneration of myelinated fibres, I have also carried out experiments on regenerated rat saphenous nerves to determine the proportions of these fibres that had grown across the injury site and that had resupplied the skin at several recovery times. The overall findings were that, by 6 months at least, the surviving unmyelinated fibre population had negotiated the injury site as well as the myelinated group and that the extent of reinnervation of the skin by these two groups of fibres was comparable.

CONCLUSION

After transection and regeneration of the rat saphenous nerve there is a substantial loss of unmyelinated fibres whereas there does not appear to be any loss of myelinated fibres. Of the unmyelinated fibres that survive, about 80% manage to grow into the distal stump. Six months after nerve injury the extent of innervation of the saphenous nerve field by regenerated polymodal nociceptor afferents is only about 50% of the normal.

ACKNOWLEDGMENT

This work was supported by the M.R.C.

REFERENCES

Aldskogius,H., Arvidsson,J. & Grant,G.(1985). The reaction of primary sensory neurons to peripheral nerve injury with particular emphasis on transganglionic changes. Brain Research Reviews,10,27-46.

Arvidsson,J., Ygge,J. & Grant,G.(1986). Cell loss in lumbar dorsal root ganglia and transganglionic degeneration after sciatic nerve resection in the rat. Brain Research, 373,15-21.

Brenan,A.(1982). Plasma extravasation following antidromic stimulation of cutaneous nerves in the rat. Journal of Physiology,327,7-8P.

Brenan,A.(1984). A dye technique for the determination of the distribution of cutaneous nerves in the rat. Journal of Anatomy,138,593-594.

Devor,M., Govrin-Lippmann,R., Frank,I. & Raber,P.(1985). Proliferation of primary sensory neurons in adult rat dorsal root ganglion and the kinetics of retrograde cell loss after sciatic nerve section. Somatosensory Research, 3,139-167.

Horch,K.W. & Lisney,S.J.W.(1981). On the number and nature of regenerating myelinated axons after lesions of cutaneous nerves in the cat. Journal of Physiology,313,275-286.

Janig,W. & McLachlan,E.(1984). On the fate of sympathetic and sensory neurons projecting into a neuroma of the superficial peroneal nerve in the cat. Journal of Comparative Neurology,225,302-311.

Jenq,C-B. & Coggeshall,R.E.(1984). Effects of sciatic nerve regeneration on axonal populations in tributary nerves. Brain Research,295,91-100.

Jenq,C-B. & Coggeshall,R.E.(1985). Numbers of regenerating axons in parent and tributary peripheral nerves in the rat. Brain Research,326,27-40.

Kenins,P.(1981).Identification of the unmyelinated sensory nerves which evoke plasma extravasation in response to antidromic stimulation. Neuroscience Letters,25,137-141.

Lisney,S.J.W.(1986). The proportions of unmyelinated afferent and sympathetic postganglionic fibres in normal and regenerated cat sural nerves. Journal of Physiology, 372,19P.

Shea,V.K. & Perl.E.R.(1985). Regeneration of cutaneous afferent unmyelinated (C) fibers after transection. Journal of Neurophysiology,54,502-512.

Effects of Injury on Trigeminal and Spinal Somatosensory Systems, pages 115–124

INJURY OF SOMATOSENSORY AFFERENTS BY CAPSAICIN: SELECTIVITY AND FAILURE TO REGENERATE.

B. Lynn, A. Pini & R. Baranowski

Physiology Department, University College London, Gower Street, London WC1E 6BT, England

Capsaicin administration to neonatal rats causes a substantial loss of afferent C-fibres of up to 95% (Jancso et al., 1980; Scadding, 1980). In adult rats a smaller loss of about 40% of C-fibres occurs following subcutaneous injection of capsaicin (Jancso et al., 1985) or local application to nerves (Lynn& Pini, 1985; Lynn, 1986). In the adult guinea pig a single capsaicin injection has been reported to produce axonal swelling within 5 min and to cause clear signs of axonal degeneration over the next 12 hours (Papka et al., 1984). In adult rats swelling of mitochondria and other signs of injury are present in dorsal root ganglion cells 1-2 hours after a single capsaicin injection (Jancso et al., 1985) and persist for at least 42-60 days (Joo et al., 1969; Chiba et al., 1986). Direct application to nerve trunks also causes immediate local swelling of C-fibres (Marsh, 1985) and at 1-4 days signs of degeneration and possible regeneration are present near the treatment site (Handwerker et al.,1984)

The cytochemical and functional effects of capsaicin are long-lasting. Peptidergic nerve profiles were still depleted 1 year after injection in the guinea pig (Papka et al., 1984). Our studies following local application to cutaneous nerves in the rat have also shown an enduring C-fibre loss (Lynn, 1986) and these studies have now been extended to 1 year. In this paper we will first review our recent morphological results on nerves from 6 weeks to 1 year after local treatment with capsaicin. Electrophysiological experiments showing the classes of fibres affected will then be considered. Finally the largely irreversible nature of the changes following capsaicin treatment will be compared with recently published data on the recovery of somatosensory C-fibres from physical injury.

AXON NUMBERS AND MORPHOLOGY

Short pieces of the saphenous nerve were removed from the treatment site 6 weeks to 1 year following a 30 min application of 1% capsaicin in olive oil or olive oil alone and from the same level in the unoperated contralateral leg. Additional nerve samples were also removed from points 10-20 mm distal and 5-15 mm proximal to the treatment site and from the equivalent levels in the contralateral leg in some

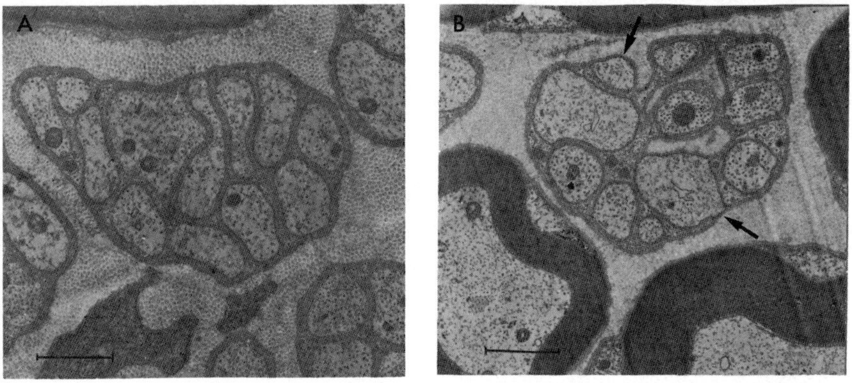

Fig 1. Electron micrographs of transverse sections of bundles of C-fibres in rat saphenous nerve. A, contralateral control nerve. B, nerve treated one year previously with 1% capsaicin. Arrows indicate exposed sections of axolemma. Scale 1 μm.

experiments. The nerves were fixed by immersion in Karnowsky's solution (2.7% gluteraldehyde, 1.3% paraformaldehyde) overnight following which they were placed in 1% osmic acid for 3 hrs and embedded in epon. Transverse sections were cut, stained with uranyl acetate and Sato's stain (lead citrate, nitrate and acetate) and examined by electron microcospy. In a few instances sections were mounted on slot grids and total numbers of A fibres were counted. In all cases sample fields were photographed and prints made at 5600X magnification. The total numbers of A and C-fibres in these fields were counted to determine the

C:A fibre ratio. Fields including a total of about 100 A fibres were counted for each nerve. In most nerves the perimeters of 160-200 C-fibres were measured from prints at 13,300X using the computerised system described by Biscoe et al. (1982).

No changes were seen in A-fibre numbers but the proportion of C-fibres was consistently reduced in treated nerves to 61.6% (±2.8%,s.e.,n=13) of the value in untreated contralateral nerves or in nerves treated with olive oil alone. No significant differences in the proportion of C-fibres in treated nerves were seen at different times from 6 weeks to 1 year or at points in the nerve 1-2 cm proximal or distal to the treatment site.

A feature of capsaicin treated nerves was the presence of substantial numbers of very small profiles. Measurements of the perimeters of 200 C-fibres from each of 3 treated nerves at 1 year gave perimeters averaging 2.62 μm (± 0.97μm, s.d.) compared with an average of 2.98 μm (± 0.81 μm) for 200 axons from each of 3 contralateral control nerves. A detailed study of 2 pairs of nerves at 1 year revealed that 6.0% of 811 C-fibres examined in treated nerves had axolemma exposed directly to the extracellular matrix (See Fig 1B) compared with only 1.6% of 623 fibres in contralateral control nerves. The normal situation is for C-fibres to be completely enclosed within the mesaxon formed by infolding of the Schwann cell. In addition, 1.5% of C-fibre profiles shared a mesaxon with 1 or more other fibres. No such structures, which presumably arise from branching axons, were seen in the control nerves. These abnormal profiles may indicate that even after one year some fibres are still attempting to regenerate towards the skin.

ELECTROPHYSIOLOGICAL RESULTS AT 6 WEEKS TO 1 YEAR AFTER TREATMENT

Recordings were made from the nerve at a point approximately 2 cm proximal to the treatment site using fine platinum wires. Pairs of stimulating electrodes were placed on the nerve just proximal to the treatment site and about 1 cm distal to it. Conduction could thus be assessed independently for an untreated proximal segment of nerve and for the treated segment. Compound action potentials (c.a. ps) were recorded to assess the total numbers of conducting axons. The peak-to-peak amplitudes of the fastest (Aαβ) component and the slowest (C) component were measured and in some experiments the slowest A component (Aδ) was also measured. Following this the nerve was microdissected to record from single units isolated by using the proximal electrical stimulus as the maximal search stimulus. Conduction of single units through the original treatment zone was assessed by applying maximal shocks to the distal electrodes. Finally the skin was searched with mechanical and thermal stimuli to try to find cutaneous fields for all units that were excited from the distal electrodes and to classify them into the major types normally present.

Table 1. Amplitudes of the major components of the compound action potential in rat saphenous nerves treated 6 weeks to 1 year previously with 1% capsaicin or with vehicle alone (olive oil). Mean ± s.e.; number of nerves in brackets.

		Capsaicin		Olive oil	
Stimulation proximal to treatment site	Aα, mV	12.4 ± 1.1	(19)	8.9 ± 1.1	(8)
	Aδ *, μV	365 ± 66	(6)	465 ± 88	(4)
	C, μV	173 ± 25	(19)	284 ± 33	(8)
Stimulation distal to treatment site	Aα, mV	6.2 ± 0.8	(19)	3.76 ± 0.49	(8)
	Aδ *, μV	216 ± 18	(18)	141 ± 23	(8)
	C, μV	43 ± 6	(19)	100 ± 21	(8)

* Slowest Aδ component only, conduction velocity 6-14 m/sec.

The compound action potential data is summarised in Table 1. The Aαβ components were unusually large in the treated nerves, a trend that seems likely to reflect random fluctuations in recording conditions since there was no evidence from the morphometric studies for changes in A-fibres following capsaicin treatment. The slowly conducting Aδ component was similar in control and treated nerves. However, consistent with the morphology, a large fall in the C-component was present both for stimulation proximal (fall to 61%) and distal (fall to 43%) to the original treatment site.

Most (95%) of the single A and C units that responded to electrical stimulation proximal to the treated zone also fired to electrical stimulation distal to it. This is not significantly different from control nerves where 92% were fired from both stimulus sites and indicates that no residual effect on nerve conduction was present at the treatment site itself 6 weeks to 1 year after capsaicin application. Conducion velocity of C-fibres was similar in treated and control nerves (0.77 ± 0.08 m/sec, n = 11 and 0.73±0.04, n = 8 respectively). There was a greater spread of C-fibre conduction velocities within a given treated nerve but since this was not accompanied by any overall slowing the result is not what would be predicted from the morphological picture which showed many very small C-fibres. It seems possible that some of these small profiles may not extend far along the nerve and so would not be apparent in the electrophysiological sample. If this were the case, it might also explain why the fall in c.a.p. size for distal stimulation is rather greater than the fall in C-fibre numbers.

Of the units with axons conducting through the treated zone, the proportion of C-fibres with cutaneous receptive fields was only 49.9% (±5.6%, s.e., average of 14 nerves) at 6 weeks to one year after capsaicin treatment. This is significantly fewer than in control nerves, where 74.3% (±5.5%, n = 6) of C-units had cutaneous fields. No changes were seen in the proportion of A-fibre units with cutaneous fields which averaged 88% in 14 treated nerves and 83% in the 7 controls.

The total sample of 66 units with cutaneous fields isolated from treated nerves comprised 33 (50%) polymodal nociceptors, 15 (23%) sensitive mechanoreceptors or thermoreceptors and 18 (27%) insensitive mechanoreceptors. The proportion of polymodal nociceptor units is reduced by 37% compared with control levels whilst the relative proportions of other types of unit, both sensitive and insensitive, are raised. The properties of the surviving units were normal. For example, C-polymodal nociceptor thresholds for heating at 1°C/sec were 49.4°C (±1.75, n = 21) for units from treated nerves and 47.7°C (±1.65, n = 16) for controls. Thresholds for punctate mechanical stimulation with Von Frey bristles were also similar for units from treated nerves (1.13 ± 0.09 log mN, n = 31) and controls (1.19 ± 0.11 log mN, n = 21).

OVERVIEW OF LONG-TERM EFFECTS OF CAPSAICIN

The morphological and electrophysiological data demonstrate that around half of all the C-fibres are missing from nerves treated with capsaicin. Amongst the surviving fibres approximately twice the normal proportion (50%) are inexcitable. It seems likely that these fibres are sympathetic efferents which are known to be unaffected by neonatal treatment with capsaicin (Cervero & McRitchie, 1982) and which comprise about one quarter of the C-fibres in distal nerves to hairy skin in the cat (Blumberg & Janig, 1982; McLachlan & Janig, 1983). The inverse relation between the overall fibre loss and the increase in the proportion of efferents is consistent with there being no change in the number of efferents following capsaicin application to the nerve. It this is the case, then the fall in numbers of unmyelinated afferents must be rather greater than 50%.

Within the surviving afferents there is an increase in the relative proportion of non-polymodal types of unit. Again, the simplest explanation is that the numbers of such units are not affected by capsaicin treatment of the nerve. Polymodal units, on the other hand, form an unusually small proportion of all units in treated nerves. In fact a selective reduction in the polymodal group to 1/3 - 1/6 of control levels would adequately fit our results. However, it should be noted that because of the small size of the total unit sample it is not possible to exclude a modest reduction in the numbers of non-polymodal afferent C-fibres. The long-term situation following direct application of capsaicin to cutaneous nerves in adult rats is thus similar to that found after adult systemic treatment, but different from the indiscriminate loss of afferent C-fibres found after neonatal capsaicin (Lynn, Carpenter & Pini, 1984).

FUNCTIONAL CHANGES AND NEUROPEPTIDE LEVELS AFTER LOCAL CAPSAICIN TREATMENT

Direct application of capsaicin to peripheral nerves causes functional and neurochemical changes comparable with those found following systemic administration. There is reduction or loss of neurogenic inflammation and of behavioural responses to heat and irritant chemicals that lasts for at least several weeks (see review by Fitzgerald,

1983). These changes are almost certainly a direct consequence of the loss of C-polymodal afferents. The amount of substance P in the skin, peripheral nerve and spinal cord also falls. There is some recovery in substance P levels at times greater then 1-2 weeks, but whether full recovery occurs has not been established (Gamse et al., 1982). Again since this peptide is found in fine afferent fibres, the observed reductions are likely to be a direct consequence of C-fibre degeneration.

The results of a number of experiments with adult capsaicin treatment have been interpreted purely in terms of the loss of neuropeptides since it was believed from early experiments that no C-fibre loss occurred (Joo et al., 1969; Jessel et al., 1978; Ainsworth et al., 1981). It is our view that substantial degeneration does occur and thus it is not possible to interpret results from adult capsaicin treatment solely in terms of discrete neurochemical changes.

FAILURE TO REGENERATE: SPECIFIC CAPSAICIN EFFECT OR GENERAL C-FIBRE PROPERTY?

The neurotoxic action of capsaicin on C-polymodal nociceptor units may be due to it reaching the cell body region, perhaps by axonal transport, and acting there. However, recent results from studies using nerve section or crush indicate that it may be sufficient simply to cause a local axonic lesion. It has been found that C-fibre numbers remain below control levels for 2-6 months after crush or section of a rat cutaneous nerve (Jenq & Coggeshall, 1984; Lisney, 1987) and substance P levels are reduced distal to a crush lesion for at least 3 months (Bisby & Keen, 1986). In the rabbit some C-fibre afferents do successfully reinnervate the skin following section, but the absolute numbers doing so have not been determined (Shea & Perl, 1985). It may be that somatosensory C-fibre afferents are generally less good at regenerating than A-fibre afferents or pre-gnaglionic autonomic C-fibres, both of which fibre groups are known to recover to normal numbers after nerve crush (Gutman and Sanders, 1943; Bray and Aguayo, 1974). Capsaicin's selective action may depend on the particular sensitivity of one fibre group (the C-polymodal afferents) to its denerative effects. The subsequent failure of many fibres to regenerate may, however, not be due to any special effect of capsaicin.

SUMMARY

1. From 6 weeks to a year following local administration of capsaicin to a cutaneous nerve in the rat a 40% loss of C-fibres has been found by electrophysiological and morphological methods.
2. The loss is highly selective for afferent C-fibres of the polymodal nociceptor type, which are reduced to only 1/3 - 1/6 of normal numbers.
3. The interpretation of experiments using capsaicin in adult rats needs to take into account the fibre loss; observed functional changes cannot be unambiguously attributed to the, possibly secondary, changes in neuropeptide levels.
4. The reasons why many polymodal C-units fail to regenerate require further investigation; it may reflect a generally poor regenerative capability of somatosensory C-fibres.

REFERENCES

Ainsworth, A, Hall, P, Wall, PD, Allt, G, Mackenzie, ML, Gibson, S, Polak, JM (1981). Effects of capsaicin applied locally to adult peripheral nerve. II. Anatomy and enzyme and peptide chemistry of peripheral nerve and spinal cord. Pain 11: 379-388.

Bisby, MA, Keen, P (1986). Regeneration of primary afferent neurons containing substance P-like immunoreactivity. Brain Research 365: 85-95.

Biscoe, TJ, Nickels, SM, Stirling, CA (1982). Numbers and sizes of nerve fibres in mouse spinal roots. Quart J. Physiol 67: 473-494.

Blumberg, H, Janig, W (1982). Changes in unmyelinated fibres including sympathetic postganglionic fibres of a skin nerve after peripheral neuroma formation. J. Autonomic Nervous System 6: 172-183.

Bray, GM, Aguayo, AJ (1974). Regeneration of peripheral unmyelinated fibres. Fate of the axonal sprouts which develop after injury. J. Anat 117: 517-529.

Cervero, F, McRitchie, HA (1982). Neonatal capsaicin does not affect unmyelinated efferent fibres of the autonomic nervous system: functional evidence. Brain Research 239: 283-288.

Chiba, T, Masuko, S, Kawano, H (1986). Correlation of mitochondrial swelling after capsaicin treatment and substance P and somatostatin immunoreactivity in small neurons of dorsal root ganglion in the rat. Neuroscience Letters 64: 311-316.

Fitzgerald, M (1983). Capsaicin and sensory neurones - a review. Pain 15: 109-130.

Gamse, R, Petsche, U, Lembeck, F, Jancso, G (1982). Capsaicin applied to peripheral nerve inhibits axoplasmic transport of substance P and somatostatin. Brain Research 239: 447-462.

Gutman, E, Sanders, FK (1943). Recovery of fibre numbers and diameters in the regeneration of peripheral nerves. J. Physiol. 101: 489-518.

Handwerker, HO, Holzer-Petsche, U, Heym, C, Welk, E (1985) C-fiber functions after topical application of capsaicin to a peripheral nerve and after neonatal capsaicin treatment. In Chahl, LA, Szolcsany, J, Lembeck, F (eds): "Antidromic Vasodilatation and Neurogenic Inflammation", Budapest: Akademiai Kiado, pp 57-78.

Jancso, G, Kiraly, E, Jancso-Gabor, A (1980). Direct evidence for an axonal site of action of capsaicin. Arch Pharmacol 313: 91-94.

Jancso, G, Kiraly, E, Joo, F, Such, G, Nagy, A (1985). Selective degeneration by capsaicin of a subpopulation of primary sensory neurons in the adult rat. Neuroscience Letters 59: 209-214.

Jenq, C-B, Coggeshall, RE (1984). Regeneration of axons in tributary nerves. Brain Research 310: 107-121.

Jessell, TM, Iversen, LL, Cuello, AC (1978). Capsaicin-induced depletion of substance P from primary sensory neurones. Brain Research 152: 183-188.

Joo, F, Szolcsanyi, J, Jancso-Gabor, A (1969). Mitochondrial alterations in the spinal ganglion cells of the rat accompanying the long-lasting sensory disturbance induced by capsaicin. Life Sciences 8: 621-626.

Lisney, SJW (1987). Studies of unmyelinated fibre regeneration in rat peripheral nerve. In Pubols, LM, Sessle, BJ (eds): "Effects of injury on spinal and trigeminal somatosensory systems", New York: Alan R Liss, pp

Lynn, B (1986). The immediate and long-term effects of applying capsaicin to cutaneous nerves. In Jancso, G, Szolcsanyi, J, Rethelyi, M (eds): "Capsaicin and sensory systems", Budapest: Akademiai Kaido, in press.

Lynn, B, Pini, A (1985). Long-term block of afferent fibres following capsaicin treatment in the rat. J. Physiol. 362: 19P.

Lynn, B, Carpenter, SE, Pini, A (1984). Capsaicin and cutaneous afferents. In Chahl, LE, Szolcsanyi, J, Lembeck, F (eds): "Antidromic vasodilation and neurogenic inflammation", Budapest, Akademiai Kaido, pp 83-92.

McLachlan, EM, Janig, W (1983). The cell bodies of origin of sympathetic and sensory axons in some skin and muscle nerves of the cat hindlimb. J Comp Neurol 214: 115-130.

Marsh, SJ (1985). Depolarization of rat vagal C-fibres and sensory neurones by capsaicin in vitro. J. Physiol. 360: 14P.

Papka, RE, Furness, JB, Della, NG, Murphy, R, Costa, M (1984) Time course of effect of capsaicin on ultrastructure and histochemistry of substance P-immunoreactive nerves associated with the cardiovascular system of the guinea pig. Neuroscience 12: 1277-1292.

Scadding, JW (1980). The permanent anatomical effects of neonatal capsaicin on somatosensory nerves. J. Anat. 131: 473-484.

Shea, VK, Perl, ER (1985). Regeneration of cutaneous afferent unmyelinated (c) fibres after transection. J. Neurophysiol 54: 502-511.

Effects of Injury on Trigeminal and Spinal Somatosensory Systems, pages 125–132

IMMUNOCYTOCHEMICALLY DEFINED POPULATIONS OF DORSAL ROOT GANGLION NEURONS REMAINING IN THE RAT AFTER NEONATAL CAPSAICIN

Sally N. Lawson

Department of Physiology, the Medical School, University Walk, Bristol BS8 1TD, U.K.

INTRODUCTION

The discovery of the neurotoxic actions of neonatal capsaicin on sensory neurones was first made by Jancsó et al 1977. Since then neonatal capsaicin treatment has been widely used as a selective neurotoxin for sensory C fibres and their cell bodies. However since it is not completely selective (see below) it is important to know the nature of the cells and fibres remaining after such treatment.

Neonatal capsaicin causes the loss of nerve fibres in dorsal roots (DRs). In lumbar DRs of the rat after 50 mg/kg, fibre losses of 61-69% were reported in L3, (Nagy et al 1983) and L4 (Lawson and Nickels 1980 and submitted). The same authors found losses of 87-89% in the unmyelinated fibres and of 12-18% in myelinated fibres at this dose. A permanent loss of neuronal somata in dorsal root ganglia (DRGs) is also found. Otten et al 1983 found a loss of 46% in lumbar DRGs L3, L4 and L5 after 40 mg/kg neonatal capsaicin. We have reported mean cell losses of 50% and 68% in two studies of L4 DRGs after 85 mg/kg capsaicin administered on the day after birth (day 1). We have also studied the cell sizes of the remaining neurones and used the antineurofilament antibody RT97 to distinguish between large light (LL) neurones and small dark (SD) neurones (see Lawson et al 1984). We found that about 84-90% of SD neurones and 13-34% of the LL neurones were lost (Lawson & Harper 1985, Lawson & Nickels submitted). No data is available on the proportions of LL and SD neurones remaining after 50 mg/kg, the more commonly used dose.

Single fibre recording in adult peripheral nerve after 50 mg/kg capsaicin neonatally shows that examples of every expected afferent fibre type, eg polymodal nociceptors, cold fibres etc., were represented within the remaining C fibres. There was no evidence for their proportions differing substantially from control rats (Lynn 1984, Welk et al 1984). It is, however, well documented that neurogenic inflammation and the sensitivity to noxious chemicals are considerably reduced after neonatal capsaicin (Jancso et al 1977). In the light of this functional information it would be interesting to know the immunocytochemical properties of the remaining neurones. There is known to be a substantial loss of substance P (SP) containing neurones (e.g. Otten et al. 1983). There is also a reduction in the number of neurones showing calcitonin gene-related peptide-like immunoreactivity (CGRPLI) (Skofitsch and Jacobowitz 1985). Since many SP containing neurones also display CGRPLI (Skofitsch and Jacobowitz 1985) it would be interesting to know if all capsaicin sensitive CGRP neurones also contain SP.

In this investigation several immunocytochemically defined subpopulations of SD neurones are examined to find if they are all reduced to the same extent as the whole SD population. The antibodies chosen are anti-SP and monoclonal antibody 2C5 since these both label predominantly small neurones (Hokfelt et al 1980, Lawson et al 1985) and little overlap occurs between them. Anti-CGRP labels both small and medium sized neurones (Gibson et al 1984). RT97 is included as a marker for LL cells and as has recently been demonstrated (Lawson and Waddell 1985) it also acts as a marker for DRG neurones with myelinated fibres in the rat.

METHODS

Two pairs of rats were used, one capsaicin and one vehicle injected in each case. The vehicle was 10% alcohol, 10% tween 80 in isotonic saline. The injections were made under halothane anaesthesia by K. Sharkey. Pair A were injected the day after birth (day 1) and the second pair (pair B) were injected on day 2. The two pairs of rats were anaesthetised with sodium pentobarbitone at three months and two months respectively. They were perfused through the heart with isotonic saline, followed by Zamboni's fixative at room temperature. The L4 DRGs and their DRs were removed, fixed for 1-2 hrs, then left overnight in 30% sucrose in phosphate buffer. Multiple series of 7um thick frozen sections were taken from each DRG. Each series comprised one section taken at regular intervals (usually 400um) throughout the ganglion. A control and a capsaicin series were mounted on a single slide thus reducing the possibility of random variations in technique affecting treated and control sections differentially. Each slide was incubated in the first layer containing two primary antibodies for 24-48 hrs at 4'C and in the second antibody layer for 30-60 mins at room temperature. RT97 was provided by J Wood, (for further details see Lawson et al 1984), 2C5 by BJ Randle (see Lawson et al 1985), anti-SP by P Keen (see Harmer and Keen 1986), and anti-CGRP by JM Polak (see Gibson et al 1984). Second layer antibodies used were FITC conjugated goat antimouse IgG to react with RT97, rhodamine labelled goat antirabbit IgG to react with the polyclonal antisubstance P and antiCGRP antibodies, and FITC conjugated goat antimouse IgM antibody to react with 2C5.

For each pair of treated and control DRGs one series of sections was examined from each ganglion for each antibody combination. Cross-sectional areas of all neurones with clear nuclear sections (about 95% of which had nucleoli) were measured and their immunoreactivity graded. The total number of myelinated fibres in each DR was counted in an unstained frozen section under interference contrast microscopy.

RESULTS

Table 1 shows the percentages of L4 DRG cells in each rat labelled with the antibodies used, A is rat pair A, B is rat pair B. The labelled cells are expressed as a percentage of all the cells measured in that series (%CAP, %VEH). The values for the two vehicle treated rats were similar to each other and to the values obtained from L4 DRGs of untreated 10 week old rats. However the percentages of neurones labelled by RT97 in the capsaicin treated rats were elevated (88.7% in A and 74.1% in B) due to the loss of SD or RT97 negative (-) neurones. The data available did not allow a direct estimate of the percentage of cells lost in the capsaicin treated ganglia. For the purposes of comparing the capsaicin and vehicle data the assumption was made that the absolute size of the RT97 positive (+) population was not reduced in the capsaicin treated ganglia, although there is probably a small reduction, see below. Thus for animal pair A all the actual percentages in the capsaicin rats were multiplied by the ratio of the percentage of LL cells in the vehicle to LL cells in capsaicin ganglia, that is by 46.1/88.7. These values (%CAP/VEH table 1) give a direct indication of the percentage of cells remaining since they express populations of labelled cells in capsaicin

TABLE 1: Effect of capsaicin on populations of labelled neurones

	A				B			
	%VEH	%CAP	%CAP/VEH	%DECREASE CAP/VEH	%VEH	%CAP	%CAP/VEH	% DECREASE CAP/VEH
RT97+	46.1	88.7	Assume 46.1	Assume 0	50.4	74.1	Assume 50.4	Assume 0
RT97-	53.9	10.4	5.4	90	47.4	24.7	16.8	64.6
anti-sP+	16.5	4.4	2.2	86	20.7	12.94	8.8	57.6
2C5+	28.7	3.8	2.0	93	23.5	2.8	1.9	92.0
anti CGRP+	37.2	21.5	11.0	70.5	44.4	35.5	24.1	45.7

ganglia as percentages of all cells in the vehicle treated ganglion in each pair. With the same assumption % DECREASE CAP/VEH is calculated for each antibody as 100*(%VEH-%CAP/VEH)/%VEH. This gives the calculated percentage reduction in each antibody labelled subpopulation.

It can be seen (%DECREASE CAP/VEH) that the loss of the SD, (RT97-) neurones was much greater in capsaicin rat A than capsaicin rat B. An estimated 10% of SD neurones remained in A while 35% remained in B, also see fig 1. The loss of neurones displaying SPLI (SP like immunoreactivity) was less than the overall SD cell loss in both ganglia, while the converse was true for 2C5. That is, the 2C5 neurones were apparently much more sensitive to the neurotoxic actions of capsaicin than neurones displaying SPLI. This was particularly obvious in capsaicin rat B (see fig 1) where over 40% of the normal complement of SP neurones but only 8% of the 2C5+ neurones remain, (also see fig. 2). The population of neurones displaying CGRPLI was also reduced by the capsaicin but a greater proportion of these than of SPLI+ or 2C5+ neurones remained, 30% in capsaicin rat A and 55% in capsaicin rat B (see figs. 1 and 2). The loss of CGRP neurones must include neurones which do not display SPLI. This can be seen by subtracting %CAP/VEH from %VEH, table 1. The capsaicin sensitive SPLI neurones comprised 12-14% of all neurones while the capsaicin sensitive CGRPLI neurones comprised 20-26% of all neurones.

There were no obvious differences in cell size distributions, see fig.1, for SPLI and RT97+ neurones after capsaicin but the few remaining 2C5+ neurones were above the SD cell size range and also showed CGRPLI. The loss of CGRPLI neurones was particularly from the SD cell size range.

FIGURE 1: SIZE DISTRIBUTIONS OF LABELLED NEURONES.

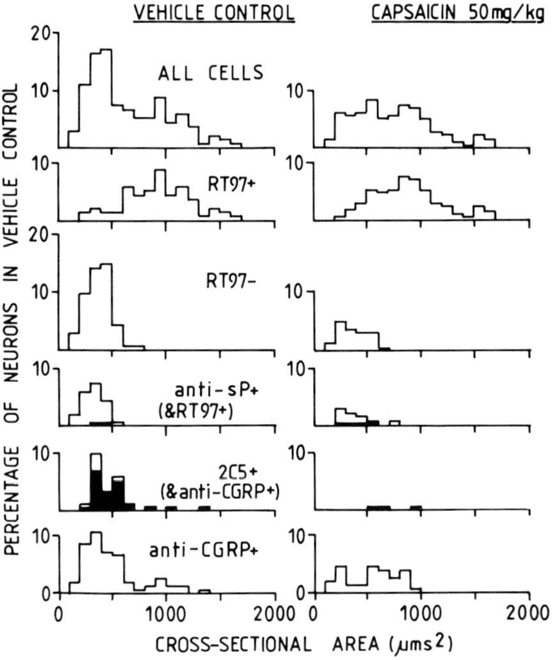

LEGEND: Histograms of neuronal cross-sectional areas from L4 DRGs of vehicle and capsaicin treated rats, pair B. It was assumed that the RT97+ cell population was the same size in both rats and the populations in the capsaicin rat adjusted accordingly. In fact the capsaicin histograms are probably overestimated by 2-10%, see text. Open histograms are cells labelled by one antibody. Solid histograms show the cells labelled by two antibodies as indicated. Labels on left apply also to right, ALL CELLS etc.

The capsaicin DR myelinated fibre counts were 4226 in A and 4643 in B, about 5% lower than the vehicle DR counts (4431 in A and 4879 in B). Compared with counts of many vehicle treated DRs (Lawson and Nickels submitted) the loss was about 10% in A and 2% in B. Our previous data (Lawson in press, Lawson and Nickels submitted) indicate a close parallel between the percentage loss of myelinated fibres and of LL cells. Thus calculations for capsaicin treated DRGs in table 1 and fig 1 made on the assumption of no LL cell loss are probably overestimates by 2-10%. This does not affect the validity of comparing the estimated percentage losses of each population with each other and with that of the SD population.

FIGURE 2: Immunoreactivity to anti-CGRP and 2C5 Antibodies

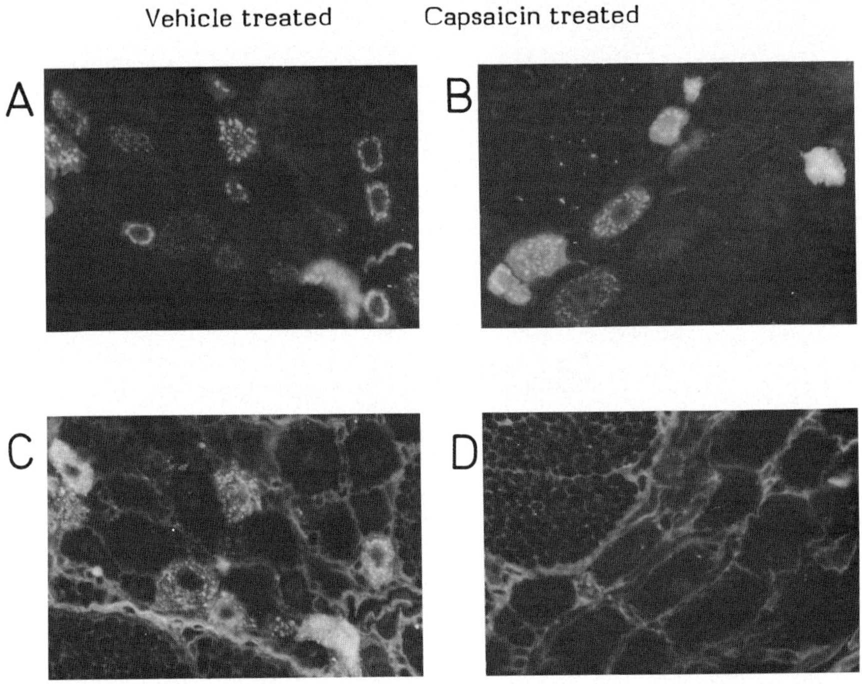

LEGEND: Immunofluorescence on 7um frozen sections of L4 DRGs. A and B, CGRPL1 (rhodamine filter), C and D, 2C5 immunofluorescence (FITC filter). A and C are the same section from vehicle treated rat B; B and D are the same section from capsaicin treated rat A. Note that in C (vehicle) there are at least 8 2C5 positive neurones, while only one very faint 2C5 positive neurone is visible in D (capsaicin).

DISCUSSION

The very different percentage losses of DRG neurones in the two treated rats may have resulted from a natural variability in the effectiveness of capsaicin from one animal to the next. However, in two further rats treated on day 2 with 50 mg/kg, 23 and 33% of the remaining neurones were RT97-. These values are similar to that for capsaicin rat B (25%), while the only rat injected on day 1 (capsaicin rat A) had a value of 10%. It is therefore possible that the difference in capsaicin rats A and B was due to the timing of the injections.

These preliminary results indicate that at a dose of 50 mg/kg, (the dose commonly used as a neurotoxin) not all SD (RT97-) neurones were equally affected by neonatal capsaicin treatment. Substantial proportions of neurones showing SPLI (14-40%) remained, and even greater proportions of neurones with CGRPLI (30-55%) remained. Presumably some of the functions normally served by these populations must be carried out by these remaining neurones. The very small proportion of 2C5 neurones remaining (8%) compared to the other populations is very intriguing. It might be expected that some of the physiological changes seen in adult rats treated neonatally with capsaicin will prove to be due to the loss of this subpopulation of DRG neurones.

ACKNOWLEDGEMENTS

I should like to thank J Wood, BJ Randle, P Keen and J Polak for the gifts of antibodies RT97, 2C5, anti-SP, and anti-CGRP respectively and K Sharkey for injecting the rats.

REFERENCES

Gibson SJ, Polak JM, Bloom SR, Sabate IM, Mulderry PM, Ghatei MA, McGregor GP, Morrison JFB, Kelly JS, Evans RM, Rosenfeld MG (1984). Calcitonin gene-related peptide immunoreactivity in the spinal cord of man and of eight other species. J Neuroscience 4:3101-3111

Harmer AJ, Keen P (1986) Methods for the identification of neuropeptide processing products: somatostatin and the tachykinins. Meths in Enzymol. 124:335-348

Harper AA, Lawson SN (1985). Conduction velocity is related to morphological cell type in rat dorsal root ganglion neurones.

Jancsó G, Király E, Jancsó-Gábor A (1977) Pharmacologically induced selective degeneration of chemosensitive primary sensory neurones. Nature 270:741

Hökfelt T, Johannsson O, Ljungdahl A, Lundberg JM, Schultzberg M (1980) Peptidergic Neurones. Nature 284:515-521

Lawson SN, Harper AA (1985) Neonatal capsaicin is not a specific neurotoxin for sensory C fibres or small dark cells of rat dorsal root ganglia. Symposium on Antidromic Vasodilation and Neurogenic inflammation. Akademiai, Kiado, Budapest. Eds. Chakl LA, Scolscanyi J.

Lawson SN, Harper AA, Harper EI, Garson JA, Anderton BH (1984). A monoclonal antibody against neurofilament protein specifically labels a subpopulation of rat sensory neurones. J Comp Neurol 228:263-272

Lawson SN, Harper EI, Harper AA, Garson JA, Coakham HB, Randle BJ (1985). Monoclonal antibody 2C5: a marker for a subpopulation of small neurones in rat dorsal root ganglia. Neuroscience 16:365-374

Lawson SN, Nickels SN (1980) The use of morphometric techniques to analyse the effect of neonatal capsaicin on rat dorsal root ganglia and dorsal roots. J. Physiol. 303:12P

Lawson SN, Nickels SN (submitted) The effect of neonatal capsaicin on sensory neurones in adult rats.

Lawson SN, Waddell PJ (1985) The antibody RT97 distinguishes between sensory cell bodies with myelinated and unmyelnated peripheral processes in the rat. J. Physiol 371:59P

Lynn B (1984) Effect of neonatal treatment with capsaicin on the numbers and properties of cutaneous afferent units from the hairy skin of the rat. Brain Res. 322:255-260

Nagy JI, Iversen LL, Goedert M, Chapman D, Hunt SP (1983) Dose dependent effects of capsaicin on primary sensory neurones in the neonatal rat. J Neuroscience 3:399-406

Otten U, Lorez HP, Businger F (1983). Nerve growth factor antagonises' the neurotoxic action of capsaicin. Nature 301: 515-517.

Skofitsch G, Jacobowitz DM (1985). Calcitonin gene-related peptide coexists with substance P in capsaicin sensitive neurons and sensory ganglia of the rat.Peptides 6:747-754

Welk E, Fleischer E, Petsche U, Handwerker HO (1984) Afferent C fibres in rats after neonatal capsaicin treatment. Pflügers Arch. 400:66-71

Effects of Injury on Trigeminal and Spinal Somatosensory Systems, pages 133–139

SUMMARY AND CRITIQUE

Ainsley Iggo

Department of Preclinical Veterinary Sciences, University of Edinburgh, Edinburgh EH9 1QH, UK

The opening paper presented by Margaret Byers initiated a topic of discussion that recurred at several points in the programme; namely, how confident can we be of the accuracy of the identification of neural elements in tissue prepared for electron microscopy, especially when dealing with the very fine terminals of about 0.01 µm diameter, such as are present in dentine and the epidermis? No convincing criteria that satisfied all participants could be formulated, except perhaps the extremely arduous process of serial reconstruction of the kind performed by Cauna when dealing with cutaneous C-fibre terminals. A similar problem arose in connection with the various methods of axonal labelling used to trace nerve fibres and their fine terminals, such as horseradish peroxidase or radio-labelled proteins as used by Margaret Byers. The precision of such techniques, involving transport of label was queried by Grant, since the absence of label could not be taken to prove the absence of neural tissue in, for example, re-innervation following nerve injury. Discussion centred on the restriction of label to the cell in which it had been transported. The entrapment is not necessarily complete, although apparently the small quantity that escaped by trans-cellular transfer into adjacent cells was not regarded by Byers as sufficient to invalidate the accuracy of autoradiographic labelling in her rat dentinal material.

An alternative method of labelling, born of molecular biology, was the use of immunoreactivity. Larry Kruger reported successful labelling using CRGP (calicitonin-gene related peptide) immunoreactivity that he claimed was specific to fine nerves innervating nociceptors, to give positive identification of the nerves in diverse samples of tissue, such as the tympanum and the cornea. The further development of this kind of immunoreactivity technique should add greater certainty to the positive identification of particular nerves and their terminals in cases of doubt, although a first step will have to be the production of specific labelled peptides or their antibodies.

The rapid loss of nerve tissue from the dentine, revealed by the ultrastructural studies of Matthews and colleagues, at two days after nerve section, drew the comment from Bryce Munger that such rapid loss was also characteristic of other sensory receptors, although the rate of disappearance was not the same for all varieties of sensory receptor. Recovery of dentinal innervation was evident in 12 weeks in the cat, and as stated by Byers, especially fast in rat molars. Functional studies in parallel with the histological work established a return of normal responses at a time when the normal pattern of dentinal large and small innervation processes had begun to return. This topic was more generally discussed, in relation to the recovery of function in other sensory systems. The advantage of using recognizable receptor models was stressed by Iggo in reference to cited studies using the SAI Merkel receptor in hairy skin, where Burgess, Horch and English had been able to mark individual touch domes with tattoo in intact normal skin and thereafter follow the recovery of function following nerve injury. The use of this system was cited by Mendell as offering the opportunity to test the hypothesis that re-innervation was specific, in the sense that the regenerating nerve sprout made contact with its appropriate accessory structures. Diamond reported confirmation of the results in experiments where Merkel cells had failed to be functionally re-innervated by A-delta or C-fibres, that is inappropriate afferent fibres did not sprout and form receptor terminal with Merkel cells. Such apparent peripheral specificity was not necessarily evident at the cerebral cortical level where, according to Manfred Zimmerman, maps of rapidly-adapting and slowly-adapting responses to cutaneous stimuli were distorted after peripheral nerve lesions in monkey experiments performed by Paul and Merzenich. A possibly confusing aspect of regenerating nerve sprouts was their non-specific excitation by light, brisk mechanical stimulation, expressed clinically as Tinel's sign. Careful quantitative electrophysiological testing using appropriate natural stimuli is thus necessary to establish normal restoration of function following nerve regeneration. The confidence in such analysis would be further enhanced by concurrent morphological studies on the same tissue.

The influence of acute inflammation on joint sensory receptors, reported by Robert Schmidt, drew enquiries from Marshall Devor about the possibility that a microneuroma might have been formed as a result of the injury. In response, Schmidt asserted that the effects could be produced by chemical action alone, and that the receptive fields were in any case remote from the injection site, where any injury might have been caused by the actual injection. The mechanism of sensitization, direct on the receptors, or indirect through some ancillary action, was raised by Besson, who suggested that the action of prostaglandin in the inflamed joint was indirect by sensitization of the receptors to other chemicals, such as bradykinin (BK) or substance P (SP). Schmidt considered that there was evidence for both kinds of action. In continuation of discussion of this aspect Perl commented that indomethacin and PGE-type blocking agents could suppress but not totally block the enhanced responses of sensitized C-fibres in a rabbit ear preparation and suggested that PG enhances by an indirect action. Iggo suggested, from chronic inflammation studies in rats, that the time course of aspirin action in reducing the enhanced sensitivity of joint receptors was inconsistent with PGE2 being the causative agent, and that a shorter-lived PG, such as prostacyclin, might be involved, even though, as Schmidt indicated, PGE2 and BK could both rapidly antagonize the action of aspirin. There was general agreement that agents such as BK had a longer latency of action, on close-arterial injection, than did K ions or acetylcholine. This delayed response was consistent with an indirect action on excitability, although not necessarily on cells other than the sensory nerve endings themselves.

Hyperalgesia caused by antidromic stimulation of cutaneous nerves, evoking memories of Lewis's nocifensor system, was species dependent, according to Bruce Lynn, although Campbell attributed the effect to electrical injury of the skin rather than to nerve stimulation. The use of BK to generate hyperalgesia, in intradermal doses of 10^{-10} molar by Campbell caused sensitization of heat sensitive receptors, although tachyphylaxis to BK in man could develop.

The technique used to obtain effective nerve repair in baboons could influence the rate of re-innervation recovery, according to Terzis, with those avoiding or preventing tension giving the best results. The complementary morphological results for this interesting study are not yet available so that confirmation of the actual receptor reformation could not be discussed. Ochoa commented that Pacinian corpuscles seemed to be difficult to re-innervate, but as Terzis pointed out, they form only a small proportion of the total cutaneous receptor population and might for this reason be underestimated in the re-innervation studies. In another re-innervation study by Jack Diamond, the possibility of C-fibre sprouting was tested by Evans-blue extravasation. In connection with the reflex testing techniques used, Devor questioned whether the thermal probe used by Diamond would allow discrimination of collateral sprouting as an explanation of the results. Diamond took the view that the latency of the response was very short, less than one second, and inconsistent with sprouting. Nor could the results be attributed to mediation by the A-delta fibres as suggested by Devor since capsaicin pre-treatment eliminated both the C-fibres and the response to heating.

The reorganisation of peripheral nerve projections following trigeminal nerve transections, as described by Rhoades, was not simply an example of the normal ability of sensory axons to branch shortly after leaving the ganglion and reach widely separated cutaneous receptive fields (as found originally by Adrian, Cattell and Hoagland in the frog), since his double-labelling experiments showed a very extensive branching after neonatal nerve transection that was lacking in normal animals. Goldberger then drew attention to the need to avoid age-related cell death complications in such experiments, but there was no evidence for it in the reported studies. On a related topic, Munger, dealing with the maturation of the dermatotopic map, confidently defended his choice of limited dorsal rhizotomy when questioned by Terzis. He stressed the different ages of motor and sensory differentiation, that could influence differentiation/denervation studies of Merkel cells of the kind reported by Diamond. The importance of this factor was that denervation studies made after birth could not properly be decisive if differentiation of the cellular elements had already occurred before birth, as was the case with Merkel cells. The ability of patients with skin-flap surgery, to recover sensibility appropriate to the nerve rather than the skin flap was advanced by Terzis as supporting views of sensory function advanced by Munger. Presumably, in such cases the central connections of the surviving axons would not have been compromised, and only the receptors would lie in new skin.

The problem of the re-growth of peripheral nerves in artificial tubes, as used in making nerve grafts, led to vigorous discussion, first by Kruger about the kinds of collagen that might influence axonal growth, although the presenter, Dick Coggeshall, had not seen any electron-microscopical evidence of differences. Next Erik Torebjork reported on the very beneficial effects of using a micromesh tube to direct re-growth over a nerve gap of 20 mm. Terzis also reported good results with an inter-position tube, although the distal structure was different in appearance from the proximal stump of the nerve. Iggo reported the excellent results of Andersson of Gothenberg using a mesothelial tube to form an inter-position graft, in which the structure of the re-growing axons looked normal in contrast to the highly abnormal EM appearance of axons in a plastic-tube induced neuroma. All the above studies were on peripheral nerve and it was not known how such procedures might influence regeneration of tissue from the central nervous system.

The topic of neuromas then appeared on the formal programme, although they had already frequently entered the discussions. Burchiel's report on the untoward excitatory action of the paralysing agent, gallamine, on neuromas spurred a defence from Devor, in whose recent work gallamine had been avoided. The time-scales of spontaneous activity, pseudoaffective reflexes and pain led to differences emerging among investigators - the early responsiveness of A-fibres subsiding and giving way to a later surge of background activity in C-fibres, that did not in Burchiel's work match the latency of autotomy, as apparently it did in Devor's studies. Another interesting aspect of neuromas was the uncertain incidence of pain--it being more common, according to Meyer, in neuromas associated with the extremities of the upper limbs than in the lower limbs. Janig's results on nerve lesions drew the question of an influence of sympathetic efferent axons in neuromas. He had not found any evidence for antidromic activity evoked by sympathetic orthodromic discharge, and despite the EM evidence for massive apposition of C-fibres in neuromas, no indication of cross-talk or a functional role had been found. The possibility of axonal branching and of re-growth back up the proximal stump of a neuroma was discounted by Christiane Vahle-Hinz who had made detailed quantitative axon counts in the relevant nerves.

The use of excised neuromas, as used by Zimmerman to study properties of the structure, was questioned by Lisney who pointed out the high sensitivity of neuromas to mechanical trauma and anoxia. Although there was no direct rebuttal of the possibility by Zimmerman, he cited "in situ" experiments on cat neuromas in which no major change in responsiveness to such stimuli was found during progressive dissection of the neuroma. Besson raised the issue of the "enormous" quantities of pharmacological agents used by Zimmerman. Although the figures cited did indicate very high dose levels, Zimmerman pointed out that much smaller quantities were also effective. Furthermore, there were major diffusion barriers in the excised neuromas that would have limited the effective concentrations of drugs. Campbell reported confirmatory results in primates, and Zimmerman was able to report that BK was totally ineffective when applied in the same way to normal nerve.

Lisney's results on regeneration in the rat were confirmed by Perl using the rabbit ear as the model. An interesting feature of Lisney's work was the almost total absence of spontaneous activity in nerves with "neuromas-in-continuity". Janig questioned whether there was any evidence for lowered conduction velocities and smaller ganglion size in Lisney's preparation, on the assumption of "die-back" in the nerve. Lisney agreed that there were conduction velocity changes.

The remaining formal papers of the session dealt with the effects of capsaicin, where Csillik in discussion, stressed the need to consider the time course of normal neural development when regeneration subsequent to capsaicin treatment was examined, and also queried the doses used. In reply Lynn explained that there was only a 30 minute exposure to capsaicin. In neuroma nerves there was a low proportion of capsaicin responding C-fibres, but Lynn stressed the need to re-assess old results in the light of the new findings that there are long-lasting losses of C-fibres following nerve treatment with capsaicin in adult rats. Sally Lawson, working with rats treated neonatally with capsaicin was informed by Westerman that administration of the agent during neonatal days 1 to 6 was necessary if sensory deficits were to be expressed subsequently in adult rats.

In general discussion an interesting comparative point was made by Schmidt, that Pierau had found that birds are apparently insensitive to capsaicin, and he speculated whether capsaicin was actually specific for substance P, to which Lawson replied that it was not a specific C-fibre block. Lynn, however, claimed that in neonates there was a loss of both A-delta and C-fibres, whereas in the adult there was a selective C-fibre lesion. The brief closing general discussion dealt with importance of comparative aspects, as illustrated by the apparent indifference of birds to capsaicin, a theme that was further developed by Munger in relation to sensory receptors.

II
SPINAL CORD AND BRAINSTEM

Effects of Injury on Trigeminal and Spinal Somatosensory Systems, pages 143–150

TRANSGANGLIONIC DEGENERATION IN RAT VIBRISSAE INNERVATING NEURONS

Jan Arvidsson

Department of Anatomy, Karolinska Institutet
104 01 Stockholm, Sweden

INTRODUCTION

It is now well established that transection of the peripheral branches of primary sensory neurons may lead to degeneration in their central branches (transganglionic degeneration; TGD). TGD has been observed in cranial and spinal primary sensory neurons both at light and electron microscopic levels (for review see Aldskogius et al., 1985). However, at present there is only little information as to whether TGD may occur in all or just some functional types of primary sensory neurons after a peripheral nerve injury.

The rat vibrissae hair follicles are densely innervated by various types of mechanoreceptor fibers (Andres, 1966). In a previous horseradish peroxidase study it was shown that the nerves innervating the vibrissae in the rat terminated in the trigeminal nucleus caudalis only in its magnocellular zone (corresponding to laminae III and IV of the dorsal horn), and in a highly ordered fashion (Arvidsson, 1982). In the present study nerves supplying individual vibrissae follicles were cut to investigate whether this type of lesion may lead to TGD. The study is based upon a light and electron microscopic analysis of the magnocellular zone of the trigeminal nucleus caudalis, an area where no ultrastructural studies of TGD have been made. A more comprehensive report of the findings is presented elsewhere (Arvidsson, 1986).

MATERIALS AND METHODS

Adult Sprague Dawley rats were used for this study. The nerves entering the vibrissae B1-4, C1-4 and D1-4 (Arvidsson, 1982) were exposed on one side and transected just outside the follicle. In some of these experiments intended for light microscopic analysis the C1-4 nerves were exposed but left intact as a control. The rats were perfused following a survival of 4-80 days and the brain stem containing the trigeminal nucleus caudalis was removed. Material intended for light microscopy was cut on a freezing microtome and stained with silver (Fink and Heimer, 1967). Sections cut on a Vibratome were used to select areas for ultrastructural analysis. The details of the experimental procedures are given elsewhere (Arvidsson, 1986).

RESULTS AND DISCUSSION

Light Microscopy

The first evidence of TGD in the magnocellular zone of nucleus caudalis appears at the 10th postoperative day. At this stage small amounts of granular argyrophilic structures are observed in this area, leaving the marginal zone and the substantia gelatinosa (corresponding to laminae I and II) free from degeneration. At 20 and 28 days survival there are considerable amounts of TGD in the magnocellular zone and fiber fragments are common (Fig. 1). The area of degeneration is rather broad and uninterrupted and located within areas of TGD observed previously after infraorbital nerve transection (Grant and Arvidsson, 1975; Arvidsson and Grant, 1979). These results also correlate well with the termination areas of vibrissae afferents observed in a horseradish peroxidase study (Arvidsson, 1982). The cases where the nerves in row C were exposed but left intact show two restricted areas of TGD in the magnocellular zone separated by an empty area (Fig. 2). This shows that the light microscopic TGD in nucleus caudalis is induced by transection of the vibrissae nerves and not by the skin incisions around the follicles.

Electron Microscopy

The first signs of altered terminals in the magnocellular

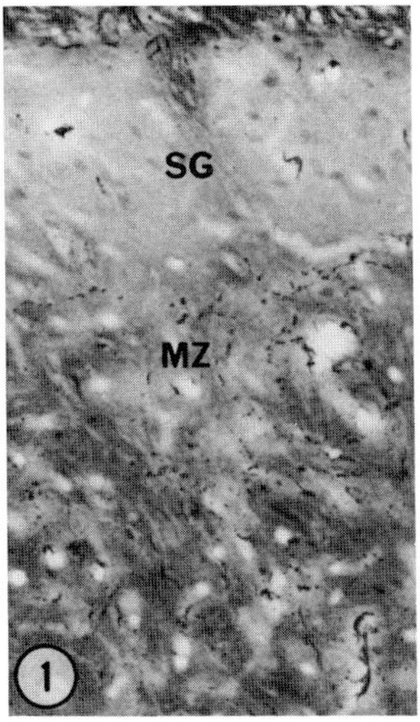

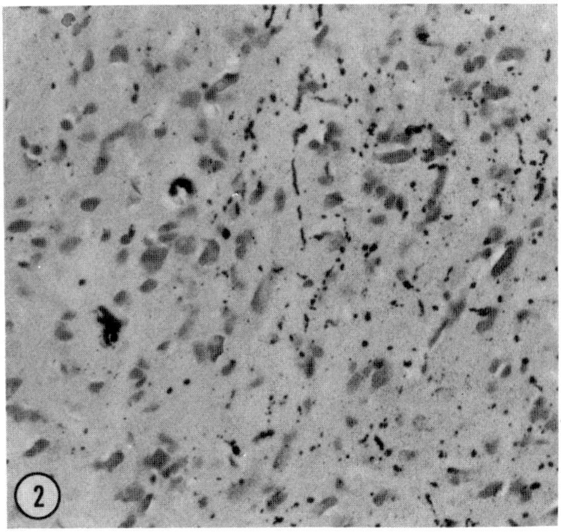

Fig. 1. Transverse Fink-Heimer stained section from nucleus caudalis. The degeneration argyrophilia is confined to the magnocellular zone (MZ) after transection of vibrissae nerves in rows B, C and D. 28 days survival. SG, substantia gelatinosa. X 170.

Fig. 2. The magnocellular zone of subnucleus caudalis showing field of degeneration representing the D row (right). Note absence of degeneration in the area representing the intact C row (left). 28 days survival. X 270.

zone appear on the 6th postoperative day, when some terminals show a slight increase in electron density (Fig. 3). These terminals often appear to contain a reduced number of synaptic vesicles and are usually presynaptic to dendrites. Terminals showing these sometimes rather subtle changes are most common at 6-8 days survival, but a few of them can be seen also 14 and 20 days postoperatively. Other terminals appear somewhat shrunken and show a moderate increase in electron density (Fig. 4). The mitochondria usually appear disrupted in these terminals, which are most common 8-10 days postoperatively. A small number of moderately darkened terminals are observed also at 14 and 20 days, but not at longer survivals. Some of these terminals proceed to a more totally darkened and shrunken state (Fig. 5).

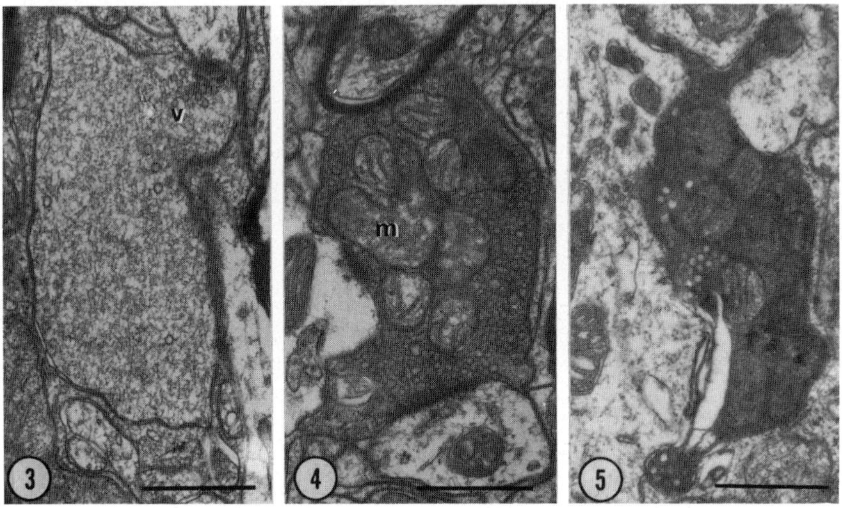

Figs. 3-7. Electron micrographs showing degenerative changes in the magnocellular zone of nucleus caudalis after transection of vibrissae nerves in rows B, C and D. Scale = 0.5 μm.
Fig. 3. Terminal showing a somewhat increased electron density and a reduced number of synaptic vesicles (v). 6 days survival.
Fig. 4. A slightly shrunken terminal with a moderate increase in electron density and mitochondria with disrupted cristae (m). 8 days survival.
Fig. 5. A dark shrunken terminal with pale round vesicles. 8 days survival.

Darkened terminals have been observed also in other studies of TGD (eg. Knyihar and Csillik, 1976; Westrum and Canfield, 1977; Arvidsson, 1979; Johnson et al., 1983). The more severely darkened terminals resemble those described in many areas during Wallerian degeneration (eg. Ralston and Ralston, 1979) and most probably represent an irreversible degenerative process.

A small number of neurofilamentous terminals are observed

8-14 days postoperatively. This type of alteration has been described also in previous studies of TGD (Arvidsson, 1979; Johnson et al., 1983; Majumdar et al., 1983). The neurofilamentous terminals are not observed at longer survivals and there is no indication that they may progress to dark terminals or that they are engulfed by glial cells. This is in accordance with a previous study of TGD in the main sensory trigeminal nucleus of the rat where it was suggested that the neurofilamentous hyperplasia may be a reversible reaction in neurons surviving the peripheral nerve transection (Arvidsson, 1979).

Degeneration in myelinated axons are observed 8-80 days postoperatively in this study. Generally the amounts and severity of axonal degeneration increase at longer survival times. Entirely electron dense axons are rather uncommon at all survival times. Disrupted myelin sheaths surrounding disintegrated axoplasmic remnants and/or empty areas are on the other hand commonly observed. These findings clearly indicate that stem axons are also involved in the process of TGD in vibrissae innervating neurons.

A very striking finding at relatively short postoperative survivals is a complex relationship between cells interpreted as microglia and terminals. Glial cell processes invaginate or surround and distort the terminal (Figs. 6 and 7). These terminals show an almost normal or more commonly a moderately increased electron density. Mitochondria usually show some disintegration in these terminals, but synaptic sites may appear unaffected even in severely distorted terminals. These events suggestive of phagocytosis by glial cells before the terminals reach a totally darkened state are very common by 8-10 days postoperatively and are observed only occasionally at longer survivals. This may explain the low number of totally darkened terminals observed in the present study. A similar glial activity has been observed also in the cat during TGD (Johnson et al., 1983).

Previous studies have shown that infraorbital nerve transection in the adult rat leads to a substantial cell loss in the trigeminal ganglion (Aldskogius and Arvidsson, 1978). The nerves innervating the vibrissae run with the infraorbital nerve, but it is not known if the vibrissae innervating neurons are among those which are lost after a peripheral nerve transection. For this reason it cannot be excluded that the degenerating terminals reflect only a partial removal of the central terminal field in surviving neurons. If the central degenerative alterations observed in this study are not related to cell death the possibility of a central

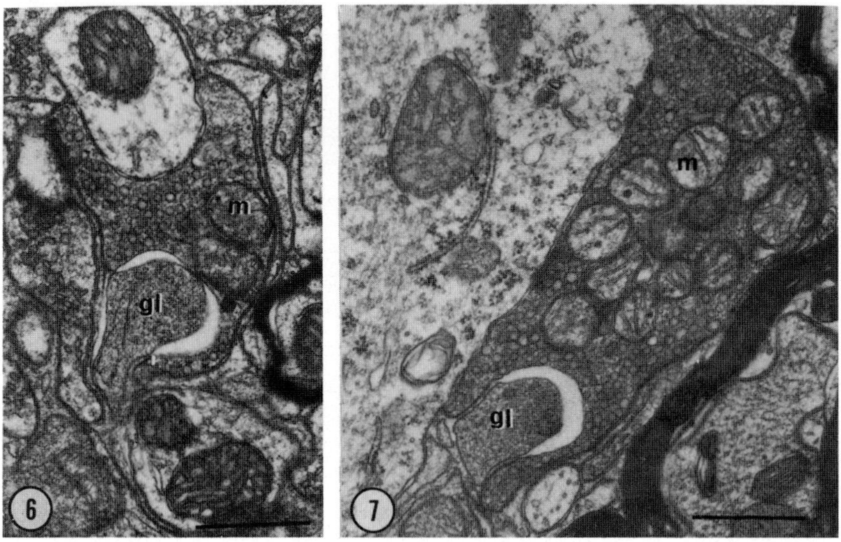

Figs. 6 and 7. Glial processes (gl) invaginating and distorting terminals with a moderate increase in electron density and disrupted mitochondria (m).
Fig. 6: 8 days survival. Fig. 7: 10 days survival.

regenerative process has to be considered. Structures interpreted as evidence for such a process have been found in the monkey dorsal horn after sciatic nerve crush (Knyihar-Csillik et al., 1985). Similar structures are not observed in this study and the degenerative alterations are therefore likely to be irreversible.

CONCLUSION

The present study has shown that peripheral nerve transection leads to degenerative alterations in the central branches of neurons innervating the vibrissae in the adult rat. These alterations can be observed both light microscopically in silver stained sections and at the ultrastructural level. The severity of many of the changes, the resemblance with Wallerian degeneration, the presence of glial phagocytosis and the absence of any evidence for regeneration altogether indicate that irreversible degenerative changes may occur in these neurons after a peripheral nerve injury.

This study was supported by the Swedish Medical Research Council, Project No. 6540 and by Harald Jeanssons stiftelse.

REFERENCES

Aldskogius H, Arvidsson J (1978). Nerve cell degeneration and death in the trigeminal ganglion of the adult rat following peripheral nerve transection. J Neurocytol 7: 229-250.

Aldskogius H, Arvidsson J, Grant G (1985). The reaction of primary sensory neurons to peripheral nerve injury with particular emphasis on transganglionic changes. Brain Res Rev 10:27-46.

Andres KH (1966). Uber die Feinstruktur der Rezeptoren an Sinushaaren. Z Zellforsch 75:339-365.

Arvidsson J (1979). An ultrastructural study of transganglionic degeneration in the main sensory trigeminal nucleus of the rat. J Neurocytol 8:31-45.

Arvidsson J (1982). Somatotopic organization of vibrissae afferents in the trigeminal sensory nuclei of the rat studied by transganglionic transport of HRP. J Comp Neurol 211:84-92.

Arvidsson J (1986). Transganglionic degeneration in vibrissae innervating primary sensory neurons of the rat: A light and electron microscopic study. J Comp Neurol 249:392-403.

Arvidsson J, Grant G (1979). Further observations on transganglionic degeneration in trigeminal primary sensory neurons. Brain Res 162:1-12.

Fink RP, Heimer L (1967). Two methods for selective silver impregnation of degenerating axons and their synaptic endings in the central nervous system. Brain Res 4:369-374.

Grant G, Arvidsson J (1975). Transganglionic degeneration in trigeminal primary sensory neurons. Brain Res 95:265-279.

Johnson LR, Westrum LE, Canfield RC (1983). Ultrastructural study of transganglionic degeneration following dental lesions. Exp Brain Res 52:226-234.

Knyihar E, Csillik B (1976). Effect of peripheral axotomy on the fine structure and histochemistry of Rolando substance: Degenerative atrophy of central processes of pseudounipolar cells. Exp Brain Res 26:73-87.

Knyihar-Csillik E, Rakic P, Csillik B (1985). Fine structure of growth cones in the upper dorsal horn of the adult primate spinal cord in the course of reactive synapto-neogenesis. Cell Tissue Res 239:633-641.

Majumdar S, Mills E, Smith PG (1983). Degenerative and regenerative changes in central projections of glossopharyngeal and vagal sensory neurons after peripheral axotomy in cats: A structural basis for central reorganization of arterial chemoreflex pathways. Neuroscience 10:841-849.

Ralston HJ, Ralston DD (1979). The distribution of dorsal root axons in laminae I, II and III of the macaque spinal cord: A quantitative electron microscopic study. J Comp Neurol 184:643-684.

Westrum LE, Canfield RC (1977). Electron microscopy of degenerating axons and terminals in spinal trigeminal nucleus after tooth pulp extirpations. Am J Anat 149:591-596.

Effects of Injury on Trigeminal and Spinal Somatosensory Systems, pages 151–158

TRANSGANGLIONIC DEGENERATION FOLLOWING DENTAL LESIONS

Lonnie R. Johnson, Lesnick E. Westrum, Michael A. Henry and Robert C. Canfield

Dept. of Surgical Dentistry, Univ. of Colorado, Denver, Colo. 80262 (L.R.J.); Depts. of Neurological Surgery/Biological Structure (L.E.W.) and Restorative Dentistry (R.C.C.), Univ. of Washington, Seattle, Wash. 98195; Facial Pain Center, Univ. of Florida, Gainesville, Fl. 32610 (M.A.H.)

INTRODUCTION

Peripheral axons innervating the teeth and supporting structures are susceptible to a variety of lesions. Axonal degeneration occurs during normal primary tooth exfoliation and permanent tooth eruption and consequent to advanced dental disease and therapeutic dental procedures. The central changes that occur with such lesions and the eventual fate of the altered elements are events that are essential for the reestablishment of central connections. The intent of this chapter is to examine the central axon and terminal changes subsequent to peripheral dental deafferentation and to compare these alterations with those induced by the application of ricin to the dental pulp.

MATERIALS AND METHODS

Twenty adult cats received pulp extirpations or tooth extractions and 10 kittens undergoing primary tooth exfoliation and permanent tooth eruption have been used for the light microscopic (LM) transganglionic degeneration studies (Westrum et al., 1976; Westrum and Canfield, 1979; Johnson and Westrum, 1980). Twenty-three adult cats and 13 kittens have been used for electron microscopy (EM) (Johnson et al., 1983, Westrum et al., 1984). Nine adult cats received intrapulpal ricin injections for the LM (Johnson et al., 1985) and EM studies (Henry et al., 1986). Following the appropriate survival time of 7-60 days for the LM and EM transganglionic degeneration studies, 3-9 months of age for the exfoliation studies and 2-8 days for the ricin studies, each animal was reanesthetized and transcardially perfused with the appropriate fixative. For LM, serial transverse frozen sections (25 µm) of the brainstem were stained with the Fink-Heimer method for degeneration. Tissue used for EM was prepared according to previously published protocols.

RESULTS LM

Following unilateral maxillary or mandibular tooth extractions or pulpectomies, LM argyrophilic degeneration is observed bilaterally in the ventral half of pars interpolaris (PI) and rostral pars caudalis (PC) (Fig. 1). The degeneration is generally heaviest on the side ipsilateral to the surgery and maximum at 30 days survival. The more dorsal areas of PI and PC are free of degeneration as are pars oralis (PO) and the main sensory nucleus (MSN).

A similar pattern of degeneration is seen during exfoliation and permanent tooth eruption (Fig. 1). At the earliest stages of primary tooth resorption (age 3 to 4 months) there is little or no argyrophilic degeneration. Significant amounts of degeneration are first seen by 5 to 6 months of age. The degeneration is bilateral and occurs in ventral PI and PC with the more rostral regions being devoid of degeneration, a pattern similar to that following dental surgery in adults (Fig. 1). The quantity of degeneration increases in the 7 month old animal, decreases by 8 months and disappears by 9 months of age.

In contrast to the restricted pattern following dental surgery or exfoliation, degenerating argyrophilic axons and terminals extend throughout the entire ipsilateral trigeminal nuclear complex (TNC) including the MSN (Fig. 2) following unilateral maxillary or mandibular intrapulpal ricin injections. This degeneration pattern is not only located in ventral PI and PC, as with dental surgery and exfoliation (compare Figs. 1 & 2) but in addition there is a major dorsal pattern in all the TNC.

RESULTS EM

Following tooth extractions or pulpectomies in adult cats and during normal primary tooth exfoliation and permanent tooth eruption, four major types of alterations are seen in terminals of the TNC: 1) electron dense degeneration, 2) neurofilamentous hyperplasia, 3) flocculent de-

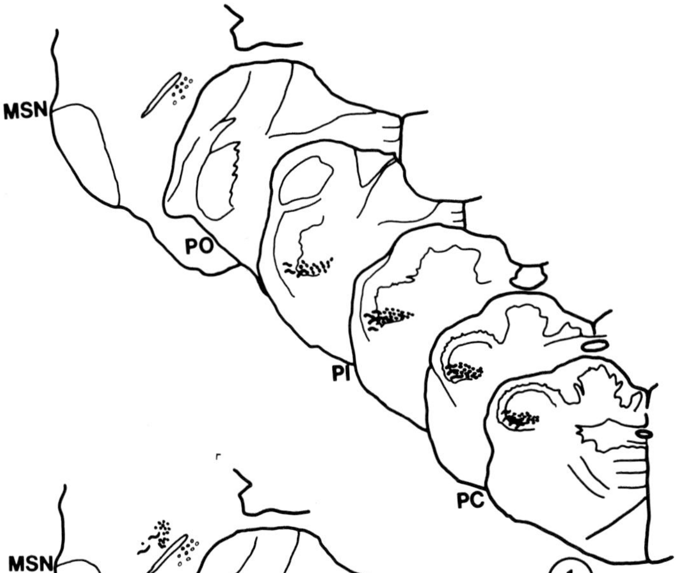

1

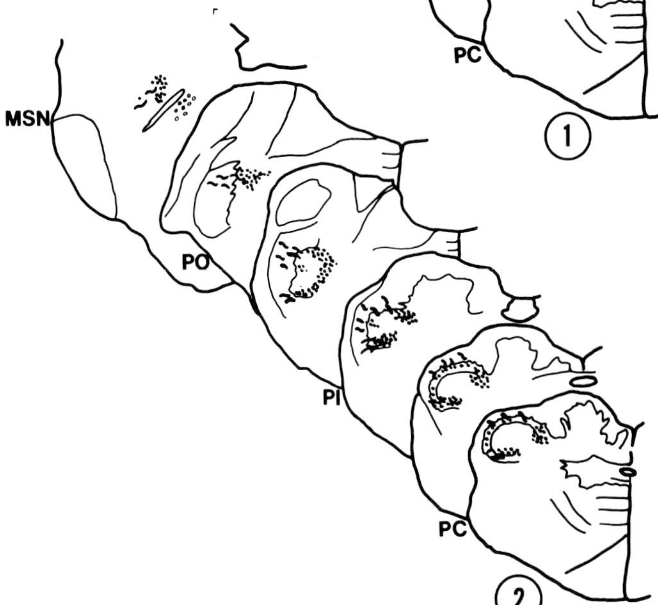

2

Fig. 1. Diagram illustrating the ipsilateral argyrophilic degeneration pattern seen following tooth extractions, pulpectomies or during tooth exfoliation and eruption. Dots = degenerating terminals, wavy lines = degenerating axons.

Fig. 2. Diagram illustrating the argyrophilic degeneration pattern seen following ricin application to ipsilateral cuspid, premolar and molar tooth pulp.

generation and 4) glycogen accumulation. Some degree of synaptic vesicle depletion is a characteristic of all four types of the alterations. Electron dense terminals (Fig. 3) have a very dense cytoplasm, altered mitochondria, clumped vesicles or the absence of vesicles, and may be shrunken or distorted. Terminals undergoing neurofilamentous hyperplasia (Fig. 4) tend to have their central portion filled with neurofilments, displacing other cytoplasmic constituents including vesicles peripherally. Flocculent alterations (Fig. 5) are characterized by a generalized increase in cytoplasmic granularity and synaptic vesicles are aggregated at the presynaptic specializations or peripherally. Following the dental lesions, terminals are seen that have abnormally large aggregates of glycogen granules (Fig. 6) that displace the reduced numbers of synaptic vesicles. In all cases the altered terminals contain round synaptic vesicles, form asymmetrical synaptic contacts and may be postsynaptic to an F terminal. No changes are seen in the postsynaptic profiles or in nearby somata indicating a lack of transynaptic effect or degeneration.

Each of these forms of terminal alteration is commonly seen in those regions that show LM argyrophilia (i.e. ventral PI and PC). However, the dense form is rare and the other forms are common in regions of dorsal MSN, PI and PC that have been shown to receive dental afferents with HRP transport techniques, but are devoid of argyrophilic LM degeneration after dental lesions or exfoliation.

Following ricin injection into the dental pulp all four types of terminal alterations are identified in various parts of the TNC. Electron dense terminals are seen not only ventrally in PI and PC, but also dorsally throughout. Altered terminals are located within ventral lateral and dorsal medial PI as well as marginalis, substantia gelatinosa and lamina V of PC. Most of the altered terminals contain round synaptic vesicles and form asymmetric contacts, but on rare occasions terminals containing flattened synaptic vesicles undergoing electron dense alterations are observed. Occasionally dendritic profiles undergoing vacuolization are also observed.

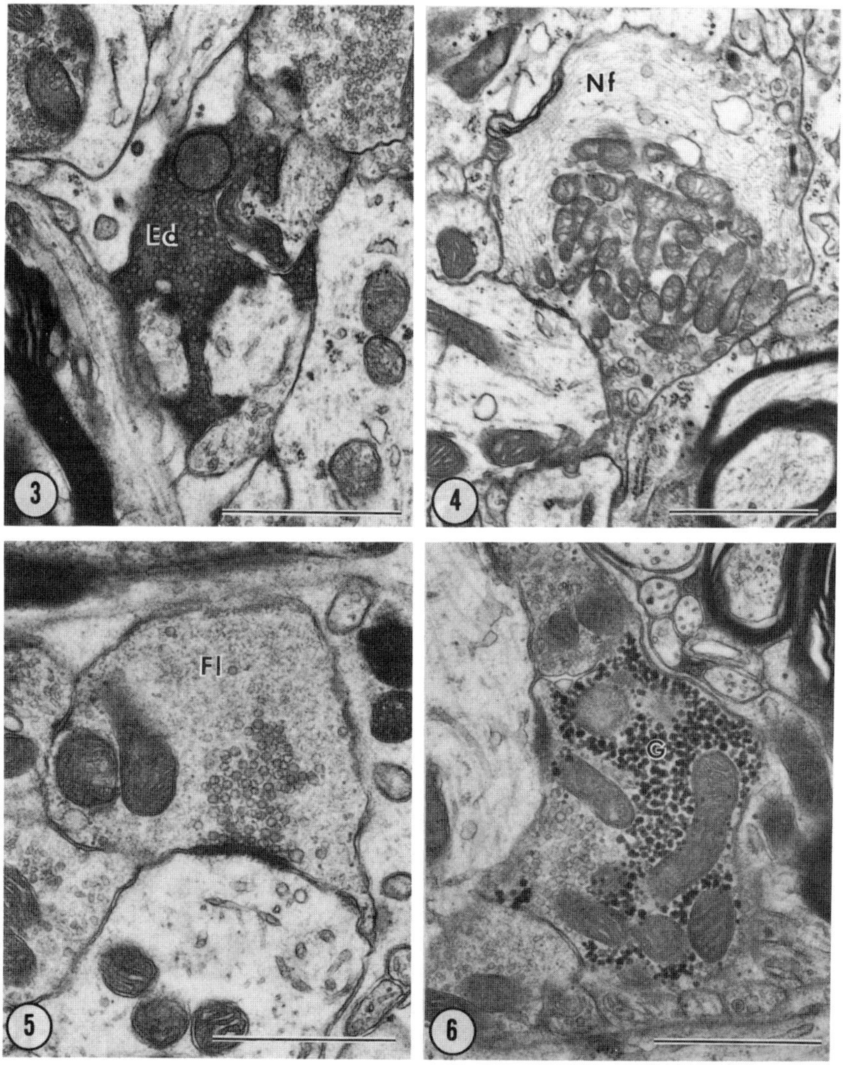

Fig. 3. Electron dense (Ed) terminal, 8 days following ipsilateral maxillary/mandibular ricin injections into tooth pulp, PI. Bar equals 1 µm throughout.
Fig. 4. Neurofilamentous hyperplasia (Nf) 10 days following ipsilateral maxillary/mandibular tooth extractions, PI.
Fig. 5. Flocculent degeneration (Fl), 7 month kitten, MSN.
Fig. 6. Glycogen accumulation (G), 29 days following ipsilateral maxillary/mandibular tooth extractions, MSN.

DISCUSSION

It is apparent from the combined results that a variety of transganglionic terminal alterations occur in response to dental deafferentation and that the occurrence of electron dense or argyophilic degeneration is site specific. In contrast to this transganglionic phenomenon, anterograde degeneration of dental afferents induced by the chromatolytic effects of ricin results in the same types of terminal alterations but without site specificity.

Following dental deafferentation neurofilamentous hyperplasia, flocculent degeneration and glycogen accumulation occur in all regions of the TNC that are known to receive dental afferents. However, electron dense or argyrophilic degeneration only occurs in the ventral portion of PI and PC. In contrast, ricin induced anterograde degeneration results in the appearance of all types of terminal alterations with no segregation of electron dense and non-dense changes as seen following a peripheral dental lesion. Thus, ricin application to dental nerves and the subsequent chromatolytic effects may be expected to cause a greater insult to the central processes of the affected ganglion cells resulting in more dramatic terminal changes. These severe central changes or the possible transneuronal transfer of the lectin may account for the transynaptic alterations observed.

The segregation of electron dense (argyrophilic) and non-dense changes following peripheral dental lesions indicates that there is a differential responsiveness of trigeminal sensory neurons and their central and collateral axons to peripheral axotomy. This hypothesis is not without precedence nor is it restricted to the trigeminal system. Arvidsson and Grant (1979) and Grant and Ygge (1982) have hypothesized that the paucity or absence of argyrophilic transganglionic degeneration in substantia gelatinosa following peripheral nerve transections may be due to the fact that a portion of the central processes of these neurons undergo non-argyrophilic changes following peripheral axotomy.

The eventual fate of the altered terminals is the critical question in regard to central repair following a peripheral lesion. At least three possible fates of the altered terminals exist: 1) they progress to the final electron dense form, 2) they are phagocytized prior to becoming electron dense, or 3) they revert to normal. A progression to the final electron dense form does not occur in the dorsal areas of the TNC following peripheral dental lesions except when the ganglion cell body is killed with ricin.

Phagocytosis of the altered terminals is also a distinct possibility. Following dental lesions all types of altered synaptic terminals completely encased in glial profiles and undergoing microphagocytosis have been seen. This phenomenon has also been described in the spinal cord dorsal horn (Ralston, 1968; Knyihar and Csillik, 1976).

The appearance and disappearance of terminal alterations seen following dental lesions temporally correlate with electrophysiologic studies (Dostrovsky et al., 1982) describing abnormal function acutely (1-4 weeks) with a return to normal function following dental lesions. This strongly indicates that the altered terminals return to normal or sprouting occurs to compensate for the effects of the lesion. This phenomenon is particularly relevant to the innervation of the teeth, since the nerves to teeth are naturally damaged during the exfoliation of the primary teeth with subsequent innervation of the succedaneous permanent teeth. Since the terminal alterations that occur during the exfoliation process are like those that occur with extractions or pulpectomies and ricin application, it may be that these alterations are transient with a return of the affected terminal to normal. Thus, the dental primary afferent system may have the ability to recover from a peripheral lesion. This plasticity would be essential for the continued normal function of the system following the exfoliation of primary teeth, as well as, following lesions of the teeth and their supporting tissues by disease or for therapeutic reasons.

REFERENCES

Arvidsson J, Grant G (1979). Further observations on transganglionic degeneration in trigeminal primary sensory neurons. Brain Res 162:1-12.

Dostrovsky JO, Ball GJ, Hu JW, Sessle BJ (1982). Functional changes associated with partial tooth pulp removal in neurons of the trigeminal spinal tract nucleus, and their clinical implications. In: B Matthews, RG Hill (eds.) Anatomical, Physiological and Pharmacological Aspects of Trigeminal Pain, Amsterdam, Excerpta Medica, pp. 293-310.

Grant G, Ygge J (1982) Somatotopic organization of the thoracic spinal nerve in the dorsal horn demonstrated with transganglionic degeneration. J Comp Neurol 202:357-364.

Henry, MA, Westrum LE, Johnson LR, Canfield RC (1986). Ultrastructure of degenerative changes following ricin application to feline dental pulps. J Neurocytol (submitted).

Johnson LR, Westrum LE (1980). Brain stem degeneration patterns following tooth extractions: visualization of dental and periodontal afferents. Brain Res 194:489-493.

Johnson LR, Westrum LE, Canfield RC (1983). Ultrastructural study of transganglionic degeneration following dental lesions. Exp Brain Res 52:226-234.

Johnson LR, Westrum LE, Henry MA, Canfield RC (1985). Toxic ricin demonstrates a dual dental projection. Brain Res 345:379-383.

Knyihar E, Csillik B (1976). Effect of peripheral axotomy on the fine structure and histochemistry of the Rolando substance: Degenerative atrophy of central processes of pseudounipolar cells. Exp Brain Res 26:73-87.

Ralston, HJ III (1968). Dorsal root projections to the dorsal horn in the cat spinal cord. J Comp Neurol 132:303-330.

Westrum, LE, Canfield RC (1979). Normal loss of milk teeth causes degeneration in brain stem. Exp Neurol 65:169-177.

Westrum, LE, Canfield RC, Black RG (1976). Transganglionic degeneration in the spinal trigeminal nucleus following removal of tooth pulp in adult cats. Brain Res 101:137-140.

Westrum, LE, Johnson LR, Canfield RC (1984). Ultrastructure of transganglionic degeneration in brain stem trigeminal nuclei during normal primary tooth exfoliation and permanent tooth eruption. J Comp Neurol 230:198-206.

Supported by NIH Grants DE 04942, NS 07144 and NS 20482.

Effects of Injury on Trigeminal and Spinal Somatosensory Systems, pages 159–165

TRANSGANGLIONIC DEGENERATION - SOME GENERAL ASPECTS

Gunnar Grant, Jan Arvidsson, Jan Ygge, Antonio Coimbra and José Castro-Lopes
Department of Anatomy, Karolinska Institutet, 104 01 Stockholm, Sweden (G.G., J.A., J.Y.) and Institute of Histology and Embryology, Faculty of Medicine, 4200 Porto, Portugal (A.C., J.C.-L.)

Transganglionic degeneration (TGD) is the kind of degeneration that affects central branches of primary afferent neurons, as a result of peripheral nerve injury. TGD has been described in the rabbit (Grant et al., 1970), rat (e.g. Grant and Arvidsson, 1975), cat (e.g. Westrum et al., 1976), opossum (Goode, 1976a,b) and monkey (Knyihár-Csillik et al., 1985). Early observations by Nageotte (1906; see Grant and Arvidsson, 1975) indicate that it exists also in man. Three general aspects of TGD will be discussed in this presentation: (i) How general is the phenomenon, and what are its morphological characteristics? (ii) What explanation can be offered for the lack, or very small amount of TGD in the substantia gelatinosa at the light microscopic level, although it has been clearly demonstrated electron microscopically? (iii) What is the relationship between TGD and sensory ganglion cell loss?

I. GENERALITY AND MORPHOLOGICAL CHARACTERISTICS OF TGD

Transganglionic axonal degenerative changes were first demonstrated in the rabbit vestibular system (Grant et al., 1970). Transection of different peripheral vestibular nerve branches in young rabbits was found to result in the appearance of argyrophilic structures in Nauta-stained sections from the vestibular nuclei. These structures were found in areas which are known to receive projections from the vestibular nerve. They were mainly granular in character, but also argyrophilic fiber-like fragments were seen. Dark degenerating myelinated axons and boutons were found at the electron microscopic level. The argyrophilic and the electron dense structures were found at postoperative survival times which were longer than would have been expected after a root transection, or after primary damage to the ganglion. This indicated an indirect or transganglionic effect on the centrally projecting branches. Later studies at the brainstem level demonstrated the occurrence of this type of degenerative reaction also in the trigeminal nuclear complex in adult rats and cats, following peripheral nerve transection (Grant and Arvidsson, 1975; Arvidsson, 1979; Arvidsson and Grant, 1979a), or nerve crush (Arvidsson and Grant, unpubl.). It has been shown to occur also after tooth extractions or tooth pulpectomies (Westrum et al., 1976; Anderson et al., 1977; Gobel and Binck, 1977; Westrum and Canfield, 1977; Johnson and Westrum, 1980) and also after removal of skin (Arvidsson and Grant, 1979b). In addition, degenerative argyrophilia has been demonstrated in the trigeminal nuclei at the age of exfoliation of the deciduous teeth in kittens (Westrum and Canfield, 1979).

At the spinal level, transganglionic degenerative changes were first described electron microscopically in the substantia gelatinosa in the adult rat (Knyihár and Csillik, 1976). Similar changes were also found in the opossum (Goode, 1976a,b). Somewhat later, at the light microscopic level Moradian and Rustioni (1977) reported degenerative changes in silver-stained sections in the cervical dorsal horn, following transection of rat forelimb nerves. In later studies at the thoracic level, we found TGD in the dorsal horn, using the Fink-Heimer method (Grant and Ygge, 1981). Like the situation in the trigeminal system (Grant and Arvidsson, 1975; Arvidsson and Grant, 1979a) TGD appeared later than the Wallerian degeneration resulting from root transection or ganglionectomy. Furthermore, the degeneration picture changed characteristically with increasing survival time. TGD was found from 13 days postoperatively, when it appeared as small argyrophilic granules in the deeper part of the dorsal horn. Some were present also in the marginal layer, but none was seen in the substantia gelatinosa. The amount of granules increased with increasing survival time, up to about 20 days. TGD was also seen at later stages, up to 53 days, which was the longest postoperative survival in that study. At these longer survival times the degeneration picture was somewhat different, with more large-sized granules and also some fiber fragments present.

Taken together, these studies had clearly demonstrated that TGD could be provoked by peripheral nerve transection both at brainstem and spinal levels, cervical as well as thoracic. On the other hand, negative findings were reported regarding degenerative argyrophilia at the lumbar level following sciatic nerve transection in adult rats (Devor and Wall, 1981; cf. also Devor et al., 1985). Because of these negative findings, and to extend our earlier results, we considered it important to investigate the lumbar level of the spinal cord (Arvidsson et al., 1986). Essentially the same findings were made as in the trigeminal system and at the thoracic level. Thus, small argyrophilic granules were found, mainly in the deep part of the dorsal horn, after short (14 days) survival, and later (from 30 days), when the overall density of the degenerating structures had increased considerably, larger granules and fiber fragments were also found. Degeneration was also found in the dorsal funiculus after short and especially longer survival times. Taken together with the previous findings, these observations on TGD at the lumbar level support the view that TGD, at least in the rat, is a general phenomenon, not restricted to a particular level of the neural axis. These findings clearly demonstrate that TGD will have to be taken into consideration, when effects of peripheral nerve lesions are discussed.

The problem as to which functional types of fibers are involved in TGD has been elucidated in part in another paper presented by one of us (J.A.) in this volume.

II. TGD IN THE SUBSTANTIA GELATINOSA

From our earlier studies on TGD it seems clear that the discrepancy between the lack or very minimal amount of argyrophilic granules in the substantia gelatinosa in silver-stained sections and the clearly degenerative changes at the electron microscopic level, cannot be accounted by either improper selection of survival times or an improper handling of the Fink-Heimer staining. One possibility would be that the degenerative changes in the substantia gelatinosa are not of the electron dense type, which has been associated with degenerative argyrophilia seen in material in which suppressive silver methods have been used. To investigate this possibility preliminary experiments have been made in which forelimb nerves have been transected in adult rats and the substantia gelatinosa at the cervical level investigated ultrastructurally (Coimbra, Castro-Lopes, Grant and Arvidsson, unpublished observations). The observations made so far indicate a loss of synaptic vesicles in the central (C 1) terminals without an increased electron density of the axoplasm, at survival times ranging from 3 to 30 days. Dense degeneration of the type occurring after dorsal rhizotomy has only rarely been found. If these findings would be representative for TGD in the substantia gelatinosa, a reasonable explanation could be offered for the lack, or very small amount of argyrophilic granules in this part of the dorsal horn; namely, that the degeneration is not, or only to a minimal extent of the electron dense type.

III. TGD AND SENSORY GANGLION CELL LOSS

Loss of sensory ganglion cells following peripheral nerve transection has been documented at brainstem as well as at spinal levels. Aldskogius and Arvidsson (1978) demonstrated such cell loss in the rat trigeminal ganglion, following infraorbital nerve transection, and Glover (1982) noted it in the cat inferior vagal ganglion after vagotomy. Furthermore, Savy et al. (1981) found nerve cell loss in the trigeminal ganglion of newborn mice following coagulation of vibrissae follicles. Later studies at spinal level have shown a similar loss of sensory ganglion cells in the cat (Risling et al., 1983), kitten (Aldskogius and Risling, 1981) and rat (Ygge and Aldskogius, 1984; Arvidsson et al., 1986), following peripheral neurectomy. In addition, cell loss has been demonstrated both in the adult guinea pig (Rich et al., 1984), the 1-day-old rat (Yip et al., 1984) and in the kitten (Aldskogius and Risling, 1981) following peripheral nerve crush. Such a loss of sensory ganglion cells following peripheral nerve lesions must be an important factor behind TGD (cf. Aldskogius et al., 1985). However, TGD could also be the result of a retraction of central collateral branches of surviving primary sensory neurons. Future studies will hopefully help solve the problem as to what extent either or both of these factors contribute to TGD.

Supported by the Swedish Medical Research Council, Projects No. 553 (G.G.) and 6540 (J.A.), and by the Center of Experimental Morphology of Oporto University (A.C. and J.C.-L.).

REFERENCES

Aldskogius H, Arvidsson J (1978). Nerve cell degeneration and death in the trigeminal ganglion of the adult rat following peripheral nerve transection. J Neurocytol 7:229-250.

Aldskogius H, Risling M (1981). Effect of sciatic neurectomy on neuronal number and size distribution in the L7 ganglion of kittens. Exp Neurol 74:597-604.

Aldskogius H, Arvidsson J, Grant G (1985). The reaction of primary sensory neurons to peripheral nerve injury with particular emphasis on transganglionic changes. Brain Res Rev 10:27-46.

Anderson KV, Rosing HS, Pearl GS (1977). Physiological and anatomical studies revealing an extensive transmedian innervation of feline canine teeth. In Anderson DJ, Matthews B (eds): "Pain in the Trigeminal Region", Amsterdam, N.Y.: Elsevier/North Holland, pp 149-160.

Arvidsson J (1979). An ultrastructural study on transganglionic degeneration in the main sensory trigeminal nucleus of the rat. J Neurocytol 8:31-45.

Arvidsson J, Grant G (1979a). Further observations on transganglionic degeneration in trigeminal primary sensory neurons. Brain Res 162:1-12.

Arvidsson J, Grant G (1979b). Degeneration of trigeminal primary sensory neurons after skin removal. Soc Neurosci Abstr 5:703.

Arvidsson J, Ygge J, Grant G (1986). Cell loss in lumbar dorsal root ganglia and transganglionic degeneration after sciatic nerve resection in the rat. Brain Res 373:15-21.

Devor M, Wall PD (1981). Effect of peripheral nerve injury on receptive fields of cells in the cat spinal cord. J Comp Neur 199:277-291.

Devor M, Govrin-Lippmann R, Frank I, Raber P (1985) Proliferation of primary sensory neurons in adult rat dorsal root ganglion and the kinetics of retrograde cell loss after sciatic nerve section. Somatosensory Res 3:139-167.

Glover RA (1982). Chronological changes in acid phosphatase activity within neurons and perineuronal satellite cells of the inferior vagal ganglion of the cat induced by vagotomy. J Anat 134:215-225.

Gobel S, Binck JM (1977). Degenerative changes in primary trigeminal axons and in neurons in nucleus caudalis following tooth pulp extirpations in the cat. Brain Res 132: 347-354.

Goode GE (1976a). The substantia gelatinosa of the American opossum. Fine structure and changes after dorsal rhizotomy and peripheral lesions. Anat Rec (Abstr) 184:412-413.
Goode GE (1976b). The ultrastructural identification of primary and suprasegmental afferents in the marginal and gelatinose layers of lumbar spinal cord following central and peripheral lesions. Soc Neurosci Abstr 2:975.
Grant G, Ekvall L, Westman J (1970). Transganglionic degeneration in the vestibular nerve. In Stahle J (ed): "Vestibular Function on Earth and in Space", Wenner-Gren symposium No 15 Oxford, New York: Pergamon Press, pp 301-305.
Grant G, Arvidsson J (1975). Transganglionic degeneration in trigeminal primary sensory neurons. Brain Res 95:265-279.
Grant G, Ygge J (1981). Somatotopic organization of the thoracic spinal nerve in the dorsal horn demonstrated with transganglionic degeneration. J Comp Neur 202:357-364.
Johnson LR, Westrum LE (1980). Brainstem degeneration patterns following tooth extractions: visualization of dental and periodontal afferents. Brain Res 194:489-493.
Knyihár E, Csillik B (1976). Effect of peripheral axotomy on the fine structure and histochemistry of the Rolando substance: degenerative atrophy of central processes of pseudounipolar cells. Exp Brain Res 26:73-87.
Knyihár-Csillik E, Rakic P, Csillik B (1985). Fine structure of growth cones in the upper dorsal horn of the adult primate spinal cord in the course of reactive synapto-neogenesis. Cell Tiss Res 239:633-641.
Moradian GP, Rustioni A (1977). Transganglionic degeneration in the dorsal horn and dorsal column nuclei in adult rats. Anat Rec (Abstr) 187:660.
Nageotte J (1906). The pars intermedia or nervus intermedius of Wrisberg, and the bulbo-pontine gustatory nucleus in man. Rev Neurol Psychiat 4:473-488.
Rich KM, Yip HK, Osborne PA, Schmidt RE, Johnson Jr EM (1984). Role of nerve growth factor in the adult dorsal root ganglia neuron and its response to injury. J Comp Neur 230: 110-118.
Risling M, Aldskogius H, Hildebrand C (1983). Effects of sciatic nerve crush on the L 7 spinal roots and dorsal root ganglia in kittens. Exp Neurol 79:176-187.
Savy C, Margules S, Farkas-Bargeton E, Verley R (1981). A morphometric study of mouse trigeminal ganglion after unilateral destruction of vibrissae follicles at birth. Brain Res 217:265-277.

Westrum LE, Canfield RC (1977). Light and electron microscopy of degeneration in the brainstem spinal trigeminal nucleus following tooth pulp removal in adult cats. In Anderson DJ, Matthews B (eds): "Pain in the Trigeminal Region", Amsterdam, New York: Elsevier, pp 171-179.

Westrum LE, Canfield RC (1979). Normal loss of milk teeth causes degeneration in brainstem. Exp Neurol 65:169-177.

Westrum LE, Canfield RC, Black RG (1976) Transganglionic degeneration in the spinal trigeminal nucleus following removal of tooth pulps in adult cats. Brain Res 101:137-140.

Ygge J, Aldskogius H (1984). Intercostal nerve transection and its effect on the dorsal root ganglion. A quantitative study on ganglion cell numbers and sizes. Exp Brain Res 55:402-408.

Yip HK, Rich KM, Lampe PA, Johnson Jr EM (1984). The effects of nerve growth factor and its antiserum on the postnatal development and survival after injury of sensory neurons in rat dorsal root ganglia. J Neurosci 4:2986-2992.

Effects of Injury on Trigeminal and Spinal Somatosensory Systems, pages 167–174

EFFECTS OF CHEMICAL CONVULSANTS ON CHRONIC TRANSSYNAPTIC DESTRUCTION OF MEDULLARY DORSAL HORN NEURONS FOLLOWING INFERIOR ALVEOLAR NEUROTOMY IN ADULT RATS

Tomosada Sugimoto

2nd Department of Oral Anatomy,
Osaka University
Faculty of Dentistry, Suita, Osaka 565

INTRODUCTION

Painful sequelae of peripheral nerve injuries are often considered attributable to ectopic spike generation by injured primary neurons. This appears true because, for example, infiltration with local anesthetics and surgical removal of painful neuromata usually relieve pain, at least temporarily. However, it is also likely that the CNS mechanism of pain perception is so altered that it can operate without noxious input from the periphery. For example, posterior rhizotomy, which aims at a complete and permanent interruption of primary input, often fails in pain relief, while leaving the rest of the rhizotomized body segment totally anesthetic. Thus, it appears that the source of posttraumatic pain shifts from the injured primary neurons to the higher order neurons in the CNS.

Transection of a peripheral nerve is known to affect the physiology and morphology of dorsal horn neurons in laboratory animals. Dorsal horn neurons disconnected from receptive fields begin to respond to stimuli applied to the body surface areas remote from their original receptive fields (Devor and Wall, 1978, 1981a, b; Lisney, 1983). Morphologically, peripheral axotomy of primary neurons by neurotomy and tooth pulp extirpations causes chronic transsynaptic destruction of small dendrites in the spinal and medullary dorsal horns (Knyihar-Csillik and Csillik, 1981; Gobel, 1984; Sugimoto and Gobel, 1984).

The transsynaptic destructive effect of transection of the inferior alveolar nerve was enhanced by systemic administration of strychnine and can be observed at the light microscopic level (Sugimoto et al., 1984). With this strychnine-enhancement, the destructive trans-synaptic effect of the inferior alveolar neurotomy occurs between 15 and 30 days postoperatively (Sugimoto et al., 1986). The present study examines the effects of systemically administered strychnine, picrotoxin, bicuculline and L-allylglycine on this transsynaptic neuronal destruction following transection of the inferior alveolar nerve in adult rats. A preliminary report has appeared (Sugimoto, et al., 1985).

MATERIALS AND METHODS

A total of 19 male adult rats (b.w. $\geq$200g) of the Sprague-Dawley Strain were used. Twelve animals underwent unilateral transection of the inferior alveolar nerve under general anesthesia with pentobarbital sodium (40 mg/kg, i.p.). The buccal skin was incised, the masseter muscle was split and retracted, and a small amount of bone was burred off to expose the inferior alveolar nerve within the mandibular canal. The nerve was ligated distally to the mandibular foramen and transected distally to the ligature. The proximal stump of the nerve with the ligature was returned to its original position and muscle and skin were sutured. Following various postoperative intervals, strychnine (1mg/kg), picrotoxin (0.5 mg/kg), bicuculline (2 mg/kg) or L-allylglycine (55.7 mg/kg) was intraperitoneally injected daily for 1-23 days. The combination of postoperative interval and duration of drug administration was so determined that it allowed the drugs to affect the animals when the transsynaptic destructive effect of neurotomy, which was enhanced by strychnine, was operating (15-30 days postoperatively, Sugimoto et al., 1986).

Seven animals were used for control experiments. Three of these underwent unilateral transection of the nerve and were histologically examined without convulsant-treatment. Four animals did not receive the nerve transection but were injected with strychnine or L-allylglycine.

Approximately 18 h after the final injection (or after an appropriate postoperative survival period for the control experiments without convulsant-treatment) animals were anesthetized with ether or pentobarbital sodium, and transcardially perfused with 1% glutaraldehyde, 1% formaldehyde and 0.05 mM $CaCl_2$ in 0.12 M phosphate buffer (pH 7.3). The brain stem was osmicated in phosphate-buffered 2% OsO_4, dehydrated in a graded series of alcohols and embedded in an epoxy resin. Tissue blocks were so trimmed and oriented that they yielded transverse sections of the brain stem at the rostral level of the medullary dorsal horn. In addition to the medulla, the hippocampus and cervical enlargements from some of the animals were also embedded. One-μm sections were cut with a glass knife attached to a LKB ultratome and stained with toluidine blue.

RESULTS

Seven days of strychnine-treatment at a postoperative interval of 23 days (four animals) and 23 days of strychnine-treatment at an interval of 7 days (two animals) yielded many dark neurons, which stained deeply with toluidine blue, in the medullary dorsal horn ipsilateral to the neurotomy (Fig. 1A). Both nucleoplasm and cytoplasm stained deeply, but it was the homogeneously elevated nucleoplasmic stainability that served as an unequivocal criterion for distinguishing dark neurons from healthier neurons. Since some neurons with moderately dark cystoplasm had morphologically intact nuclei, the elevated cytoplasmic stainability did not serve as a reliable criterion unless it was extreme. The dark neurons were found in the dorsal part of the medullary dorsal horn (Fig. 1B) which has been reported to receive dense primary innervation from the transected nerve (Jacquin et al., 1983; Sugimoto et al., 1984). Dark neurons were not found in the spinal dorsal horn of these animals at the level of the cervical enlargement. No dark neuron was seen in the medullary dorsal horn following strychnine administration alone (for 7 or 23 days) or transection alone (survival period=15, 25 or 30 days).

When administered for 23 days at an interval of 7 days, both picrotoxin (two animals) and bicuculline (two animals) failed to produce a dark neuron. This was not due to failure of these drugs to reach their targets in the CNS because hippocampal neurons were found damaged by these drugs. L-allylglycine, however, induced extensive neuronal

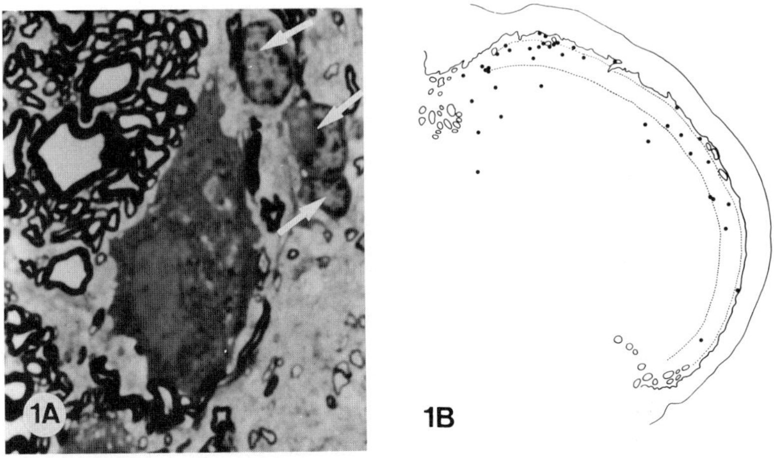

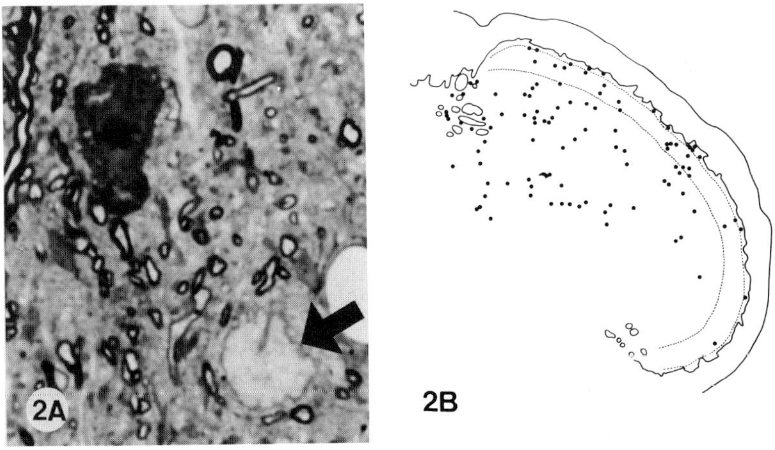

Figures 1 and 2. A photomicrograh (A, X 1,700) and camera lucida drawing (B, X 29) from a single toluidine blue-stained 1 µm section of the medullary dorsal horn ipsilateral to the inferior alveolar nerve transection. Broken lines indicate laminae I/II and II/III borders. Fig. 1: Strychnine administration for 7 days at a postoperative interval of 23 days. The dark neuron can be distinguished from oligodendroglia (arrows) which have conspicuous heterochromatin. Fig. 2: L-allylglycine administration for 2 days at a postoperative interval of 2 days. Elevated stainability easily distinguishes the dark neuron from a nearby healthier neuron (arrow). (Figs. 1B and 2B have been reproduced from Sugimoto et al. 1985, by courtesy of Elsevier Science Publishers.)

damage in the medullary dorsal horn. One day (one animal) or 2 days (one animal) of administration of this drug at a postoperative interval of 20 days revealed many dark neurons in the dorsal part of the medullary dorsal horn (Fig. 2A). These dark neurons were morphologically indistinguishable from those produced by strychnine, but there was a tendency that the proportion of the dark neurons distributed in deeper layers (laminae III/IV) was greater for L-allylglycine than for strychnine (compare Figs. 1B and 2B). Since two days of L-allylglycine-treatment alone did not produce a dark neuron, these dark neurons are considered to be the result of a synergistic interaction between chronic neurotomy and the drug (as was also the case for strychnine).

DISCUSSION

In view of the topographic distribution of dark neurons which roughly coincided with the central terminal field of the inferior alveolar nerve primary afferents (Jacquin et al., 1983), the destructive effect of neurotomy is considered to have been exerted trans-synaptically. This transsynaptic effect appears excitatory in nature because it was enhanced by convulsants strychnine and L-allylglycine.

Despite being separated from their original receptive fields, peripherally axotomized primary neurons may acquire ectopic spike generation (Wall and Gutnich, 1974a,b; Govrin-Lippman and Devor, 1978; Devor and Janig, 1981; Korenman and Devor, 1981) and ephaptic transmission (Seltzer and Devor, 1979; Blumberg and Janig, 1982; Lisney and Pover, 1983) within neuromata. Since peripherally axotomized primary neurons maintain their synaptic connections for at least 1 month (Sugimoto and Gobel, 1982), it is probable that ectopic activity was transmitted to the second order neurons in the medullary dorsal horn and caused the observed neuronal damage. The posttransectional time window, in which strychnine produced dark neurons (Sugimoto et al., 1986), fell within the posttransectional period that is associated with many injured primary neurons with ectopic activities (Scadding, 1981). Further evidence for ectopic spike generation as a cause of transsynaptic destruction is that topical application of axonal transport blockers, which reduces the ectopic electrical activity of injured primary neurons, prevents strychnine-enhanced transsynaptic destruction of medullary dorsal horn neurons following inferior alveolar neurotomy (Sugimoto et al., 1986).

Since picrotoxin and bicuculline did not enhance the transsynaptic destruction, L-allylglycine appears to have enhanced the transsynaptic destruction by removing the inhibition mediated at GABAb sites. Absence of effects of picrotoxin and bicuculline in this study can be explained by chronic impairment of GABAa sites by peripheral axotomy because these two drugs enhanced the acute transsynaptic destruction caused by injury discharge (in preparation).

Starting at the end of the first posttransectional week, primary afferent depolarization (PAD) of peripherally axotomized primary neurons evoked by conditioning stimuli to nearby healthy primary neurons begins to decrease in amplitude (Horch and Lisney, 1981; Wall, 1982; Woolf and Wall, 1982). This reduction is not attributable to transganglionic destruction of central terminals of injured primary neurons because conditioning stimuli applied to the injured primary neurons evoke normal PAD in nearby healthy primary neurons (Wall and Devor, 1981). Since PAD is considered to be mediated at GABAa sites (Mokha et al., 1983), reduction of PAD is probably due to failure in synthesis of GABAa receptors and/or related ionophores by injured primary neurons. The rate of protein synthesis by primary neurons may be reduced after peripheral axotomy (Hall, 1982).

In view of the above, the direct cause of strychnine- and L-allylglycine-enhanced transsynaptic destruction following chronic neurotomy is considered to be the ectopic spike discharge at the site of transection. In addition, impairment of presynaptic GABAa sites appears to facilitate the destructive effect of ectopic spike discharge. The ectopic spike discharge and impairment of GABAa sites may be involved in transsynaptic destruction without enhancement by convulsants (Gobel, 1984; Sugimoto and Gobel, 1984). Modulation of this posttraumatic transsynaptic destruction is possible in many ways, e.g., one can facilitate or interfere with the peripheral mechanism of ectopic spike generation, or one can pharmacologically modify segmental inhibition as well as descending controls of dorsal horn neurons. It may be thereby possible to treat and/or prevent some posttraumatic sensory disorders.

REFERENCES

Blumberg H, Janig W (1982) Activation of fibers via experimentally produced stump neuromas of skin nerves: ectopic transmission or retrograde sprouting?. Exp Neurol 76:468-482.

Devor M, Janig W (1981) Activation of myelinated afferents ending in a neuroma by stimulation of the sympathetic supply in the rat. Neurosci Lett 24:43-47.
Devor M, Wall PD (1978) Reorganization of spinal cord sensory map after peripheral nerve injury. Nature (Lond) 275:75-76.
Devor M, Wall PD (1981a) Effect of peripheral nerve injury on receptive fields of cells in the cat spinal cord. J Comp Neurol 199:277-291.
Devor M, Wall PD (1981b) Plasticity in the spinal cord sensory map following peripheral nerve injury in rats. J Neurosci 1:679-684.
Gobel S (1984) An electron microscopic analysis of the trans-synaptic effects of peripheral nerve injury subsequent to tooth pulp extirpations on neurons in laminae I and II of medullary dorsal horn. J Neurosci 4:2281-2290.
Govrin-Lippman R, Devor M (1978) Ongoing activity in severed nerves: source and variation with time. Brain Res 159:406-410.
Hall ME (1982) Changes in synthesis of specific proteins in axotomized dorsal root ganglia. Exp Neurol 76:83-93.
Horch KW, Lisney SJW (1981) Changes in primmary afferent depolarization of sensory neurons during peripheral nerve regeneration in the cat. J Physiol (Lond) 313:287-299.
Jacquin MF, Semba K, Egger MD, Rhoades RW (1983) Organization of HRP-labeled trigeminal mandibular primary afferent neurons in the rat. J Comp Neurol 215:397-420.
Knyihar-Csillik E, Csillik B (1981) Selective 'labelling' by transsynaptic degeneration of substantia gelatinosal cells: an attempt to decipher intrinsic wiring in the Rolando substance of primates. Neurosci Lett 23:131-136.
Korenman EMD, Devor M (1981) Ectopic adrenergic sensitivity in damaged peripheral nerve axons in the rat. Exp Neurol 72:63-81.
Lisney SJW (1983) Changes in the somatotopic organization of the cat lumbar spinal cord following peripheral nerve transection and regeneration. Brain Res 259:31-39.
Lisney SJW, Pover CM (1983) Coupling between fibres involved in sensory nerve neuromata in cats. J Neurol Sci 59:255-264.
Mokha SS, McMillan JA, Iggo A (1983) Dorsal root potentials in the cat: effects of bicuculline. Brain Res 259:313-318.
Scadding JW (1981) Development of ongoing activity, mechanosensitivity, and adrenaline sensitivity in severed peripheral nerve axons. Exp Neurol 73:345-364.
Seltzer Z, Devor M (1979) Ephaptic transmission in chroni-

cally damaged peripheral nerves. Neurology 29:1061-1064.
Sugimoto T, Gobel S (1982) Primary neurons maintain their central axonal arbors in the spinal dorsal horn following peripheral nerve injury: an anatomical analysis using transganglionic transport of horseradish peroxidase. Brain Res 248:377-381.
Sugimoto T, Gobel S (1984) Dendritic changes in the spinal dorsal horn following transection of a peripheral nerve. Brain Res 321:199-208.
Sugimoto T, Takemura M, Okubo J, Sakai A (1984) Subconvulsive dose of strychnine enhances the transneuronal effect of peripheral sensory nerve transection. Brain Res 323:320-325.
Sugimoto T, Takemura M, Okubo J, Sakai A (1985) Strychnine and L-allylglycine but not bicuculline and picrotoxin induce transsynaptic degeneration following transection of the inferior alveolar nerve in adult rats. Brain Res 341:393-398.
Sugimto T, Takemura M, Sakai A, Ishimaru M (1986) Topical application of colchicine, vinblastine and vincristine prevent strychnine-enhanced transsynaptic degeneration in the medullary dorsal horn following transection of the inferior alveolar nerve in adult rats. Pain (in press).
Wall PD (1982) The effect of peripheral nerve lesions and of neonatal capsaicin in the rat on primary afferent depolarization. J Physiol (Lond) 329:21-35.
Wall PD, Devor M (1981) The effect of peripheral nerve injury on dorsal root potentials and on transmission of afferent signals into the spinal cord. Brain Res 209: 95-111.
Wall PD, Gutnick M (1974a) Properties of afferent nerve impulses originating from a neuroma. Nature (Lond) 248:740-743.
Wall PD, Gutnick M (1974b) Ongoing activity in peripheral nerves: the physiology and pharmacology of impulses originating from a neuroma. Exp Neurol 43:580-593.
Woolf CL, Wall PD (1982) Chronic peripheral nerve section diminishes the primary afferent A-fibre mediated inhibition of rat dorsal horn neurons. Brain Res 242:77-85.

Effects of Injury on Trigeminal and Spinal Somatosensory Systems, pages 175–187

TRANSGANGLIONIC REGULATION OF PRIMARY CENTRAL SENSORY TERMINALS IN THE UPPER DORSAL HORN

Bert Csillik

Department of Anatomy, University Medical School, H-67o1 Szeged, Hungary

In contrast to earlier dubitations, the effects of peripheral nerve lesion upon central nervous structures are becoming part of our textbook knowledge. Now a basic rule of neurobiology seems to emerge which apparently governs the functional structure of primary central afferent terminals in the spinal cord and in the medulla. Since the structural and functional integrity of these terminals appear to be subjected to infrastructural signals (but not to afferent impulses) arriving from the peripheral nerve terminals, we coined the term "transganglionic regulation" to describe this system. In some respects, transganglionic regulation seems to disobey the law of the trophical entity of the neuron, as formulated at the turn of the century by the classics of neuroanatomy. On the other hand, it can be regarded a logical consequence of the general theorem of cytology regarding the organization of the eukaryotic cell. The objective of this present paper is to summarize the experimental facts supporting the theory of transganglionic regulation and to ponder the possibility of the extrapolation of this principle to other cell types in the central nervous system.

MATERIAL AND METHODS

Investigations were performed on young adult CFY albino rats of both sexes; the number of animals used throughout the studies this summary is based upon, is approximately 65o. Marker techniques used to demonstrate one or the other cell population in dorsal root ganglia, as well as their central and peripheral terminals, are summarized in Table 1. For details regarding the methodology of the marker techniques, see References. Experimental surgery was performed under pentobarbital anesthesia.

Table 1. Markers for primary nociceptive neurons

Enzyme histochemistry:	
FRAP	(Knyihàr-Csillik and Csillik 1981)
TMPase	(Knyihàr-Csillik et al, 1986)
Immune histochemistry:	
Substance P	(Hökfelt et al, 1976)
Somatostatin	(Seybold and Elde 198o)
Cholecystokinin	(Tuchscherer and Seybold 1985)
Lectin histochemistry:	
Fucose and Galactose terminated glycoconjugates	(Fischer and Csillik 1985) (Streit et al, 1985)

RESULTS AND DISCUSSION

(1) Normal distribution. All three groups of the genuine cytochemical markers (enzymes, neuropeptides and lectin-binding glycoconjugates) are localized in small to medium-sized nerve cells of dorsal root ganglia and cranial sensory ganglia, as well as in their peripheral processes (e.g. in the cornea) and in their central terminals, which are located in the upper dorsal horn of the spinal cord and in the homologuous structures of the medulla, resp. Coexistence of some of the markers is probable, though not obligatory; some of them

show a marked species-specificity. Thus for example FRAP and TMPase are located in the very same small-sized cell population in dorsal root ganglia and their peripheral and central terminals (these latter in the substantia gelatinosa Rolandi) exert FRAP and TMPase enzyme activity. In contrast, the central terminals of the substance P-positive dorsal root ganglion cells, which also belong to one of the small-sized groups, are located mainly, though not exclusively, in Lamina I of the dorsal horn. The disparateness of FRAP and substance P cells has been emphasized by Nagy and Hunt (1981); recent studies, however, appear to be less unequivocal (Dalsgaard et al., 1984). Finally, BBS and RCA lectin-binding glycoconjugates in the rat are located in cells and terminals identical to those exhibiting FRAP and TMPase activity; whereas in man, UEA-1 lectin-binding glycoconjugates are located in medium-sized dorsal root ganglion cells and in their central terminals in Lamina IIi and III.

(2) Effect of peripheral nerve injury. The first signs following mechanical injury (transection, crushing, or ligature) of a peripheral sensory nerve (Fig. 1) are identical to those seen after perineural application of a microtubule inhibitor (Csillik and Knyihar, 1975, 1986). In this respect it is important to note that perineurally applied Vinca alkaloids (Vinblastin, Vincristin, Leurosin, etc.), known to be the most potent microtubule inhibitors, induce structural, cytochemical, and functional alterations of the primary central sensory terminals even in those extremely small amounts (10^{-8} M Vinblastin or 10^{-9} M Vincristin) which do not induce Wallerian degeneration of the peripheral nerve (Fitzgerald et al., 1984). It is therefore evident that the blockade of the axoplasmic transport mechanism, rather than the structural impairment of the peripheral axon itself, is responsible for the alterations induced in the upper dorsal horn. Indirect evidence suggests that the very cause of these alterations is a failure of the fast retrograde axoplasmic transmission to provide infrastructural information from the peripheral terminal to the cell body

(Csillik et al, 1982). This is, however, not due to the lack of nerve impulse conduction in the affected axons, since neither the application of local anesthetics (Knyihár-Csillik and Csillik 1981) nor that of tetrodotoxin (Wall et al, 1982) will induce any alterations in the central terminals.

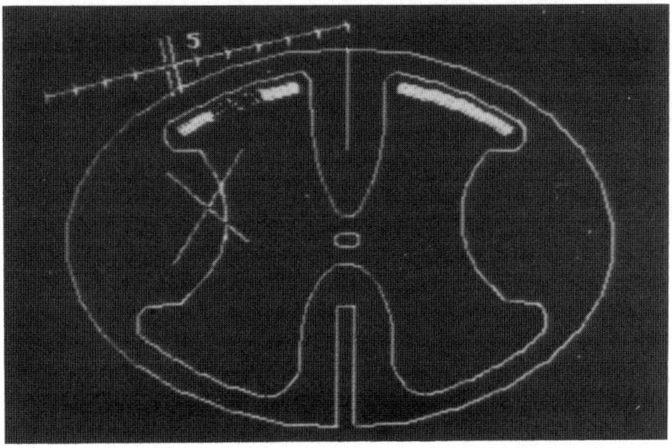

Figure 1. Depletion of TMPase from the substantia gelatinosa of the rat, after transection of the sciatic nerve. Computer graphics used for quantitative evaluation of serial sections (Bezzegh et al, 1986).

(3) Stages of transganglionic alterations. It seems that at least three different stages can be clearly distinguished with successively increasing severity, which ensue after peripheral nerve lesions in structure and function of the upper dorsal horn. Stage 1 is a mild form of transganglionic atrophy, ensuing after a nerve crush or after microtubule inhibition (Léránth et al, 1984); it is characterized by depletion of marker enzymes and neuropeptides from the affected central terminals. As soon as peripheral axonal regeneration is completed (or more properly, as soon as the retrograde axoplasmic transport mechanism is re-established), central terminals are revived by replenishment of marker enzymes and neuropeptides (Fig. 2).

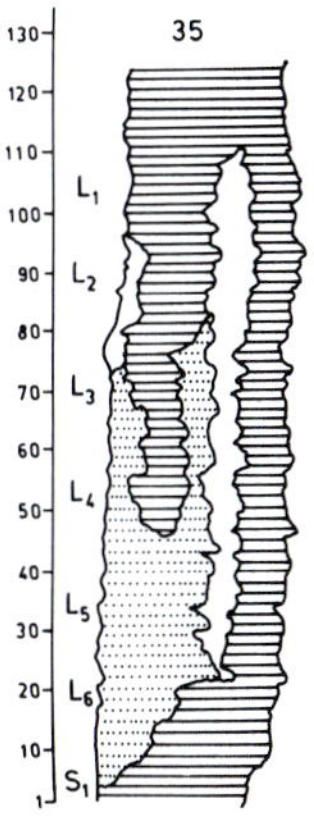

Figure 2. Replenishment of FRAP 35 days after crushing the sciatic nerve. Reconstruction of the rat lumbar intumescence on the basis of transverse serial sections. Hatch marked area: normal FRAP activity; dotted area: replenished FRAP activity; empty area: depleted (not yet replenished) (Ferencsik 1986).

- Stage 2 is a more severe form; it ensues if retrograde axoplasmic transport fails to be re-established within a few weeks, but the nerve cells in the dorsal root ganglion still do not die. Electron dense shrinkage and labyrinth formation characterizes the central terminals in this stage (Fig. 3) which is, however, still reversible. Thus, if peripheral regeneration succeeds in completing the infrastructural continuity of the neuron, new axonal sprouts equipped with axonal growth cones appear in the upper dorsal horn. These axonal sprouts establish new synapses with perikarya, dendrites and dendritic growth cones of substantia gelatinosal cells (Fig. 4) that formerly underwent transsynaptic dedifferentiation (Knyihár-Csillik et al, 1985). The net result of Stage 2 is, therefore, a re-structuring of the formerly disrupted wiring in the dorsal horn.
-Finally, Stage 3, the most severe form, is irreversible. This ensues if peripheral axons fail to succeed in regenerating and, consequently, their parent cells in the dorsal root ganglion die. Consequently, central terminals undergo a straightforward Wallerian degeneration; the outcome of Stage 3 is gliosis in the upper dorsal horn. These alterations are identical to those described by Grant and his school under the term "transganglionic degeneration" (Grant 197o; Grant and Arvidsson 1975; Aldskogius et al, 1985)

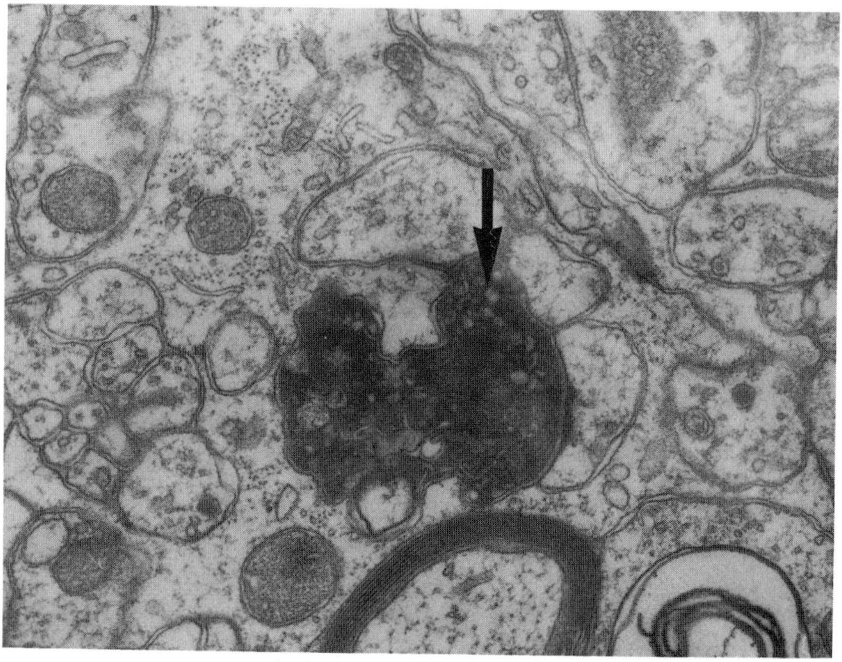

Figure 3. Osmiophilic pattern of transganglionic degenerative atrophy of a primary central terminal in the monkey upper dorsal horn, 1 month after transection of the sciatic nerve.

Main characteristic of stages 1-3 are summarized in Table 2. In terms of neurophysiology, every stage is characterized by a detriment of the dorsal root potential (DRP) which is evident from an increased latency and a decreased amplitude. After stages 1 and 2, respectively, replenishment and/or regeneration of terminals is accompanied by restitution of DRP (Pór 1985). However, this fails to take place during stage 3.

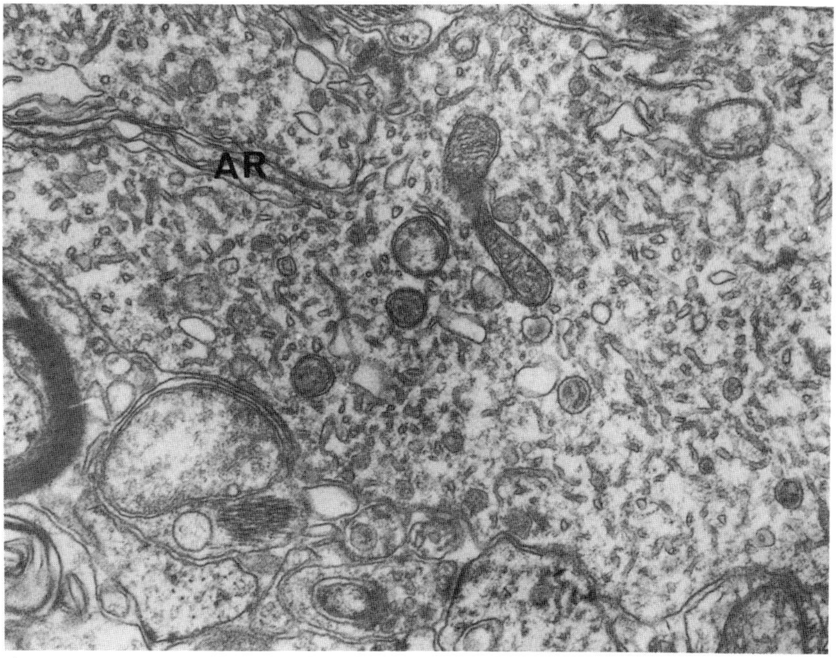

Figure 4. Axonal growth cone in the upper dorsal horn of an adult monkey 3 months after crush injury of the sciatic nerve. AR: axoplasmic reticulum (Knyihár-Csillik et al, 1985).

(4) Role of nerve growth factor (NGF) in the maintenance of primary central afferent terminals in the upper dorsal horn. Since the pioneering studies of Rita Levi-Montalcini, literally thousands of publications appeared in the literature dealing with various aspects of this 13 kD polypeptide; for details, see the excellent review by Thoenen and Barde (198o). From our point of view, however, most important is the discovery that in adult animals, NGF is continuously being taken up by sensory nerve endings and carried, by means of a fast retrograde axoplasmic transport mechanism, to nerve cell bodies located in the dorsal root ganglia (Stoeckel et al, 1975). Here, by intervention of a hitherto unknown second messenger,NGF stimulates and regulates the synthesis of neuroproteins and neuropeptides destined for the central

and peripheral terminals. Our early prediction that blockade of retrograde axoplasmic transport in the peripheral sensory nerve might be responsible for the transganglionic alterations (Csillik et al, 1982) already indicated the involvement of NGF in the transganglionic regulatory process.

Table 2. Transganglionic alterations

	Duration	Characteristics	Outcome	Terminology
Stage 1	weeks	depletion of markers; osmiophobic EM pattern of terminals	reversible: replenishment of terminals	TDA
Stage 2	weeks or a few months	osmiophilic, shrunken EM pattern of terminals, labyrinth formation	reversible: regeneration of terminals	TDA
Stage 3	several months	death of DRG cells: Wallerian degeneration of terminals	irreversible: gliosis	TD

Direct proofs in favour of this theory accumulated during the last few years. Three sets of experiments should be briefly mentioned in this context:

4.1. Application of an anti-NGF serum around a peripheral nerve induces TDA in the ipsilateral, segmentally related upper dorsal horn; depletion of marker enzymes (FRAP, TMPase) is similar to that seen after microtubule inhibition (Fig. 5).

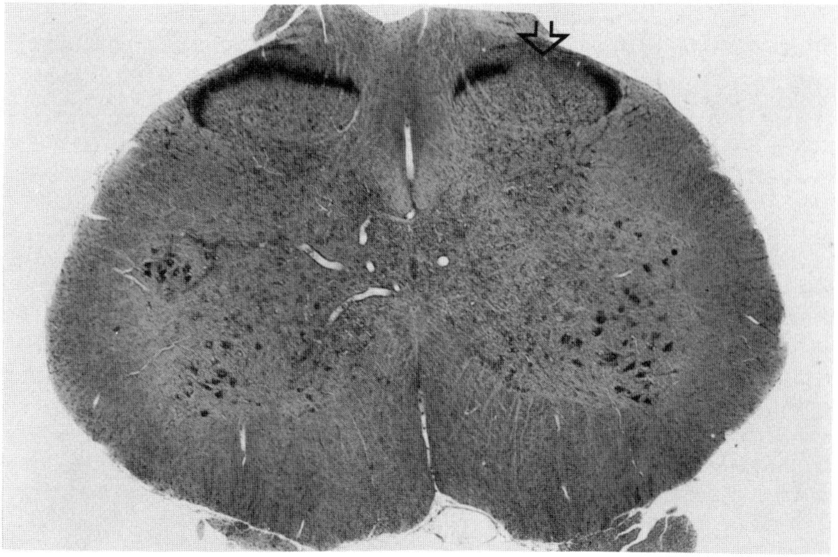

Figure 5. Effect of anti-NGF serum on FRAP activity in the substantia gelatinosa of the rat, 2 weeks after perineural application. Arrow points to the site of depletion.

4.2. Threshold concentration of locally applied Vinblastin needed to induce TDA is identical to that blocking retrograde transport of isotope-labelled ^{125}I-NGF in the sciatic nerve (Csillik, Schwab, Thoenen 1985).

4.3. NGF applied at the proximal stump of a transected peripheral nerve prevents or delays depletion of the marker enzyme FRAP and that of substance P from the related central sensory terminals in the upper dorsal horn (Csillik 1984).

CONCLUSION

Central terminals of primary sensory neurons are subjected to regulation by trophic substance(s) provided by the retrograde axoplasmic transport. Blockade of retrograde transport in the peripheral sensory axon results in a reversible TDA or in irreversible transganglionic degeneration, respectively, of primary central afferent terminals. Transganglionic alterations are due to the lack of nerve growth factor; however, the lack of other trophic factors may also contribute to this effect.

By extrapolation, it can be hypothesized that not only the pseudounipolar cells of dorsal root ganglia, but also other neurons may be subjected to some kind of transcellular regulation. In addition to other offshoots of the neural crest (sympathetic and parasympathetic nerve cells of autonomic ganglia), the principle of regulation by retrogradely transported trophic factors of the metabolic activity of the cell body, and consequently, of a transcellular regulation of other processes of the same neuron, may apply also to intrinsic neurons of the central nervous system deriving from the neural tube proper. Prestige (1967) suggested the role of a maintenance factor in the survival of spinal motoneurons; recent studies by Unsicker et al (1986) seem to indicate that a wide variety of polypeptides may contribute to the trophism of various cells of the CNS. It is an intriguing possibility that, per analogism of the primary sensory neuron, regeneration and synaptoneogenesis of disabled axons and axon terminals of intrinsic CNS cells might be induced by application of appropriate neurotrophic factors to the corresponding dendritic field - a challange for clinically oriented neurobiologists.

ACKNOWLEDGEMENT. This work was supported by Grant No. o6/4-o1/449 from the Hungarian Ministry of Health and No. o5-o65 from the Hungarian Academy of Sciences. NGF and anti-NGF were kindly donated by Prof. H. Thoenen (Max-Planck-Institute, München-Martinsried).

REFERENCES

Aldskogius H, Arvidsson J, Grant G (1985). The reaction of primary sensory neurons to peripheral nerve injury with particular emphasis on transganglionic changes. Brain Res 10: 27-46.

Bezzegh A, Knvihár-Csillik E, Böti Zs, Tajti J, Záborszky Z, Csillik B (1986). A computer-aided analysis of the effect of peripheral nerve transection on TMPase activity of substantia gelatinosa Rolandi. Z mikrosk-anat Forsch (Leipzig), 100: 161-165.
Csillik B (1984). Nerve growth factor regulates central terminals of primary sensory neurons. Z mikrosk-anat Forsch (Leipzig) 98: 1S 11-16.
Csillik B, Knyihár E (1975). Degenerative atrophy and regenerative proliferation in the rat spinal cord. Z mikr-anat Forsch (Leipzig),89:1o99-11o3.
Csillik B, Knyihár-Csillik E (1986). The Protean Gate. Plasticity of the Primary Nociceptive Analyzer. Academy Publishing House, Budapest.
Csillik B, Knyihár-Csillik E, Tajti J (1982). Blockade of retrograde axoplasmic transport induces transganglionic degenerative atrophy of central terminals of primary nociceptive neurons. Acta Biol Acad Sci Hung 33: 149-156.
Csillik B, Schwab ME, Thoenen H (1985). Transganglionic regulation of central terminals of dorsal root ganglion cells by nerve growth factor (NGF). Brain Res 331: 11-15.
Dalsgaard C-J, Ygge J, Vincent SR, Ohrling M, Dockray GJ, Elde R (1984). Peripheral projections and neuropeptide coexistence in a subpopulation of fluoride-resistant acid phosphatase reactive spinal primary sensory neurons. Neurosci Lett 51: 139-144.
Ferencsik M (1986). Depletion and replenishment of fluoride-resistant acid phosphatase (FRAP): temporospatial alterations in substantia gelatinosa Rolandi (in Hungarian). Kisérletes Orvostudomány 38: 44-5o.
Fischer J, Csillik B (1985). Lectin-binding: A genuine marker for transganglionic regulation of human primary sensory neurons. Neurosci Lett 54: 263-267.
Fitzgerald M, Woolf CJ, Gibson SJ, Mallaburn PS (1984). Alterations in the structure, function and chemistry of C fibers following local application of vinblastine to the sciatic nerve of the rat. J Neurosci 4: 43o-441.

Grant G (197o). Neuronal changes central to the site of axon transection. A method for identification of retrograde changes in perikarya, dendrites and axons by silver impregnation. In WJH Nauta, SOE Ebbesson (eds), Contemporary Research Methods in Neuroanatomy, Springer, Berlin, pp 173-185.

Grant G, Arvidsson J (1975). Transganglionic degeneration in trigeminal primary sensory neurons. Brain Res 95: 265-279.

Hökfelt T, Elde R, Johansson O, Luft R, Nilsson G, Arimura A (1976). Immunohistochemical evidence for separate populations of somatostatin-containing and substance P-containing primary afferent neurons. Neuroscience 1: 131-136.

Knyihár-Csillik E, Csillik B (1981). FRAP: Histochemistry of the Primary Nociceptive Neuron. Gustav Fischer, Stuttgart, Progr Histochem Cytochem 14: 1-137.

Knyihár-Csillik E, Bezzegh A, Böti Zs, Csillik B (1986). Thiamine monophosphatase: A genuine marker for transganglionic regulation of primary sensory neurons. J Histochem Cytochem 34:365-371.

Knyihár-Csillik E, Rakic P, Csillik B (1985). Fine structure of growth cones in the upper dorsal horn of the adult primate spinal cord in the course of reactive synapto-neogenesis. Cell Tiss Res 239: 633-641.

Léránth Cs, Csillik B, Knyihár-Csillik E (1984). Depletion of substance P and somatostatin in the upper dorsal horn after blockade of axoplasmic transport. Histochemistry 81: 391-4oo.

Nagy JI, Hunt SP (1982). Fluoride-resistant acid phosphatase-containing neurons in dorsal root ganglia are separate from those containing substance P or somatostatin. Neuroscience 7: 89-98.

Pór I (1985). Alterations of dorsal root potential in the course of transganglionic degenerative atrophy. Acta Physiol Hung 65: 255-262.

Prestige MC (1967). The control of cell number in the lumbar spinal ganglia during the development of Xenopus laevis tadpoles. J Embryol Exp Morph 17: 453-471.

Seybold V, Elde R (198o). Immunohistochemical studies of peptidergic neurons in the dorsal horn of the spinal cord. J Histochem Cytochem 28: 367-37o.
Stoeckel K, Schwab M, Thoenen H (1975). Specificity of retrograde transport of nerve growth factor (NGF) in sensory neurons: a biochemical and morphological study. Brain Res 89: 1-14.
Streit WJ, Schulte BA, Balentine JD, Spicer SS (1985). Histochemical localization of galactose-containing glycoconjugates in sensory neurons and their processes in the central and peripheral nervous system of the rat. J Histochem Cytochem 33: 1o42-1o52.
Thoenen H, Barde Y-A (198o). Physiology of nerve growth factor. Physiol Rev 6o: 1284-1335.
Tuchscherer MM, Seybold VS (1985). Immunohistochemical studies of substance P, cholecystokinin-octapeptide and somatostatin in dorsal root ganglia of the rat. Neuroscience 14: 593-6o5.
Unsicker K, Reichert-Preibsch H, Pettmann G, Labourdette G, Sensenbrenner M (1986). Astroblasten- und Fibroblasten-Wachtumsfaktoren (AGF 1, 2; FGF acidic, basic) sind trophe Faktoren für Neurone des peripheren und zentralen Nervensystems. Anat Ges Abstr (Lübeck) 81: 183.
Wall PD, Mills R, Fitzgerald M, Gibson SJ (1982). Chronic blockade of sciatic nerve transmission by tetrodotoxin does not produce central changes in the dorsal horn of the spinal cord of the rat. Neurosci Lett 3o: 315-32o.

Effects of Injury on Trigeminal and Spinal Somatosensory Systems, pages 189–196

BRAINSTEM EFFECTS OF NATURALLY OCCURRING DENTAL DEAFFERENTATION IN KITTENS

James W. Hu, James G. Broton, Yvonne Lenz, Etsuo Shohara and Barry J. Sessle

Faculty of Dentistry, University of Toronto, Toronto, Canada M5G 1G6

INTRODUCTION

We have previously demonstrated that tooth pulp deafferentation in the adult cat may cause statistically significant but reversible changes in the functional properties of brainstem neurons of trigeminal (V) subnucleus oralis that are consistent with observations in the adult spinal somatosensory system (see Dostrovsky et al, this volume). One feature that earmarks the V as opposed to the spinal somatosensory system, however, is the occurrence of a natural deafferentation process: in the young cat, the primary (deciduous) teeth exfoliate and are replaced by the permanent teeth. Resorption of the primary teeth is associated with degeneration of the peripheral sensory nerve endings in the tooth pulp and supporting periodontal tissues. However, only limited study has been made of the central consequences of this peripheral V deafferentation process. For this reason, plus our own observations of pulp deafferentation-induced functional changes of V brainstem neurons in the adult cat, we wished to determine if changes occur in these neurons during this process of natural dental deafferentation.

METHODS

Twenty-eight kittens at the "mixed" dentition stage and 24 adult cats were studied. The majority of kittens had known birth dates; others were in well-defined stages of exfoliation of their primary teeth and eruption of permanent teeth, and their ages could thus be approximated by post-mortem x-ray examination (Shapiro, 1930; Westrum et al, 1984). For the electrophysiological studies, 11 of the kittens were divided into two groups. One group (n=6; 3-4 months of age) still had firmly implanted primary canines but their primary incisors had been shed. The other group (n=5; 5-6 months) had erupted permanent canines, their posterior primary teeth were in the process of exfoliation and their permanent posterior teeth were erupting. The adult cats studied electrophysiologically had a full complement of clinically healthy permanent teeth and showed no evidence of previous injury to the mouth or face: 11 underwent coronal pulpotomy of the mandibular ipsilateral canine, premolar and molar teeth 7-15 days before the electrophysiological recording session; 10 control cats did not receive any such experimental manipulation. The data from these 10 control and 11 deafferented cats are the same as those presented previously (Dostrovsky et al, this volume).

Methods for electrophysiological recording of single neurons were identical to those described by Dostrovsky et al (this volume), and were standardized and similarly applied to all four groups of anesthetized animals. One to four pair(s) of electrodes were implanted in ipsilateral and contralateral (deciduous or permanent) canine tooth pulps in order to activate pulp afferents (single pulse, 0.1 msec, 0.01-5 mA); electrical stimuli were also applied to oral mucosa and facial skin. One or two anteroposterior planes at the level of subnucleus oralis were studied, with several microelectrode tracks made in each plane. Once a unit was isolated and the presence or lack of spontaneous activity established, we determined its mechanoreceptive field and response properties to electrical and mechanical stimuli, e.g. light touch, brush, pinch with serrated forceps, tapping with a blunt probe (Sessle and Greenwood, 1976; Dostrovsky et al, this volume). At the conclusion of the experiment, the animal was perfused and the brainstem prepared for histological reconstruction of recording sites.

To determine if indeed the afferents of the deciduous pulp in the young kitten project to the ipsilateral V brainstem complex and terminate in regions comparable to those of afferents from permanent teeth of the adult, an additional 17 kittens and 3 adult cats were used for horseradish peroxidase (HRP) labeling experiments. All 17 kittens (aged 2-4 months) had firmly implanted deciduous canines. Under barbiturate anesthesia (Nembutal, 35 mg/kg), one canine pulp was exposed by carefully removing the coronal enamel and dentin, and 1-2 ul of concentrated 50% HRP was applied within this opening and left for 1-3 hours. After this time, the exposed pulp was closed with dental cement. After 48 hours, the animals were given a lethal dose of anesthetic, perfused, and brainstem tissue was processed by the TMB method of Mesulam (e.g. see Arvidsson and Gobel, 1981; Marfurt and Turner, 1984).

RESULTS

The most dense terminal HRP labeling of deciduous pulp afferents was in the rostral and dorsal part of subnucleus oralis and in lamina I (medial two-thirds) of subnucleus caudalis. Less-dense terminal labeling was also found in the area bordering lamina IV and lamina V of caudalis, and also in the main sensory nucleus and caudal end of subnucleus interpolaris. A comparable pattern was noted for the pulp afferent projection of the permanent teeth in adults.

The electrophysiological studies revealed that low threshold mechanoreceptive neurons predominated in the subnucleus oralis of the kittens as well as in the adult animals. Most neurons in kittens and adult control cats had a mechanoreceptive field localized to one V division and showed other comparable response features (Table 1). The somatotopic organization of the subnucleus in the kitten was also similar to that in the adult, i.e. an inverted, medially facing head (e.g. Dubner et al, 1978). However, in adult control cats and the older kittens, many (approximately 50%) of the neurons having a dental input received convergence of both pulpal and periodontal afferent inputs as determined by electrical stimulation of the pulp and tactile stimulation of the teeth, whereas few (16%) of such neurons in the younger group of kittens received both inputs. The latencies (mean±SD,msec) of the deciduous pulp-evoked responses were also much longer in the group of younger kittens (13.6±9.0) than the permanent pulp-evoked responses in the adults (8.0±4.8) and older kittens (8.5±6.0). In contrast, the latencies of neuronal responses evoked by electrical stimulation of the cutaneous/mucosal receptive field were comparable in adult cats (5.5±3.6), older kittens (4.3±2.6) and younger kittens (4.1±1.4).

Neuronal properties (extent of the mechanoreceptive field, incidence of spontaneous activity, and habituating responses to brisk tap) were similar for both groups of kittens and adult control cats but contrasted with those noted in adult deafferented cats. Whereas the mechanoreceptive field extent of the majority of neurons in kittens and control cats was restricted to one V division, most neurons in pulp-deafferented cats had a mechanoreceptive field spanning two or three divisions. Both kittens and adult control cats also had an incidence of spontaneously active or habituating tap-sensitive neurons which was much lower than that of adult pulp-deafferented cats (Table 1).

TABLE 1. Receptive Field and Response Properties of Neurons in V Subnucleus Oralis

	Kitten 3-4 mos. (124)	Kitten 5-6 mos. (113)	Adult Cat Control (318)	Adult Cat Deafferented (350)
Mechanoreceptive Field:				
Restricted to One V Division	70%	61%	64%	46%
Spanning Two or Three V Divisions	30%	39%	36%	54%
Spontaneous Activity	11%	12%	9%	27%
Habituating Response to Tap	0%	0%	1%	11%

(numbers in parentheses refer to number of neurons studied)

DISCUSSION

Our anatomical findings of the projection sites of deciduous pulp afferents represent the first documentation of the brainstem pathways for these afferents in kittens. The sites noted are in general agreement with our own and earlier findings (Arvidsson and Gobel, 1981; Marfurt and Turner, 1984; Johnson et al, 1985; Shigenaga, 1986) of the distribution and termination sites in the V brainstem complex of pulp afferents of permanent teeth in adults. The rostral part of subnucleus oralis and lamina I of subnucleus caudalis showed the heaviest projection, and the former was the part of the complex which we explored electrophysiologically.

The electrophysiological study also represents the first such approach to this area. In the kitten, oralis neuronal properties were in general comparable to those which we noted in adult control cats and to those observed in previous studies of adult animals (e.g. see Sessle and Greenwood, 1976; Dubner et al, 1978). The only notable difference between kittens and adults was the lower incidence of dental convergence and the longer latency of neuronal responses to electrical stimulation of the canine pulp in the younger kittens. Thus, our electrophysiological study indicates that subnucleus oralis of kittens is a mature somatosensory system, and the similarity of the pulp projection sites in the kitten and adult is consistent with this view. In this regard it is noteworthy that in their study of facial somatosensory inputs to neurons located in the basal ganglia, Schneider et al (1985) concluded that the 3-month-old kitten has an adult-like pattern of neuronal receptive field properties. Related preliminary studies in our laboratory in subnucleus caudalis also suggest that mechanoreceptive field properties of caudalis units are similar in kittens and adults (Hu, unpublished data).

There are several possible explanations for our observations that the oralis neuronal properties of kittens and normal adult cats are comparable but differ from those of pulp-deafferented adult cats. Naturally occurring dental deafferentation exhibits several noticeable differences from the pulpal deafferentation which we experimentally induced in the adults. First, the two processes are not equivalent in terms of the afferents involved. In the resorption of the primary teeth, the peripheral endings of periodontal as well as pulp afferents undergo degeneration whereas in the endodontic procedure applied to the permanent teeth, we caused damage only to the pulp afferent endings. Thus deafferentation in the adults would have affected pulp afferents belonging primarily, although not exclusively, to A-delta and C-fiber spectra involved in nociceptive mechanisms, whereas in the kittens large and small-diameter periodontal afferents conveying tactile as well as nociceptive information would have been affected (e.g. Dubner et al, 1978; Byers, 1984). The central consequences of a deafferentation of "mixed" (large and small afferents) nerves may be different from that occurring with the deafferentation involving primarily small-diameter afferents (Dubner et al, 1978) which for example contain higher or lower concentrations of certain neurochemicals having central actions (see below).

Second, the damage to deciduous pulp afferents is a gradual process compared to the single, "synchronized" damage inflicted on the permanent pulp by the endodontic procedure which in the adult induces central changes that are short-lived and last for no more than 1-2 months (Dostrovsky et al, this volume). Deafferentation associated with exfoliation occurs over several months, and is a sequential process: resorption and shedding of primary incisors, then canines, and then molars. This gradual, staged process may allow the brainstem ample time for recovery from each stage. Certain trophic agents having higher (or lower) concentrations in the kitten than the adult may be critical factors which enable the developing V brainstem complex to deal more effectively with the changes accompanying dental deafferentation. For example, a wide range of neuropeptides (e.g. substance P, somatostatin) occurring in dental afferents (Byers, 1984; Olgart, 1985) could be candidates for this hypothetical neurotrophic action, and Fitzgerald et al (1985) have demonstrated that nerve growth factor may act to reverse some effects of deafferentation on central neurons. Such substances in dental afferents may normally be transported centrally to preserve the normal receptive field properties of V brainstem neurons. They might be markedly diminished after pulpotomy, thus resulting in the changes we observed in the adult, whereas in the kitten the gradual sequential exfoliation of the teeth may cause a less substantive loss of these substances.

Another possibility to account for the similarity in oralis neuronal properties of kittens and normal adult cats is that exfoliation of primary teeth is not associated with any substantial degeneration or alteration of the central portion of dental afferents. This is consistent with the sparse degeneration in the proximal portion of dental nerves of kittens despite the substantial degeneration taking place in the distal portion of the nerves (Fried, 1982). Westrum et al (1984) have described degenerating neural profiles in the V brainstem complex of the kitten at the mixed dentition stage, and have attributed them to changes in the central endings of deciduous dental primary afferents undergoing degeneration. Perhaps these changes are not of sufficient magnitude to be reflected in substantive electrophysiological changes, given the staged process of exfoliation (see above), although it still remains to be demonstrated that the central degeneration seen in the kitten is indeed related to dental deafferentation and not, for example, to central changes and reorganization occurring in other peripheral, or central, inputs to the V brainstem complex at this age. It is curious that the degeneration which Westrum et al reported may occur at sites inconsistent with the somatotopic pattern of distribution of dental afferents described in other investigations in the adult (Arvidsson and Gobel, 1981; Marfurt and Turner, 1984; Johnson et al, 1985; Shigenaga, 1986) and in the present anatomical and physiological investigations of deciduous pulp afferents in the kitten.

Surprisingly, little study has been directed to the pattern and interrelationships of the innervations of deciduous and permanent teeth. There is also very little clinical data obtained from experimentally controlled studies in children which address the possible changing sensitivity of the deciduous and permanent teeth as the former exfoliate and the latter erupt. Likewise, little attempt has been made to address the related, fundamental issue of whether or not the permanent tooth is supplied by collaterals of the same afferent fibers that supply its predecessor (or adjacent tissues, e.g. Lisney and Matthews, 1978), or by a new set of afferents which innervate the permanent tooth after the afferents supplying the deciduous tooth have degenerated. The apparent lack of substantial morphological changes in central dental nerves (Fried, 1982) and of changes in the properties of V brainstem neurons reported here at the mixed dentition stage is more consistent with the possibility that the same afferent may supply both deciduous and permanent teeth. A greater research focus is needed in this unique model system for an improved understanding of the neuroplasticity and clinical sensitivity of dental structures in the maturing V somatosensory system.

This research was supported by U.S. NIH Grant DE 04786 and Can. MRC Grant MT 4918.

REFERENCES

Arvidsson J, Gobel S (1981). An HRP study of the central projections of primary trigeminal neurons which innervate tooth pulps in the cat. Brain Res 210:1-16.

Byers MR (1984). Dental sensory receptors. Int Rev Neurobiol 25:39-94.

Dubner R, Sessle BJ, Storey AT (1978). "The Neural Basis of Oral and Facial Function." New York: Plenum.

Fitzgerald M, Wall PD, Goedert M, Emson PC (1985). Nerve growth factor counteracts the neurophysiological and neurochemical effects of chronic sciatic nerve section. Brain Res 332:131-141.

Fried K (1982). Development, degeneration and regeneration of nerve fibres in the feline inferior alveolar nerve and mandibular incisor pulps. Acta Physiol Scand Suppl 504:1-28.

Johnson LR, Westrum LE Henry MA, Canfield RC (1985). Toxic ricin demonstrates a dual dental projection. Brain Res 345:379-383.

Lisney SJW, Matthews B (1978). Branched afferent nerves supplying tooth-pulp in the cat. J Physiol (London) 279:507-517.

Marfurt DF, Turner DF (1984). The central projections of tooth pulp afferent neurons in the cat as determined by the transganglionic transport of horseradish peroxidase. J Comp Neurol 223:535-547.

Olgart LM (1985). The role of local factors in dentin and pulp in intradental pain mechanisms. J Dent Res 64:572-578.

Sessle BJ, Greenwood LF (1976). Inputs to trigeminal brain stem neurones from facial, oral, tooth pulp and pharyngolaryngeal tissue: I. Response to innocuous and noxious stimuli. Brain Res 117:211-226.

Shapiro HH (1930). Growth and time correlations between ossification centers in the long bones and calcification centers in the mandibular dentition of the cat. Int J Orthod 16:690-702.

Schneider JS, Levine MS, Hull CD, Buchwald NA (1985). Development of somatosensory responsiveness in the basal ganglia in awake cats. J Neurophysiol 54:143-154.

Shigenaga Y (1986). Personal Communication.

Westrum LE, Johnson LR, Canfield RC (1984). Ultrastructure of transganglionic degeneration of brain stem trigeminal nuclei during normal primary tooth exfoliation and permanent tooth eruption in the cat. J Comp Neurol 230:198-206.

Effects of Injury on Trigeminal and Spinal Somatosensory Systems, pages 197–204

EFFECTS OF TOOTH PULP DEAFFERENTATION ON TRIGEMINAL BRAINSTEM NEURONES

Jonathan O. Dostrovsky, Barry J. Sessle and James W. Hu

Department of Physiology, Faculty of Medicine and Faculty of Dentistry, University of Toronto, Toronto, Canada

INTRODUCTION

As other papers in this symposium have indicated, spinal deafferentation may be associated with functional, morphological, and neurochemical changes at various levels of the adult spinal somatosensory system. These changes have been viewed on one hand as a reflection of the central neural potential for regeneration and plasticity, and on the other hand as processes important in the pathophysiology of chronic pain. In contrast, there have been few studies of effects of deafferentation in the adult trigeminal (V) somatosensory system. However, Gobel (1984) has recently shown that extirpation of the tooth pulp results in morphological alterations in brainstem neurones of the V spinal tract nucleus. We therefore decided to test for possible physiological correlates of these morphological changes induced by removal of this sensory input to the brain that is predominantly, if not exclusively, related to nociception (Dubner et al., 1978).

MATERIALS AND METHODS

The coronal tooth pulps of the right maxillary or mandibular canine, premolar and molar teeth in adult cats were removed, and the coronal pulp chamber was then filled and sealed off with dental cement by routine aseptic endodontic procedures. A histological examination of the deafferented teeth at the end of the experiments revealed no evidence of neuroma formation, infection or extensive inflammation in the remaining apical part of the pulp.

After recovery, each cat was then studied electrophysiologically at a single post-operative time that varied between 3 days and 2 years; additional unoperated cats served as controls. A quantitative mapping of the V subnucleus oralis and/or subnucleus caudalis was undertaken and data were collected in the same manner for control and deafferented cats; 4 of these experiments were carried out "blind" in control and operated cats by those of us who were not aware of the tooth pulp condition (intact or not) of the animal. The cats were anaesthetized with alpha-chloralose (60mg/Kg, 59 cats) or electrolytically decerebrated (3 cats). Neurone activity was recorded extracellularly (Hu et al., 1981; Sessle and Hu, 1981) by a microelectrode stereotaxically introduced into the right V spinal tract nucleus in a series of vertical microelectrode tracks made in 0.25-0.5 mm transverse steps at one or more anteroposterior planes; in 13 cats the left subnucleus oralis was also examined. Electrical stimuli were delivered to 4-6 tooth pulps, ipsilateral supraorbital, maxillary and mandibular skin, and ipsilateral mucosa of anterior palate, maxillary and mandibular buccal alveolar ridges, and tongue dorsum, and natural tactile and noxious mechanical or heat stimuli were applied bilaterally to skin and intraoral sites (Hu et al., 1981). By such approaches we were able to classify each neurone as low-threshold mechanoreceptive (LTM), wide dynamic range (WDR) or nociceptive-specific (NS).

To determine if the observed changes in receptive field or response properties of oralis neurones in deafferented cats were associated with an alteration in the powerful central inhibitory influence that nucleus raphe magnus (NRM) normally exerts on these neurones (Dubner et al., 1978; Sessle and Hu, 1981), bipolar concentric electrodes were stereotaxically placed in histologically confirmed sites within NRM in 24 deafferented cats and 8 control cats, and conditioning effects of NRM stimulation (20 msec train of 0.2 msec pulses at 400 Hz) tested on near-threshold responses of single oralis neurones evoked by oral-facial test stimuli (Sessle and Hu, 1981).

RESULTS

Nearly all the ipsilateral (1750) and contralateral (220) oralis neurones recorded were LTM neurones; only a small number were WDR and NS (n=13). In contrast many of the 600 caudalis neurones were WDR and NS (n=131).

Differences between control and deafferented animals were apparent in the 'blind' experiments and in both anaesthetized and unanaesthetized (decerebrate) preparations. In control animals, approximately one-third of the ipsilateral oralis neurones (exclusive of neurones with localized ophthalmic receptive fields) had a mechanoreceptive field localized within the mandibular division and one-third had a receptive field localized within the maxillary division; only 37% had a receptive field involving two or all three V divisions. In contrast, in animals deafferented 7-15 days prior to neurone recording, these proportions were almost completely reversed; compared with control animals, the incidences of neurones having a receptive field limited to the V division in which the deafferentation had occurred or a field involving two or three V divisions were significantly decreased, and increased, respectively ($p<0.05$, F-test). These changes were associated with a loss of the fine detail of the orderly 'inverted-head' pattern of topographic representation that normally characterizes oralis (Dubner et al., 1978), but they progressively returned towards control values (Fig. 1).

In deafferented animals, there was no significant difference in the incidence of oralis nociceptive neurones, but the incidence of spontaneously active neurones significantly increased (Fig. 1); however, the mean firing frequency of 2.5 Hz was not different from control levels. There was also a statistically significant increase (Fig. 1) in the incidence of ipsilateral oralis neurones which could only be excited by a brisk tap applied to ipsilateral oral or facial sites and which rapidly habituated to subsequent taps. The use of an electronically controlled mechanical stimulator revealed that, in contrast to rapidly adapting LTM neurones (mean maximal following-frequency 6.6 Hz), these habituating tap-sensitive neurones could not respond to repetitive rectangular tactile stimuli (e.g. mean frequency 0.3 Hz) and showed complete lack of entrainment by sinusoidal stimuli.

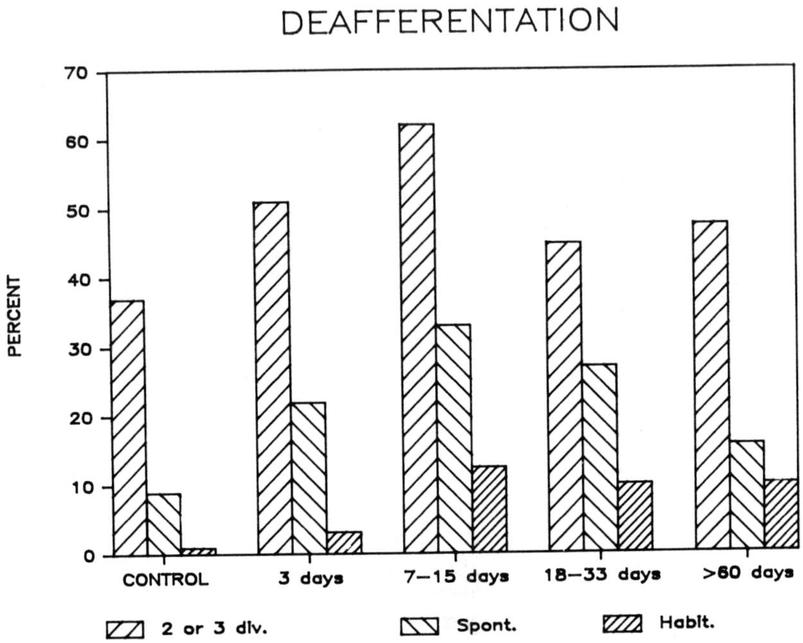

Fig. 1: Incidence of ipsilateral oralis neurones having a LTM field involving 2 or 3 V divisions, spontaneous activity or habituating tap-sensitivity in control or deafferented cats. Note the statistically significant increase in the 7-15 day deafferented group, and the progressive return towards control values (linear trend analysis).

There were no statistically significant differences in the incidence or latency of responses electrically evoked from the various sites tested (see Methods) between control and deafferented cats, e.g. for tongue, 44% in control and 45% in deafferented cats. Of particular note was the high incidence (45%) of ipsilateral oralis neurones in control animals that could be activated by electrical stimuli applied to V regions outside, as well as within, their carefully delineated LTM field; the incidence was reduced (to 20%) in 7-15 day deafferented cats.

Effects of NRM conditioning stimulation were tested on the responses of 60 ipsilateral oralis neurones recorded in control animals and 216 recorded in 7-33 day-deafferented animals. The incidence, time course and threshold of NRM-induced suppression of either pulp or skin/mucosal-evoked responses in ipsilateral oralis were comparable in control and deafferented animals, e.g. approximately 92% of the neuronal responses could be suppressed in the control and deafferented groups and there were no significant differences (ANOVA, two-tailed; $p>0.05$) between the groups in the threshold for NRM-induced suppression of either pulp or skin/mucosal-evoked responses.

Although smaller, changes comparable to those noted in the ipsilateral subnucleus were also apparent in the contralateral oralis, and the incidences of neurones with a mechanoreceptive field limited to the deafferented V division and of spontaneously active neurones were significantly increased over control. In the ipsilateral subnucleus caudalis, we also observed in the 7-15 day deafferented group a marked increase in the incidence of both LTM and nociceptive (WDR and NS) neurones showing spontaneous activity or a mechanoreceptive field involving 2 or 3 V divisions.

DISCUSSION

These quantitative studies indicate that the sensory loss caused by tooth pulp deafferentation can produce marked changes in receptive field properties and activity of V spinal tract neurones of the adult cat. These changes are statistically significant at 7-15 days post-operatively, and are reversible. Compared with most other deafferentation studies, only a very small part (<5%) of the peripheral afferent input to the central region examined was eliminated and it involved an input which is predominantly if not exclusively nociceptive (Dubner et al., 1978). Moreover, the pulp input comprises only part of the afferent synaptic drive to most if not all of the pulp-driven neurones since the great majority also respond to cutaneous or other non-pulp intraoral sites (e.g. Sessle and Greenwood, 1976; Hu et al., 1981). Thus the striking deafferentation effects observed were associated with only a partial loss of sensory input to the neurones and may have been directed at those neurones normally receiving a pulp afferent input.

In accordance with earlier observations in V subnuclei caudalis and interpolaris (Anderson et al., 1971; Black, 1974), an increased incidence of spontaneously active neurones was noted in deafferented animals although the mean firing frequency was not higher than in control animals. We have additionally shown statistically significant yet reversible alterations in response properties, receptive field extent, and disruption of somatotopic organization. A morphological correlation apparently exists for our findings since transneuronal alterations in V spinal tract neurones have been noted (Gobel, 1984) 14-60 days after partial removal of pulps comparable to those similarly removed in the present study.

We cannot completely discount peripheral factors contributing to some of the observed changes although our findings do not support this possibility (e.g. no evidence of neuroma formation). In the spinal somatosensory system, central mechanisms have been viewed as being the major contributors to deafferentation-induced changes, and as pointed out elsewhere in this symposium, sprouting or unmasking of existing afferent connections have been especially emphasized. While we cannot rule out the former as a contributing factor, our data favour an unmasking of existing afferent connections. In normal animals we have found a surprisingly high degree of convergence of cutaneous, mucosal, dental, muscle, or visceral afferents on V spinal tract neurones (Sessle and Greenwood, 1976; Sessle et al., 1986) and in the present study we also noted extensive V cutaneous/mucosal inputs to oralis. Yet it is particularly noteworthy that the proportions of the different electrically evoked inputs and their latencies were comparable in control and deafferented animals except for V regions outside the LTM field. Collectively, these data suggest that the changes in neuronal mechanoreceptive field and response properties associated with deafferentation may have involved unmasking of inputs that normally occur from outside the neurone's mechanoreceptive field. This view is consistent with spinal cord data indicating that many central neurones may receive inputs that can be evoked by electrical stimulation but not by natural stimuli, and that these inputs may become operative and result in activation of these neurones by natural stimuli in pathophysiological situations such as deafferentation (Wall, 1983). It has been suggested that these inputs are normally held in check by afferent inhibition or by central modulatory mechanisms involving for example the NRM; however, we found no alteration as a result of pulp deafferentation in the threshold, time course or incidence of raphe-induced inhibition of responses in oralis neurones.

Our data underscore the marked potential for plasticity and reorganization of the adult V brainstem system. Since the permanent teeth do not erupt and assume a sensory function until well after other sensory systems are established, there may be a greater potential for neuroplasticity and regeneration existing in the dental representation of the V system of the young adult than in other sensory systems (also see Hu et al., this volume). Our data also show that both subnuclei oralis and caudalis may be subject to deafferentation-induced functional changes. Subnucleus caudalis has long been considered the major brainstem nociceptive relay in the V system (see Dubner et al., 1978), and oralis has also been recently implicated in orofacial nociceptive mechanisms. The association of both subnuclei with nociceptive processes, plus the findings of deafferentation-induced changes in spinal nociceptive pathways and the clinical association of deafferentation with pain (e.g. Sunderland, 1978; Tasker, 1984), raises the possibility that changes in central V somatosensory pathways of the type described here after dental deafferentation procedures may contribute to the development of chronic orofacial pain conditions. Nonetheless, we saw no gross evidence of abnormal nocifensive behaviours in the pulp-deafferented animals (cf. Black, 1974), and there appears to be a low prevalence of chronic orofacial pain in humans despite the high incidence of dental deafferentation (through tooth extraction, endodontic therapy etc.). Such observations may be related to our findings that most of the brainstem changes are reversible and are particularly striking in the cat only 1-2 weeks after pulp deafferentation. Additional factors (e.g. further deafferentation, infection) may have to be superimposed to produce permanent functional alterations that may have relevance to the development of chronic pain, and these factors should be considered in future studies of V deafferentation.

The study was supported by NIH grant DE04786.

REFERENCES

Anderson LS, Black RG, Abraham J, Ward AA (1971). Neuronal hyperactivity in experimental deafferentation. J Neurosurg 35:444-452.

Black RG (1974). A laboratory model for trigeminal neuralgia. Adv Neurol 4:651-659.

Dubner R, Sessle BJ, Storey AT (1978). "The Neural Basis of Oral and Facial Function." New York: Plenum.

Gobel S. (1984). An electron microscopic analysis of the trans-synaptic effects of peripheral nerve injury subsequent to tooth pulp extirpations on neurons in laminae I and II of the medullary dorsal horn. J Neurosci 4:2281-2290.

Hu J, Dostrovsky JO, Sessle BJ (1981). Functional properties of neurons in cat trigeminal subnucleus caudalis (medullary dorsal horn). I. Responses to oral-facial noxious and nonnoxious stimuli and projections to thalamus and subnucleus oralis. J Neurophysiol 45:173-192.

Sessle BJ, Greenwood LF (1976). Inputs to trigeminal brain stem neurones from facial, oral, tooth pulp and pharyngolaryngeal tissues: I. Responses to innocuous and noxious stimuli. Brain Res 117:211-226.

Sessle BJ, Hu JW, (1981). Raphe-induced suppression of the jaw-opening reflex and single neurons in trigeminal subnucleus oralis, and influence of naloxone and subnucleus caudalis. Pain 10:19-36.

Sessle BJ, Hu JW, Amano N, Zhong G (1986). Convergence of cutaneous, tooth pulp, visceral, neck and muscle afferents onto nociceptive and non nociceptive neurones in trigeminal subnucleus caudalis (medullary dorsal horn) and its implications for referred pain. Pain, in press.

Sunderland S (1978). "Nerves and Nerve Injuries." Edinburgh: Churchill Livingstone, 2nd Ed.

Tasker RR (1984). Deafferentation, In Wall PD, Melzack R (eds): "Textbook of Pain." Edinburgh: Churchill Livingstone, pp 119-132.

Wall PD (1983). Alterations in the central nervous system after deafferentation: connectivity control. In Bonica JJ, Lindblom U, Iggo A (eds): "Advances in Pain Research and Therapy, Vol. 5." New York: Raven, pp. 677-689.

Effects of Injury on Trigeminal and Spinal Somatosensory Systems, pages 205–214

ABSENCE OF INTRAMEDULLARY SPROUTING IN TRIGEMINAL PRIMARY AFFERENT AXONS CAUDAL AND ROSTRAL TO A PARTIAL MEDULLARY HEMISECTION

Brian H. Hallas, William E. Renehan, Bradley G. Klein and Mark F. Jacquin

Department of Neuroscience
New York College of Osteopathic Medicine
Old Westbury, New York 11568

INTRODUCTION

It is well known that when the CNS is damaged, few if any axons grow into or through the site of the lesion. Clinicians have taken advantage of this failure to regenerate to produce long-term denervations of the CNS, particularly for relief from chronic pain. A trigeminal (V) tractotomy procedure (Sjoqvist operation), which partially divides the V spinal tract and brainstem complex in its caudal extent near the obex, and therefore isolates subnucleus caudalis from its V primary afferent inputs and rostral subnuclei, has been used to produce varying amounts of orofacial analgesia, with minor effects on tactile sensations (Sjoqvist, 1938; Kunc, 1970, 1979; Kerr, 1979; Schvarcz, 1979). However, neuralgia returns in a significant percentage of tractotomy patients (Kunc, 1979; Schvarcz, 1979). It is, therefore, likely that postoperative CNS reorganization is responsible for restitution of neuralgic symptoms. The latter could reflect alterations in the morphology of V primary afferent axons or postsynaptic cells, subsequent to tractotomy. In the present study we have examined the effects of V tractotomy upon the morphology of V primary afferent axons at points rostral and caudal to tractotomy in barbiturate-anesthetized adult rats. Anterograde bulk-labelling and intra-axonal recording and HRP labelling procedures were used.

RESULTS

Twenty-one to 50 days subsequent to a transverse section through the lateral medulla, the ipsilateral V ganglion was exposed and injected with HRP (Jacquin and Rhoades, 1985). Figure 1A illustrates an extensive lesion which encompassed all of the V spinal tract and nucleus, at the level of the obex, while 1B shows an absence of anterograde label caudal to the site of the lesion. The presence of heavy and dense HRP reaction product rostral to the lesion (Fig. 2), but not caudal, suggests that V primary afferents do not regenerate past the point of a total V tractotomy performed in adult rats.

Tractotomized adult rats have also provided data bearing upon two other important issues:
1) The capacity for renewed growth in <u>non</u>injured V primary afferents; and 2) the capacity for renewed growth in the intact collaterals of severed V primary afferents; i.e. growth of new collaterals from axons proximal to the point of transection.

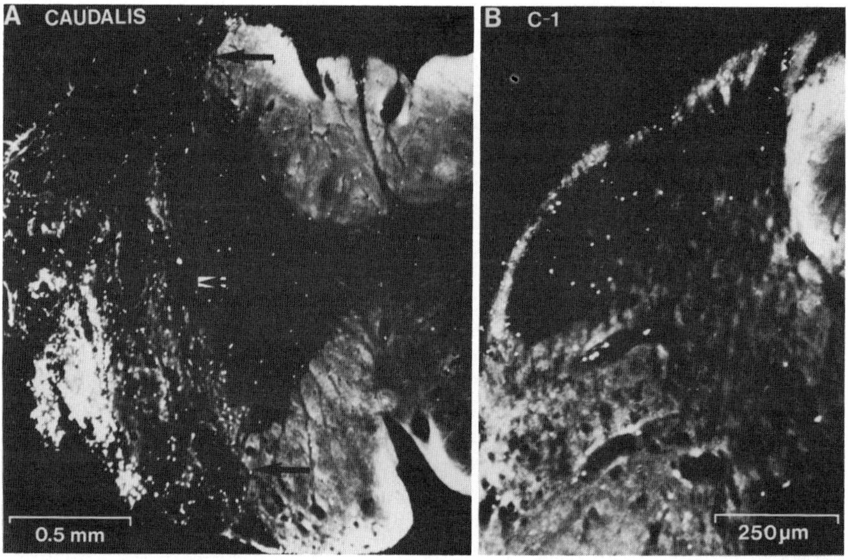

Figure 1. A: Dark-field photomicrograph illustrating the extent of a complete V tractotomy (arrows) which included all of the V spinal tract and nucleus at the level of the caudal medullary dorsal horn. Rostral to the lesion, anterograde HRP label from the V ganglion was extremely heavy (see Fig. 2). Caudal to the lesion (B), there were no labelled fibers.

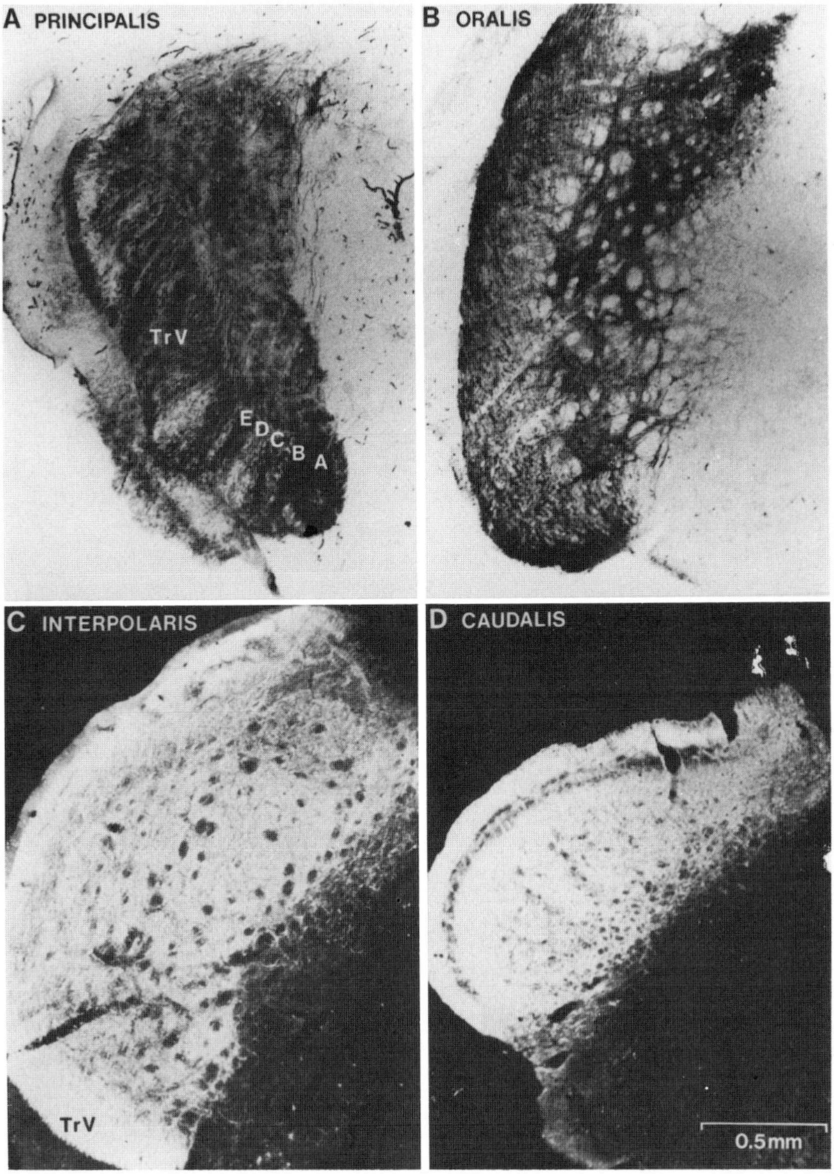

Figure 2. Anterograde HRP labelling from the V ganglion to brainstem regions rostral to tractotomy performed 35 days earlier. The lesion site is shown in Figure 1. Note that the label is patchy in ventral maxillary regions in all subnuclei, except oralis (B). TrV - trigeminal spinal tract.

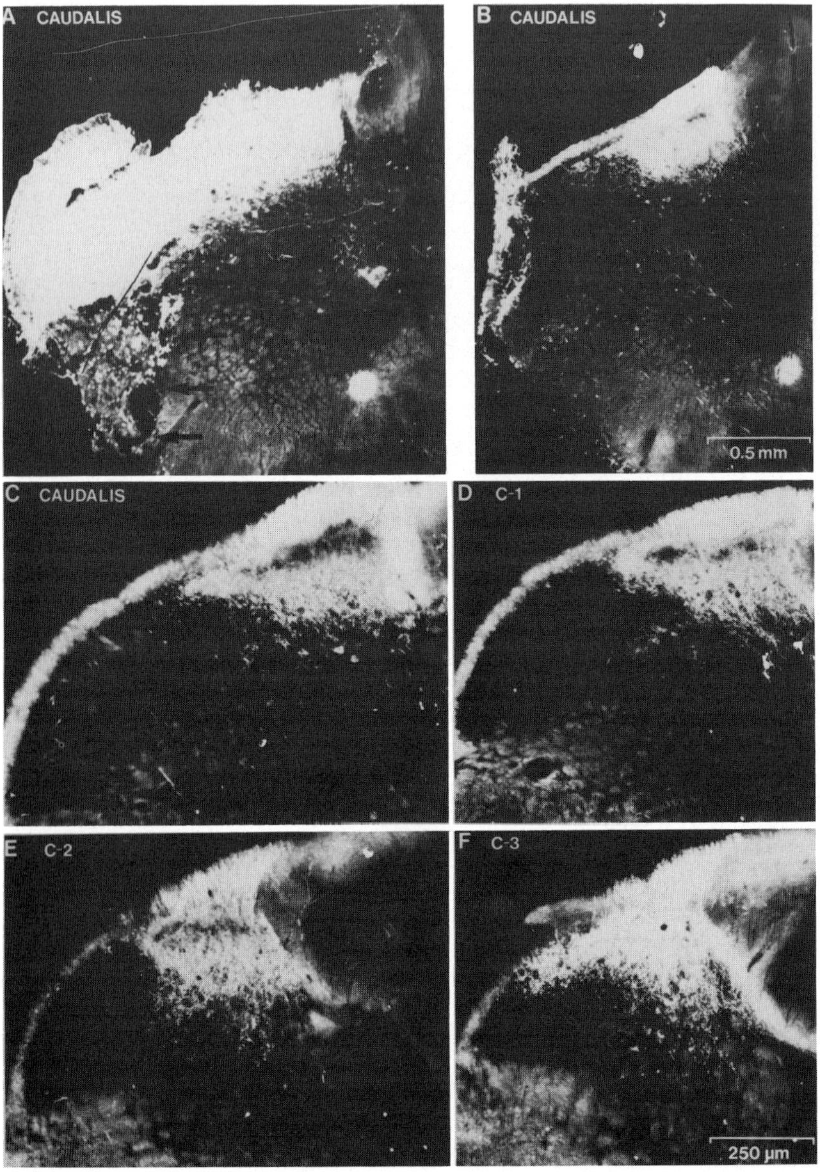

Figure 3. Central projections of the V nerve to the medullary (A-C) and cervical (D-F) dorsal horns, as revealed by anterograde HRP transport. Arrows in A indicate the medial extent of the lesion performed one month earlier. Dorsomedial mandibular fibers were spared and they maintain a dorsomedial trajectory.

Tractotomy and Projections of Noninjured V Primary Afferents

The anterograde label shown in Figure 3 suggests that a partial tractotomy does not result in an exuberant projection from spared V primary afferents. The lesion was restricted to maxillary and ophthalmic portions of the V spinal tract and nucleus, sparing dorsomedially located mandibular regions. Subsequent HRP injections into the V ganglion revealed that in caudal subnucleus caudalis (Fig. 3C), C-1 (Fig. 3D), C-2 (Fig. 3E), and C-3 dorsal horn (Fig. 3F), labelled fibers maintained their dorsomedial trajectory and termination zone. Portions of the dorsal horn which normally receive maxillary and ophthalmic fibers were devoid of label. Thus, mandibular fibers appeared normal in their termination pattern, while lesioned axons did not extend beyond the point of tractotomy. In this regard, our results are consistent with those of Rodin et al. (1983) and Rodin and Kruger (1984) who have documented an absence of collateral sprouting in both spared spinal dorsal root and partially hemisected adult cats. Our results are also consistent with those of Kerr (1975) who found no evidence of extension of cervical primary afferents into the chronically denervated V brainstem complex of adult cats.

All of the above, and the results of recent studies using peripheral nerve section (e.g. Jacquin and Rhoades, 1985), suggest a rather fixed projection of noninjured somatosensory primary afferents to the V brainstem complex, irrespective of the type of denervation employed. However, there are sampling and sensitivity problems inherent to anterograde bulk-transport procedures. For example, subtle alterations in central arbor morphology may go undetected. We have, therefore, carried out a series of intra-axonal recording and labelling experiments to assess possible anomalies in the morphology of spared V primary afferents, caudal to a partial tractotomy in adult rats. Figure 4 illustrates our results for spared vibrissa primary afferents in caudalis, two months subsequent to a partial tractotomy encompassing mandibular and maxillary regions. Normal-looking arbors were observed in topographically appropriate portions of caudalis. Preliminary quantitative analyses indicate that arbor area, number of collaterals, and the number of boutons per collateral fall within normal ranges for these afferent fiber types in caudalis (Jacquin et al., 1986a). Moreover, arbors from spared guard hair and hairy skin afferents also could not be distinguished from normal. These data therefore provide further support for the notion that

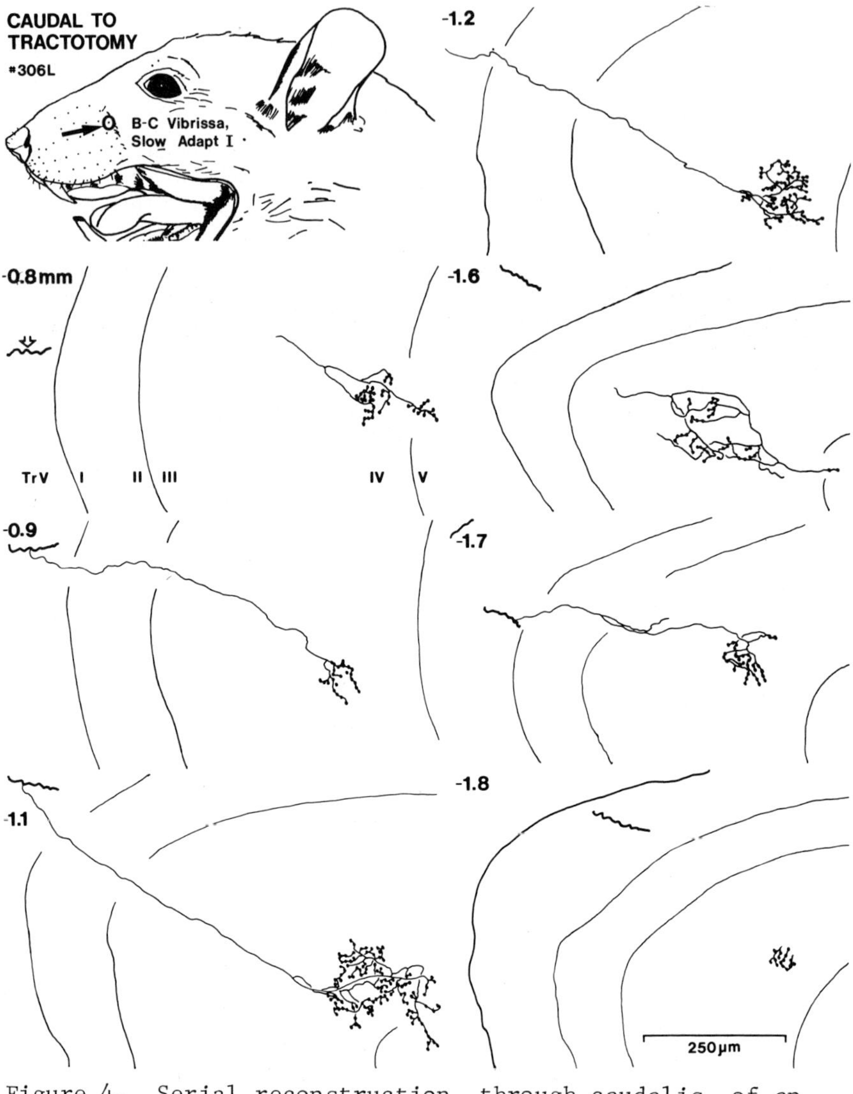

Figure 4. Serial reconstruction, through caudalis, of an intra-axonally labeled vibrissa-sensitive primary afferent which was spared in a partial V tractotomy through mandibular and maxillary regions. This lesion was made at the caudalis-interpolaris border 50 days earlier. All arbors in left caudalis are shown in transverse sections from rostral (-0.8 mm) to caudal caudalis (-1.8 mm). Laminae I-V are indicated by thin smooth lines. These data should be compared with the normative data provided in Jacquin et al. (1986a).

partial surgical isolation of caudalis from V primary afferent input is not accompanied by collateral sprouting in spared axons caudal to the lesion, though it remains to be determined if nociceptive fibers respond to such a lesion.

Tractotomy and Projections of Injured V Primary Afferents

Figure 2 illustrates the central projections of the V nerve to regions rostral to a complete transection through the V spinal tract and nucleus at the level of the obex. The pattern and distribution of labelled primary afferents were indistinguishable from those of normal adult rats (compare with Bates and Killackey, 1985; Jacquin and Rhoades, 1983, 1985). Most notably, maxillary regions contained a series of rostrocaudally oriented terminal columns that corresponded in pattern to the vibrissae on the face. This pattern was most conspicuous in principalis (letters in Fig. 2A correspond to the rows of vibrissae which are normally represented here), caudal interpolaris, and rostral caudalis. Though HRP bulk-labelling of afferent terminals does not allow for detailed analysis of collaterals proximal to the lesion, we interpret the presence of a normally segmented maxillary projection, one that is isomorphic with the pattern of the vibrissae on the face, as evidence that V axons maintain their normal collateral pattern proximal to a central maxillary lesion. Growth of new collaterals, or expansion of the terminal fields of existing collaterals, would have either masked the "barreloid" primary afferent pattern, should the new collaterals have entered the usually terminal-free regions between patches, or enlarged the maxillary terminal area, should the new collaterals have maintained their "barreloid" configurations. Neither of these possibilities was obvious in our material.

Figure 5 illustrates the results of our intra-axonal labelling studies rostral to axotomy at the level of the obex. Fibers were heavily labelled to the point of tractotomy, at which point their descent through the V spinal tract ended abruptly. The following therefore represents the morphology of V primary afferent collaterals rostral to the point of their severance at the level of the obex. In interpolaris, vibrissa afferents gave rise to circumscribed, transversely oriented, arbors in topographically appropriate locations (Fig. 5). Maxillary guard hair fibers had arbors with a similar configuration, though with fewer boutons than vibrissa afferents (not illustrated). Hairy skin afferents had a more

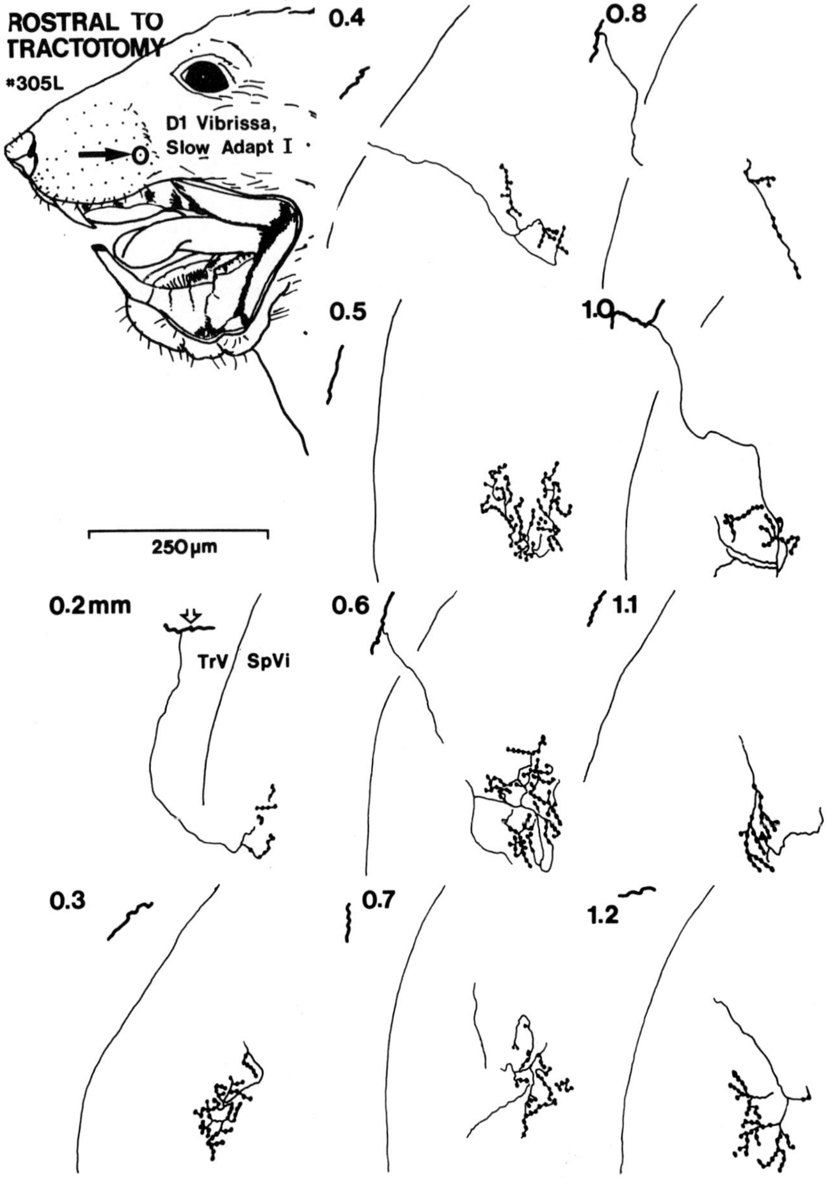

Figure 5. Serial reconstruction of a vibrissa primary afferent rostral to the point of axotomy at the level of the obex. All sections are from subnucleus interpolaris. The lesion was made 35 days prior to labeling of this axon. Its morphology looks normal (compare with Fig. 2 of Jacquin et al., 1986b).

tortuous "stringy" appearance (not illustrated). These structure-function relationships exist normally (compare with Jacquin et al., 1986b). These data therefore suggest that tractotomy does not result in collateral sprouting in axotomized V primary afferents. Taken together with the above-described data on spared afferents, we conclude that V primary afferents do not alter their gross morphology following V tractotomy in adult rats.

CONCLUSIONS

Primary afferent reorganization may not be responsible for the restitution of nociceptive function following partial V tractotomy at the level of the obex in humans. Neuralgic recurrences could reflect the normally present nociceptive input to more rostral V brainstem subnuclei (Jacquin et al., 1986c), central sprouting from cervical primary afferents, renewed growth of postsynaptic dendrites and/or axons, or unmasking of normally inhibited inputs to postsynaptic neurons rostral or caudal to the lesion.

ACKNOWLEDGEMENTS

Supported by NIH grant #DE07662 and the American Osteopathic Association. Thanks to H. Lowe for technical help.

REFERENCES

Bates CA, Killackey HP (1985). The organization of the neonatal rat's brainstem trigeminal complex and its role in the formation of central trigeminal patterns. J Comp Neurol 240:265-287.

Jacquin MF, Rhoades RW (1983). Central projections of the normal and "regenerate" infraorbital nerve in adult rats subjected to neonatal unilateral infraorbital lesions: A transganglionic horseradish peroxidase study. Brain Res 269:137-144.

Jacquin MF, Rhoades RW (1985). Effects of neonatal infraorbital lesions upon central trigeminal primary afferent projections in rat and hamster. J Comp Neurol 235:129-143.

Jacquin MF, Renehan WE, Mooney RD, Rhoades RW (1986a). Structure-function relationships in rat medullary and cervical dorsal horns. I. Trigeminal primary afferents.

J Neurophysiol 55:1153-1186.
Jacquin MF, Woerner D, Szczepanik AM, Riecker V, Mooney RD, Rhoades RW (1986b). Structure-function relationships in rat brainstem subnucleus interpolaris. I. Vibrissa primary afferents. J Comp Neurol 243:266-279.
Jacquin MF, Renehan WE, Klein BG, Rhoades RW (1986c). Axon arbors from nociceptive, hairy skin, glabrous skin, guard hair, periodontal, lingual mucosa, and vibrissa primary afferents in rat trigeminal subnucleus interpolaris. Anat Rec 214:60A.
Kerr FWL (1975). Neuroplasticity of primary afferents in the neonatal cat and some results of early deafferentation of the trigeminal spinal nucleus. J Comp Neurol 163:305-329.
Kerr FWL (1979). Craniofacial neuralgias. In Bonica JJ, Liebeskind JC, Albe-Fessard DG (eds): "Advances in Pain Research and Therapy," Vol 3, New York: Raven Press, pp 283-296.
Kunc Z (1970). Significant factors pertaining to the results of trigeminal tractotomy. In Hassler R, Walker AE (eds): "Trigeminal Neuralgia," Stuttgart: Georg Thieme Verlag, pp 90-100.
Kunc Z (1979). Vertical trigeminal partial nucleotomy. In Bonica JJ, Liebeskind JC, Albe-Fessard DG (eds): "Advances in Pain Research and Therapy," vol 3, New York: Raven Press, pp 325-330.
Rodin BE, Kruger L (1984). Absence of intraspinal sprouting in dorsal root axons caudal to a partial spinal hemisection: A horseradish peroxidase study. Somato Res 2:171-192.
Rodin BE, Sampogna S, Kruger L (1983). An examination of intraspinal sprouting in dorsal root axons with the tracer horseradish peroxidase. J Comp Neurol 215:187-198.
Schvarcz JR (1979). Stereotactic spinal trigeminal nucleotomy for dysesthesic facial pain. In Bonica JJ, Liebeskind JC, Albe-Fessard DG (eds): "Advances in Pain Research and Therapy," Vol 3, New York: Raven Press, pp 331-336.
Sjoqvist O (1938). Studies on pain conduction in the trigeminal nerve. A contribution to the surgical treatment of facial pain. Acta Psychiat Neurol Scand 1:1-139.

Effects of Injury on Trigeminal and Spinal Somatosensory Systems, pages 215–225

ON MECHANISMS OF SOMATOTOPIC PLASTICITY

Marshall Devor

Department of Zoology, Life Sciences Institute
Hebrew University of Jerusalem, Jerusalem 91904
Israel

INTRODUCTION

In recent years a large number of electrophysiological studies have been published demonstrating plastic reorganization of somatotopic maps within the CNS following partial deafferentation. The bulk have used a standard paradigm, originally introduced by Wall and Egger (1971). First a two-dimensional somatotopic map is defined. Then afferent input to a part of the map is deleted by surgical or other treatments in the periphery or the central nervous system (CNS). The experimental observation common to most of the studies is that cells that lost their normal functional drive (receptive field, RF) acquire a new RF in the nearest neighboring part of the somatotopic map. Somatotopic reorganization of this sort has been observed at all levels of the somatosensory system (spinal dorsal horn, dorsal column nuclei, trigeminal nuclei, deep tectum, ventrobasal thalamus and neocortex) and occurs not only in neonates, but also in fully mature mammals, including primates and probably including man (Kaas et al., 1983; Devor, 1984). It is not yet known, however, to what extent RF shifts in 2nd and 3rd order maps reflect local processes versus the relay of changes in 1st order maps. In the present chapter I will discuss current concepts of the neural process(es) underlying somatotopic plasticity. The discussion is based principally on a single model, somatotopic reorganization of the distal hindlimb map in the dorsal horn following transection of the sciatic and saphenous nerves in adult cats and rats (Devor and Wall, 1978,1981a,1981b; Lisney,1983; Fitzgerald et al.,1985)[1]. In this model, medial dorsal horn neurons with RF's on the foot and toes acquire, over a period of days to weeks, novel and somatotopically inappropriate RF's on the thigh, perineum and lower back . The principles involved, however, are relevant to the other models as well.

WHAT SIGNALS SOMATOTOPIC REORGANIZATION ?

After some types of deafferentation, dorsal rhizotomy for example (e.g.Basbaum and Wall, 1976), the central synaptic terminals of the cut dorsal root fibers undergo rapid and near-synchronous anterograde degeneration. Terminal degeneration, however, does not appear to be a prerequisite for the induction of somatotopic reorganization. Following nerve section, for example, the central terminals of peripherally axotomized primary afferent neurons do not undergo rapid and massive degeneration. It is true that some proportion of sensory cell somata undergo retrograde degeneration eventually and as part of this process their central synaptic endings die (Devor et al.,1986; Arvidsson et al., 1986). However, new proximal RF's emerge well beforehand (Devor and Wall, 1981b), and indeed can be found in large numbers at a time when the central terminals of the peripherally axotomized neurons are still functioning normally (Wall and Devor, 1981; Wall et al., 1982).

Short of frank degeneration, it is well known that the central terminals of peripherally axotomized neurons undergo changes in their ultrastructural appearance and histochemistry (Csillik and Knyihar-Csillik, 1986), and the timing of these changes often meshes well with the time of appearance of novel RF's . So far, however, the role of these trophic changes is uncertain. One of the dramatic biochemical changes in the rat dorsal horn following nerve section, for example, is the virtual disappearance of fluoride resistant acid phosphatase (FRAP) from the affected synaptic terminals in the substantia gelatinosa. This occurs at almost the exact time that novel RF's emerge among the immediately subjacent cells. However, an almost identical loss of FRAP occurs after nerve crush, and this lesion does not induce somatotopic reorganization (Devor and Wall, 1981b).

[1] Pubols (1984), using procedures different in several important repects, failed to observe somatotopic remapping in cat dorsal horn.

One of the most appealing candidate signals is blockage of impulse activity along the injured nerve. The evidence so far, however, is not encouraging. First, and paradoxically, nerve section does not silence afferent input into the deafferented part of the spinal map. In rats at least, both the developing nerve-end neuroma, and the dorsal root ganglia, produce massive ectopic impulse activity during exactly the period of somatotopic reorganization, albeit in a pattern obviously different from normal (Devor, 1984). Second, tetrodotoxin block of nerve conduction in the absence of mechanical injury does not appear to induce it. (Wall et al., 1982). Recent data based on axoplasmic trans-transport block and on NGF treatment suggest a possible role for trophic signalling (Devor,1983; Fitzgerald et al.,1985).

DO RF'S ACTUALLY MOVE ?

When a cell that originally had a restricted peripheral RF acquires a novel proximal one, the obvious interpretation is that the RF shifted spatially. An alternative , however, is that the RF simply expanded up the leg. Of course the distal part of the expanded "virtual" RF is not expressed because the nerves serving distal skin have been cut - the net outcome, a proximal RF. The evidence on shift versus expansion is not yet definite. In nerve injured rats and cats we often observed reorganized cells with relatively small proximal RF's surrounded by still innervated skin (Devor and Wall, 1981a,b). In such cells the case for RF shift seems good. However, since dorsal horn neurons in intact animals may have structured RF's with islands of high sensitivity surrounded by low (eg.Devor and Wall, 1981a), it is possible that in certain excitability states an expanded RF would take the form of a proximal island. New evidence from primate cortex after digit amputation shows smooth translations of the forelimb map without obvious expansion of average RF size, and this certainly favours the idea of spatial RF shift (Merzenich et al.,1984).

LONG-RANGE SPROUTING

When new functional connectivity is observed it is natural to infer the growth of new anatomical links. For the hindlimb map in dorsal horn the required direction of growth can be well specified. For medial dorsal horn cells that acquire novel proximal (thigh) RF's, the shortest trajectories are lateralward growth of dendrites, or medialward growth of thigh afferent axons. Both of these routes can be ruled out with some confidence (Devor et al., 1986). There is an alternative trajectory for growth in the rostrocaudal axis, but here the distances that would have to be traversed are much larger, and again, the experiments that have been done so far show no sign of it. Note that "long range" in the present context need not mean many millimeters. The sprout need only cross some definable somatotopic border, the distance involved being related to the grain of the map. In our preparation (the mediolateral axis of spinal cord) we have never attempted to define a map that resolves more than two points (vis. proximal versus distal hindlimb) and doubt that it would even be possible to define more than three or four. "Long-range" is therefore measured in 100's of microns. In a more precisely mapped system (eg. the brainstem whisker map) to cross a definable topographic border may take less distance, while in a less precisely mapped system (eg.the rostrocaudal spinal axis) it it may take substantially more.

SOMATOTOPICALLY INAPPROPRIATE CONNECTIONS

In the absence of evidence for long-range sprouting one must consider the possibility of preexisting connections that are somatotopically inappropriate. If such connections exist, of course, it would then be necessary to explain why they are not normally expressed. In our preparation, there are abundant anatomical structures that could, in principle, convey information mediolaterally across the dorsal horn. These include local interneurons, the mediolateral axonal plexus of many 2nd order spinal projection neurons, and cells with wide dendritic arbors that reside primarily, but not exclusively, in the deeper layers of the dorsal horn (see Devor et al., 1986). Unfortunately, analytical approaches to local polysynaptic networks are exceedingly difficult, and this motivates a search for circuits in which the somatotopically inappropriate input reachs 2nd order dorsal horn neurons monosynaptically. For our preparation, this means thigh afferent terminals directly on cells in the medial dorsal horn.

For deep cells, and some lamina I neurons with wide ranging dendrites, this presents no special problem in principle, although the detailed relationship of afferent axons to 2nd order neurons is not really known for any cell type. Even for cells in laminae II - IV , however, there is frequently a short latency response to electrical stimulation of thigh nerves suggesting that here,too, there may be substantial monosynaptic input from somatotopically inappropriate afferents (Devor and Wall, 1981a). Response latency to peripheral stimulation is a notoriously uncertain diagnostic for synaptic chain length, however. What is needed is anatomical evidence. And indeed, such evidence has begun to emerge (see Devor et al.,1986). For example, light and electron-microscopic studies using transganglionic transport of lectin-conjugated HRP from nerves of the thigh in intact rats have recently uncovered a population of relatively large diameter axons that sweep through the medial dorsal horn on their way laterally, forming axodendritic synaptic contacts along the way. These are good candidates for somatotopically inappropriate terminals, although the case cannot be made with certainty until the postsynaptic dendrites are identified. But are there mechanisms that could cause such latent somatotopically inappropriate connections to be expressed?

THE EFFECTIVENESS OF SYNAPTIC CONTACTS AT DRIVING POSTSYNAPTIC NEURONS AND THE MATTER OF "SHORT RANGE SPROUTING"

Single afferent fibers typically apply more than one synaptic bouton to 2nd order sensory neurons (eg.Brown and Noble, 1982), and it is the compound synaptic current from all terminals invaded by any particular action potential that determines the local synaptic efficacy of a fiber on its target cell. But local synaptic efficacy is not enough. Numerous factors are involved in determining how much the compound synaptic current of a single afferent will contribute to the creation of an action potential. These include, for example, the location of the synapse(s) on the dendritic arbor, dendritic cable properties, dendritic and spine excitability, current shunting, the excitability of the spike initiation zone itself etc. etc. Furthermore, the effectiveness of a given afferent fiber is influenced by its own history of activity and the activity of neighboring synapses, both other afferents activated along with it, local circuit interneurons, and descending control circuits. At present, the determinants controlling synaptic efficacy can be evaluated only roughly, even using the most advanced computer simulation techniques (eg.Segev et al., 1985) ; to unravel the matter in vivo will be a major challenge in the coming years (Redman and Walmsley, 1983). Consider two extremes: for Ia afferent input to spinal motorneurons the

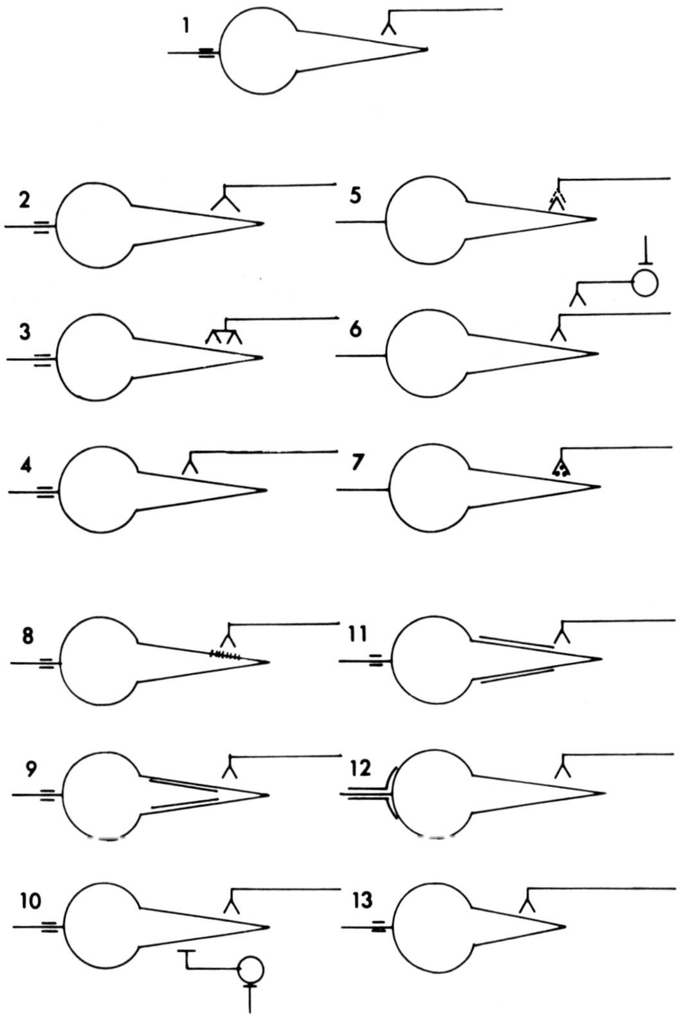

Figure 1. A sample of pre- (2-7) and postsynaptic (8-13) factors capable of modulating effective synaptic strength. (1) reference axodendritic synapse. (2) expansion of terminal. (3) short-range sprouting. (4) synaptic translocation (5) narrowed synaptic cleft. (6) presynaptic disinhibition. (7) increased transmitter release. (8) receptor number and kinetics. (9) dendritic conductance and shunting. (10) postsynaptic disinhibition. (11) dendritic and spine excitability. (12) ecxitability of spike initiation zone. (13) dendritic retraction.

perikaryal EPSP generated by a single fiber is usually measured in tens of microvolts (presumably for some such fibers the EPSP is so small as to be undetectable in the baseline noise), while in the case of spinocervical tract neurons a single action potential in a single afferent may produce repetitive firing of the postsynaptic neuron (Mendell et al.,1976; Brown et al.,1973).

Virtually all of the factors that come into play in determining the effectiveness of a synaptic input channel are potentially under dynamic control within short, intermediate or long time frames. Figure 1 illustrates twelve such mechanisms, six presynaptic and six postsynaptic. Many more could be generated. Note that in this context the local duplication ("sprouting") of new synaptic endings (panel 3 in Fig.1) may constitute just one more mechanism for strengthening preexisting synaptic links (see chapter by M. Murray in this volume). Such "short range sprouting" stands in marked contrast to the "long range sprouting" discussed above. The key difference is whether the new contacts formed cross defineable somatotopic borders. For "long range sprouting" as defined above, they must; for "short range sprouting" they may or may not. For example, within the medial dorsal horn, a new local contact made by the short range sprouting of a thigh afferent onto the dendrite of a local medial dorsal horn cell violates the somatotopy of the medial dorsal horn and is therefore "a somatotopically inappropriate short range sprout"; the same new synapse made on a medially extending dendrite of a cell located in the lateral dorsal horn does not cross a somatotopic border and is therefore a "somatotopically appropriate short range sprout".

SPECIFIC EVIDENCE

Althought the mechanism(s) underlying somatotopic respecification in the adult mammalian CNS are not known at present, there has been steady progress at narrowing the options. The lines of attack fall roughly into three categories:

(1) <u>The search for long range sprouts:</u> In well defined systems it is possible to predict the trajectory and the length of newly outgrowing sprouts that should come into being under this option . The evidence so far has been

consistently negative (see above). Indeed, even the early claims of long distance sprouting across somatosensory maps following massive rhizotomy (Liu and Chambers, 1958) are no longer accepted by most authors (see chapter by P.Brown in this volume). Without minimizing the uncertainties of negative evidence, this now appears a less fruitful line of investigation than it once did.

(2) The search for somatotopically inappropriate connections in normal animals: Here substantial positive evidence has accummulated. In many systems it has been shown that cells with restricted functional RF's (defined by natural stimulation of the skin) respond, and often at short latency, to electrical stimulation of nerves serving skin outside the RF (Merrill and Wall, 1972; Devor and Wall, 1981a). With electrical stimulation, the synchroneity of the afferent volley is expected to augment otherwise weak synaptic links. Correspondingly, one can often define at least a minimal subliminal fringe with standard intracellular recording methods. During prolonged observations of individual dorsal horn neurons, RF borders can often be seen to expand and contract spontaneously as more then less of the fringe is expressed . Furthermore, such meanderings can be enhanced using tetanic electrical stimulation, convulsants, manipulation of anaesthetic level, and variation of afferent input and brainstem descending control (eg. Heavner 1975; Dubuisson et al.,1979; Devor and Wall, 1981a; Saade et al.,1982; McMahon and Wall, 1984). In some systems RF's may undergo somatotopic expansion and/or shift immediately upon functional deafferentation (Dostrovsky et al., 1976; Merzenich et al.,1984), although generally one has to wait days or weeks. As stated above, the anatomical substrates at the spinal level for the normally unexpressed synaptic drive indicated in these electrophysiological studies, both polysynaptic and monosynaptic, has recently begun to fall into place.

(3) Mechanism(s) that strengthen relatively ineffective synaptic drive: Although this question remains wide open, circumstantial evidence suggests that a number of different mechanisms may be at work simultaneously, each with its own characteristic time-frame (Wall, 1985). In the short term (milliseconds - seconds), pre- and especially postsynaptic inhibition is clearly important. In the intermediate term (seconds - hours), exciting new evidence concerning the gating of afferent A-fiber input by cumulative activity in afferent C-fiber drive has begun to appear (McMahon and

Wall, 1984; Wall, 1985). In the long term (hours - days) there are a number of tantalizing observations suggesting trophic regulation of the gain of dorsal horn circuitry by means of the primary afferent depolarization (PAD) mechanism (Wall and Devor, 1981; Wall, 1982) and perhaps by the regulation of synaptic density .

ACKNOWLEDGEMENTS

Supported by the United States - Israel Binational Science Foundation and the International Spinal Research Trust.

REFERENCES

Arvidsson, J, Ygge, J, Grant, G (1986). Cell loss in lumbar dorsal root ganglia and transganglionic degeneration after sciatic nerve resection in the rat. Brain Res 373:15-21.

Basbaum,AI, Wall,PD (1976). Chronic changes in the response of cells in adult cat dorsal horn following partial deafferentation: the appearance of responding cells in a previously non-responsive region. Brain Res 116:181-204.

Brown, AG, Noble,R (1982). Connexions between hair follicle afferent fibers and spinocervical tract neurons in the cat:the synthesis of receptive fields.J Physiol 323:77-91.

Brown, PB, Moraff,H, Tapper, DN (1973). Functional organization of the cat's dorsal horn: spontaneous activity and central cell response to single impulses in single type I fibers. J Neurophysiol 36: 827-839.

Csillik, B, Knyihar-Csillik, E (1986). "The Protean Gate" Budapest, Akademiai Kiado.

Devor,M (1983). Plasticity of spinal cord somatotopy in adult mammals: involvement of relatively ineffective synapses. In:" Nervous System Regeneration" B.Haber, JR Perez-Polo, GA Hashim, and A-M Giuffrida-Stella eds. New York, Liss pp 287-314.

Devor, M (1984a). The pathophysiology and anatomy of damaged nerve. in: "Textbook of Pain." London, Churchill-Livingston pp 49-64.

Devor,M (1984b). Spinal cord plasticity induced by peripheral nerve injury and some consequences for sensory dysfunction. In: " Wenner-Gren Center International Symposium 40: Somatosensory Mechanisms" C.Von Euler, O. Franzen, U. Lindblom, D. Ottoson eds. London, MacMillan pp 339-351.

Devor,M, Basbaum ,AI, Seltzer,Z (1986). Spinal somatotopic plasticity: possible anatomical basis for somatotopically inappropriate connections. In: "Development and Plasticity in the Mammalian Spinal Cord" M Goldberger, A Gorio, M Murray eds. Padova, Fidia Research Series vol.3. pp 239-253.

Devor,M.,Govrin-Lippmann,R, Frank, I, Raber,P (1986). Proliferation of primary sensory neurons in adult rat dorsal root ganglia and the kinetics of retrograde cell loss after sciatic nerve section.Somatosens Res 3:139-168.

Devor,M, Wall,PD (1978). Reorganization of spinal cord sensory map after peripheral nerve injury. Nature 275:75-76.

Devor, M, Wall, PD (1981a) The effect of peripheral nerve injury on receptive fields of cells in the cat spinal cord. J Comp Neurol 199:277-291.

Devor, M, Wall, PD (1981b). Plasticity in the spinal cord sensory map following peripheral nerve injury in rats. J Neurosci 1:679-684.

Dostrovsky, JO, Millar,J, Wall,PD (1976). The immediate shift of afferent drive of dorsal column nucleus cells following deafferentation: a comparison of acute and chronic deafferentation in gracile nucleus and spinal cord. Exp Neurol 52: 480-495.

Dubuisson,D, Fitzgerald, M, Wall, PD (1979). Amoeboid receptive fields of cells in laminae 1,2 and 3. Brain Res 177: 376-378.

Fitzgerald, M, Wall, PD, Goedert,M, Emson, PC (1985). Nerve growth factor counteracts the neurophysiological and neurochemical effects of chronic sciatic nerve section. Brain Res 332: 131-141.

Heavner,JE (1975). Jamming spinal sensory input: effects of anaesthetic and analgesic drugs in the spinal cord dorsal horn. Pain 1:239-255.

Kaas, JH, Merzenich, MM, Killackey, HP (1983). The organization of somatosensory cortex following peripheral nerve damage in adult and developing mammals. Ann Rev Neurosci 6:325-356.

Lisney, SJW (1983). Changes in the somatotopic organization of the cat lumbar spinal cord following peripheral nerve transection and regeneration. Brain Res 259:31-39.

Liu,CN, Chambers,WW (1958). Intraspinal sprouting of dorsal root axons. Arch Neurol Psychiat 79: 46-61.

McMahon, SB, Wall, PD (1984). Receptive fields of rat lamina 1 projection cells move to incorporate a nearby region of injury. Pain 19:235-247.

Mendell,LM, Munson,JB, Scott, JG (1976). Alterations of synapses on axotomized motoneurones. J Physiol 255:67-79.

Merrill,EG, Wall, PD (1972). Factors forming the edge of a receptive field. The presence of relatively ineffective afferents. J Physiol 226: 825-846.

Merzenich,M, Nelson, RJ, Stryker, MP, Cynader, MS, Schoppmann, A, Zook,JM (1984). Somatosensory cortical map changes following digit amputation in adult monkeys. J Comp Neurol 224: 591-605.

Pubols, LM (1984). The boundary of proximal hindlimb representation in the dorsal horn following peripheral nerve lesions in cats. Somatosens Res 2:19-32.

Redman,S, Walmsley,B (1983). The time course of synaptic potentials evoked in cat spinal motoneurones at identified group Ia synapses. J Physiol 343: 117-133.

Saade,NE, Banna,NR, Khoury,A, Jabbur, SJ, Wall, PD (1982). Cutaneous receptive field alteration induced by 4-aminopyridine. Brain Res 232:177-180.

Segev,I, Fleshman,JW, Miller,JP, Bunow,B (1985). Modeling the electrical behavior of anatomically complex neurons using a network analysis program: Passive membrane. Biol Cybern 53:27-40.

Wall, PD (1982). The effect of peripheral nerve lesions and of neonatal capsaicin in the rat on primary afferent depolarization. J Physiol 329: 21-35.

Wall, PD (1985). Future trends in pain research. Phil Trans R Soc Lond 308: 393-401.

Wall,PD, Devor, M (1981). The effect of peripheral nerve injury on dorsal root potentials and on transmission of afferent signals into the spinal cord. Brain Res 209:95-111.

Wall, PD, Egger, MD (1971). Formation of new connections in adult rat brains after partial deafferentation. Nature 232: 542-545.

Wall,PD, Fitzgerald,M, Gibson,SJ (1981). The response of rat spinal cord cells to unmyelinated afferents after peripheral nerve section and after changes in substance P levels. Neuroscience 6:2205-2215.

Wall, PD, Mills,R, Fitzgerald,M, Gibson, SJ (1982) Chronic blockade of sciatic nerve transmission by tetrodotoxin does not produce central changes in the spinal cord of the rat. Neurosci Lett 30:315-320.

Effects of Injury on Trigeminal and Spinal Somatosensory Systems, pages 227–238

CHANGES OF SPINAL CIRCUITRY IN RESPONSE TO ALTERATIONS OF INPUT; AN EVALUATION OF THE DEVELOPMENT AND BASIS OF CONTEMPORARY THEORIES.

P. Wilson, D.E.R. Meyers* and P.J. Snow

Mammalian Neurobiology Laboratory, Department of Anatomy, University of Queensland, St. Lucia, Queensland, 4067 Australia.

*Present Address: Laboratory of Neural Control, National Institutes of Health, Bethesda, Md 20205, U.S.A.

Neurologists have, for many years, documented both transient and permanent perceptual changes in somatic sensation, such as those occurring in amputees, In recent years attempts have been made to explore the mechanisms underlying the capacity of the central nervous system (CNS) to vary its internal connectivity. This paper represents an attempt to evaluate the research strategies and theories which have emerged from recent studies of plasticity in the mammalian spinal cord.

PLASTICITY IN THE MAMMALIAN SPINAL CORD: CONTROVERSIAL ISSUES

The present era of research into mechanisms responsible for long term changes in connectivity probably began with the first demonstration of axonal sprouting in the CNS. In 1958 Liu and Chambers claimed that chronic section of all dorsal roots but L7 (L7 spared-root preparation) caused a considerable increase in the segmental distribution and local density of projection of axons in the spared root (cf. Figs. 1a & 1b). While this much quoted paper established axonal sprouting as a phenomenon relevant to plasticity in the adult CNS, more recent workers have been unable to confirm this result, Goldberger and Murray (1978, 1982) for example, found that in the chronic L6 spared-root preparation the segmental distribution of the L6 dorsal root did not change. They did, however, note an increase in the *density* of the projection of the root to the L6 segment, particularly in lamina II and III of the lateral part of the dorsal horn. The emergent proposal from this work was that following partial deafferentation of a region of dorsal horn there is a proliferation of the arborizations and terminals of intact primary afferent axons which is restricted to the territory they already occupy (Fig. 1c) (see, however, Rodin et al., 1983). This explanation was adopted by Pubols and Goldberger (1980) to account for the reestablishment of normal receptive fields (RFs) of dorsal horn neurons (DHNs) in the lateral part of the L6 dorsal horn in the chronic L6 spared-root preparation (Fig. 1).

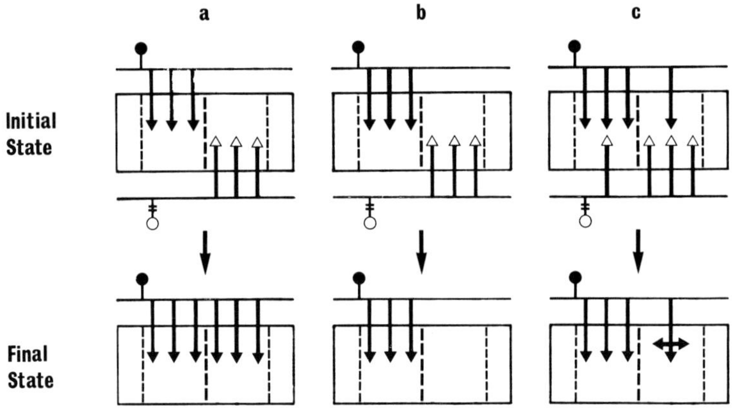

Figure 1. Diagrammatic representation of various proposed effects of chronic dorsal root section on the projection of remaining intact afferent fibers. (a) intact fibers sprout new projections into partially deafferented region. (b) no sprouting of intact fibers occurs. (c) local sprouting of intact afferents in partially deafferented regions to which they already project.

The major alternative to sprouting as a basis of plasticity in the dorsal horn has derived from the work of Wall and colleagues (reviewed by Wall, 1977, 1981 and by

Merrill and Wall, 1978). These workers suggested that longterm changes in central connectivity in the dorsal horn are due not to the formation of new connexions, but to modulation of the strength of preexisting, but "relatively ineffective" afferent connexions. The presence of such connexions may normally only be demonstrated when they are activated synchronously, as for example by electrical stimulation. They therefore play no measurable role in the synthesis of the natural RFs of DHNs, but after partial deafferentation of a region of dorsal horn their efficacy is somehow enhanced, and DHNs thereby acquire new RFs in the dermatomes of nearby spared-roots (Basbaum and Wall, 1976). Intracellular recording from DHNs in the partially deafferented region indicated that the enhancement is due in part to an increase in the strength of monosynaptic inputs from the spared-root (Mendell et al. 1978).

Experimentally, attention rapidly became centered upon the spatial relation between afferent projections and the somatotopic organization of postsynaptic neurons. Thus, in the spinal cord, it was initially important to show that afferent fibers have *somatotopically inappropriate* (SI) projections - that is, projections to regions where the extracellularly determined natural RFs of DHNs do not encompass the RFs of the afferent fibers. Such projections, which must be much less effective in firing DHNs than *somatotopically appropriate* (SA) projections were considered to be likely sites for relatively ineffective afferent terminals. Recent anatomical studies have indicated that the spinal projections of dorsal root axons are too restricted to account for the results of Wall and co-workers. Brown and Culberson (1980), for example, studied the projection of the L3 to S2 dorsal roots to laminae III and IV of the dorsal horn, and found that only those roots caudal to L4 projected to segments L7-S1. Indeed a reexamination of the somatotopic organization of DHNs (Brown and Fuchs, 1975), the extent of the dermatomes (Brown and Koerber, 1978; Kukulinsky and Brown, 1979) and the projections of hindlimb nerves (Koerber and Brown, 1982), have suggested that, within the limits of resolution attainable when comparing data from different animals, afferent fibers project only to those regions where their RFs are represented in the RFs of DHNs.

By definition, SI projections must be ineffective in firing DHNs during natural stimulation. However, the presence of a S1 projection really only represents a known *potential* source of input to a DHN. The presence of subliminal inputs to neurons and the regulation of these by a number of well-documented biophysical and pharmacological mechanisms are phenomena recognized throughout the CNS. Thus the finding of subliminal inputs to DHNs, as described by Wall and colleagues, does not necessarily support the theory that the strengthening of relatively ineffective afferent input from S1 afferent fibers underlies plasticity in the dorsal horn.

The first direct evidence that S1 projections might be involved in dorsal horn plasticity came with the demonstration that chronic section of a peripheral nerve produced quite dramatic changes in dorsal horn somatotopy. Section but not crush of nerves supplying the distal part of the hindlimb in the cat or rat caused DHNs in the medial part of the dorsal horn, which normally have distal RFs, to acquire new RFs on proximal skin (Devor and Wall, 1979, 1981a,b; Lisney, 1982,1983). These authors suggested that the reorganization of RFs was due to a strengthening of preexisting but ineffective connexions between afferents from proximal skin and medially placed DHNs (Fig. 2a). Historically, this seems a curious suggestion in light of the then recent demonstration that the terminals of group II afferent fibers are organized into narrow rostrocaudally oriented columns (for refs. see Brown, 1981), and also the limited mediolateral spread of the dendrites of DHNs (Proshansky and Egger, 1977; see also Brown, 1981).

In 1980 Barbut *et al.* showed that within 5 days of nerve section in the rat substance P disappears from the superficial dorsal horn. At the same time, there is a decrease of dorsal root potentials (DRPs) in the rat (Wall and Devor, 1980), a reduction of primary afferent depolarization (PAD) in the cat (Horch and Lisney, 1980) and a decrease in the A-fiber mediated inhibition of A- and C- fiber evoked excitation of DHNs (Woolf and Wall, 1982). These changes did not occur if nerves were crushed, and not cut. Finally, it was reported that adult rats treated neonatally with the neurotoxin capsaicin, which destroys most unmyelinated primary afferents, also had reduced PAD and a disturbed somatotopic organization of DHNs (Wall, 1982; Wall et al. 1982). Changes of somatotopy also occurred after application of capsaicin to peripheral nerve (Wall and Fitzgerald, 1982). These findings led Wall (1985) to suggest that nerve section prevented the transmission of trophic substances (perhaps peptides) to the dorsal horn via C-fibers. This results in a breakdown of normal inhibitory mechanisms which control the RFs of DHNs, and a consequent unmasking of relatively inaffective afferent terminals. Unfortunately, the experimental basis for this global explanation for the central effects of nerve section is now largely controversial for (a) attempts to replicate the effects of distal denervation on somatotopy in three different laboratories have failed (Brown et al. 1984; Pubols, 1985; Wilson, 1984 and in preparation) and (b) it has been shown that neonatal capsaicin does not affect PAD or DRPs in rats, and any effect it might have on the RFs of DHNs is restricted to those which have C-fiber input (Cervero and Plenderleith, 1984, 1985).

PLASTICITY IN THE MAMMALIAN SPINAL CORD: NEW THEORIES

In 1983 the possible existence of SI projections in the somatosensory system and their involvement in plasticity constituted an important theory, but it still remained to demonstrate them unequivocally. Meyers and Snow (1984) adopted the direct strategy of examining the morphology of the projections of single primary afferent fibers to somatotopically identified regions of the dorsal horn. In doing so they postulated that, owing to the columnar organization of group II afferent projections, SI projections might be distributed rostral or caudal of the SA projections. They found that as many as 42% of the collaterals of hair follicle afferent fibers (HFAs) were SI to the regions of dorsal horn in which they terminated. The SI projections were located rostral and caudal of the SA projections of the same fibers. The SI collaterals more than 600 µm from the SA region showed little branching and had very few synaptic boutons. That at least some of these collaterals are invaded by action potentials has been confirmed by averaging potentials generated at their terminal regions in somatotopically identified regions of dorsal horn (Meyers and Snow, 1986).

The discovery of the SI collaterals prompted us to seek their ontogenetic origin, their synaptic influence (if any) on DHNs, and their possible involvement in plasticity of the adult spinal cord. In neonatal cats the somatotopic organization of DHNs does not show the broader convergence from the periphery that might be predicted if afferents from a larger area of skin were capable of activating postsynaptic neurons (Wilson and Snow, 1985 and in preparation). Neither have we been able to detect monosynaptic input from single cutaneous afferent fibers to DHNs rostral or caudal of the SA region of each fiber (Wilson et al., 1986a).

Concerning the question of whether the SI projections might be involved in plasticity, account had to be taken of the finding that these projections were to be found rostral and caudal of the SA region. In the somatotopic map of Brown et al. (1980) the clearest rostrocaudally organized topographic representation was that of the four digits in the medial part of the dorsal horn. Because these maps lacked the precision necessary for our purposes we made extensive and detailed maps of the dorsal horn in a number of individual cats. This showed that the somatotopic representation of toes 2, 3 and 4 occupies a 3 to 4 mm length of dorsal horn, from the most medial toe rostrally to the most lateral toe caudally. The representation of each toe is delineated from that of the next by a mediolaterally oriented boundary (Wilson et al. 1986b). In order to produce changes in neural circuitry, we decided to try chronic peripheral nerve section. Accordingly, we sectioned all four digital nerves supplying toe 3, providing a restricted region of the somatotopic map in which we could identify the effects of any inputs which normally activate only those DHNs situated further rostral or caudal. To determine the position of the original boundaries between the representations of toes 2 and 3 and of toes 3 and 4 we acutely cut the same nerves in the opposite foot, the somatotopic representation of the two sides being highly symmetrical (Brown et al. 1981) and then used extracellular recording to map the RFs of antidromically identified SCT cells on both sides of the cord (Wilson et al. 1986b; Wilson and Snow, 1987). Shortly after nerve section SCT cells within a circumscribed region of the representation of the denervated toe lacked cutaneous RFs. Thirty to 70 days after nerve section many SCT cells in the region were found to have cutaneous RFs on the adjacent toes and/or on the skin around the base of toe 3. There was no evidence of mediolateral reorganization, in that SCT cells which lost their original RFs did not develop RFs on skin normally represented more laterally.

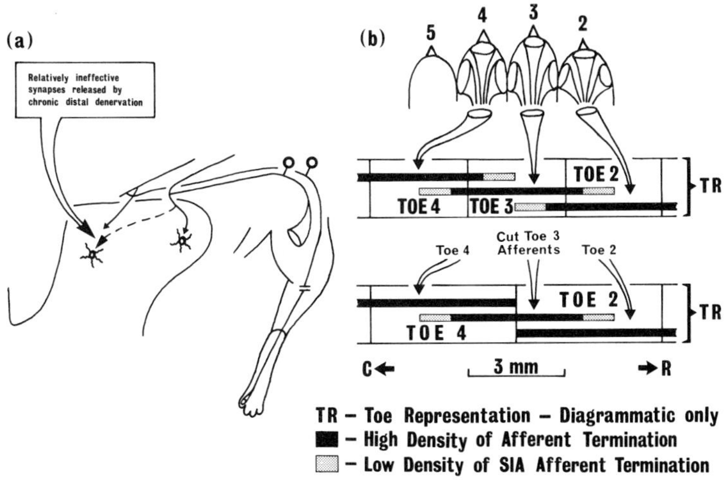

Figure 2. (a) Diagram to illustrate the mechanism of reorganization of dorsal horn somatotopy proposed by Wall and colleagues following chronic peripheral nerve section. (b) Diagrammatic representation of the afferent projection from the digits to the dorsal horn in the cat, and the proposed effect of digital nerve section. Afferents give off many arborizations in the somatotopically appropriate region, and a few sparse arborizations to somatotopically inappropriate regions rostral and caudal of this. Following denervation of toe 3 the inappropriate projections of toe 2 and 4 afferents become activated, possibly by local terminal sprouting, and are able to drive neurons in the toe 3 region. R - rostral; C - caudal.

At present there is thus evidence that reorganization of neural circuitry in the dorsal horn may occur over a rostrocaudal distance of about 1-2 mm, a distance which is equal to or greater than its width, and that in the normal cat, cutaneous afferent fibers have Sl projections which extend for at least this distance rostral and caudal of the SA region. If we wish to speculate that these two observations are related, certain points must be taken into consideration. First, it seems unlikely that the SI projections of HFAs more than 600 μm from the SA region are sufficiently dense to enable them to activate DHNs.

Certainly a search for subthreshold monosynaptic e.p.s.p.s in SCT cells due to activation of SI afferent projections has proved unrewarding. Second, we are persuaded by the studies of Goldberger and Murray (1978, 1982) that deafferentation of a part of the dorsal horn may elicit local proliferation of preexisting terminations of intact afferent fibers. Third, given the likelihood that some kind of denervation supersensitivity develops in deafferented DHNs (Loeser and Ward, 1967) we have no difficulty in agreeing with Pubols and Goldberger (1980) and with Pubols and Brenowitz (1982) that following partial deafferentation local proliferation of the terminals of surviving afferent fibers might substantially increase their effectiveness (Fig. 2b). We thus propose that, following deafferentation of a restricted region of dorsal horn, the SI projections of the primary afferent fibers which normally effect only nearby regions, are stimulated to sprout, thereby becoming effective in exciting DHNs. The SI projections of a primary afferent can thus be regarded as *exerting a latent claim* over the territory adjacent to that occupied by its SA projections. This mechanism might also account for the reorganization seen in the Sl cortex following amputation of a single digit (Merzenich et al., 1984; Snow, Nudo, Rivers, Jenkins and Merzenich, in preparation).

REFERENCES

Barbut D, Polak JM, Wall PD (1980). Substance P in spinal cord dorsal horn decreases following peripheral nerve injury. Brain Res 205: 289-298.

Brown AG (1981). "Organization in the spinal cord." New York: Springer Verlag.

Brown AG, Brown PB, Fyffe REW, Pubols LM (1983). Effects of dorsal root section on spinocervical tract neurones in the cat. J Physiol 337: 589-608.

Brown AG, Fyffe REW, Noble R, Rowe MJ (1984). Effects of hindlimb nerve section on lumbosacral dorsal horn neurones in the cat. J Physiol 354: 375-394.

Brown AG, Fyffe REW, Noble R, Rose PK, Snow PJ (1980). The density, distribution and topographical organization of spinocervical tract neurones in the cat. J Physiol 300: 409-428.

Brown PB, Culberson JL (1981). Somatotopic organization of hindlimb cutaneous dorsal root projections to cat dorsal horn. J Neurophysiol 45: 137-143.

Brown PB, Fuchs JL (1975). Somatotopic representation of hind limb skin in cat dorsal horn. J Neurophysiol 38: 1-9.

Brown PB, Koerber H (1978). Cat hindlimb tactile dermatomes determined with single-unit recordings. J Neurophysiol 41: 260-267.

Brown PB, Koerber H, Culberson JL (1981). Somatotopic organization of cutaneous projections to cat dorsal horn. In Brown AG, Rethelyi M (eds): "Spinal Cord Sensation: Sensory Processing in the Dorsal Horn", Edinburgh: Scottish Academic Press, pp45-54.

Cervero F, Plenderleith MB (1984). Dorsal root potentials are unchanged in adult rats treated at birth with capsaicin. J Physiol 357: 357-368.

Cervero F, Plenderleith MB (1985). C-fibre excitation and tonic descending inhibition of dorsal horn neurones in adult rats treated at birth with capsaicin. J Physiol 365: 223-237.

Devor M, Wall PD (1978). Reorganization of spinal cord sensory map after peripheral nerve injury. Nature 276: 75-76.

Devor M, Wall PD (1981a). Effect of peripheral nerve injury on receptive fields of cells in the cat spinal cord. J Comp Neurol 199: 277-291.

Devor M, Wall PD (1981b). Plasticity in the spinal cord sensory map following peripheral nerve injury in rats. J Neurosci 1: 679-684.

Goldberger ME, Murray M (1978). Recovery of movement and axonal sprouting may obey some of the same laws. In Cotman CW (ed): " Neuronal Plasticity", New York: Raven Press, pp73-96.

Goldberger ME, Murray M (1982). Lack of sprouting and its presence after lesions of the cat spinal cord. Brain Res 241: 227-239.

Horch KW, Lisney SJW (1980). Changes in primary afferent depolarization of myelinated cutaneous sensory fibres during nerve regeneration in the cat. J Physiol 313: 287-299.

Koerber HR, Brown PB (1982). Somatotopic organization of hindlimb cutaneous nerve projections to cat dorsal horn. J Neurophysiol 48: 481-489.

Kukulinsky DH, Brown PB (1979). Cat L4-S1 dermatomes determined using signal averaging. Neurosci Lett 13: 79-82.

Lisney SJW (1982). Receptive fields of spinal cord dorsal horn neurones in cats shortly after peripheral nerve injury. J Physiol 325: 76P.

Lisney SJW (1983). Changes in the somatotopic organization of the cat lumbar spinal cord following peripheral nerve transection and regeneration. Brain Res 259: 31-39.

Liu CN, Chambers WW (1958). Intraspinal sprouting of dorsal root axons. Arch Neurol Psychiat 79: 46-61.

Loeser JD, Ward AA (1967). Some effects of deafferentation on neurons of the cat spinal cord. Arch Neurol 17: 629-636.

Merrill EG, Wall PD (1978). Plasticity of connection in the adult nervous system. In Cotman CW (ed): "Neuronal Plasticity", New York: Raven Press, pp97-111.

Meyers DER, Snow PJ (1984). Somatotopically inappropriate projections of single hair follicle afferent fibres to the cat spinal cord. J Physiol 347: 59-73.

Meyers DER, Snow PJ (1986). Distribution of activity in the spinal terminations of single hair follicle afferent fibers to somatotopically identified regions of the cat spinal cord. J Neurophysiol In the Press.

Proshansky E, Egger MD (1977). Dendritic spread of dorsal horn neurons in cats. Exp Brain Res 28: 153-166.

Pubols LM (1984). The boundary of proximal hindlimb representation in the dorsal horn following peripheral nerve lesions in cats: a reevaluation of plasticity in the somatotopic map. Somatosens Res 2: 19-32.

Pubols LM, Brenowitz G (1981). Alteration of dorsal horn functions by acute and chronic deafferentation. In Brown AG, Rethelyi M (eds): "Spinal Cord Sensation: Sensory Processing in the Dorsal Horn", Edinburgh: Scottish Academic Press, pp319-327.

Pubols LM, Goldberger ME (1980). Recovery of function in dorsal horn following partial deafferentation. J Neurophysiol 43: 102-117.

Rodin BE, Sampogna SL, Kruger L (1983). An examination of intraspinal sprouting in dorsal root axons with the tracer horseradish peroxidase. J Comp Neurol 215: 187-198.

Wall PD (1977). The presence of ineffective synapses and the circumstances which unmask them. Phil Trans R Soc Lond B 278: 361-372.

Wall PD (1981). The nature and origins of plasticity in adult spinal cord. In Brown AG, Rethelyi M (eds): "Spinal Cord Sensation: Sensory Processing in the Dorsal Horn", Edinburgh: Scottish Academic Press, pp297-308.

Wall PD (1982). The effect of peripheral nerve lesions and of neonatal capsaicin in the rat on primary afferent depolarization. J Physiol 329: 21-35.

Wall PD (1984). Introduction. In Wall PD, Melzack R (eds): "Textbook of Pain", Edinburgh: Churchill Livingstone, pp1-16.

Wall PD (1985). Future trends in pain research. Phil Trans R Soc Lond B 308: 393-401.

Wall PD, Devor M (1981). The efect of peripheral nerve injury on dorsal root potentials and on transmission of afferent signals into the spinal cord. Brain Res 209: 95-111.

Wall PD, Fitzgerald M (1981). Effects of capsaicin applied locally to adult peripheral nerve. I. Physiology of peripheral nerve and spinal cord. Pain 11: 363-377.

Wilson P, Snow PJ (1985). Somatotopy in the spinal cord of neonatal kittens. Neurosci Letts Suppl 19: S110.

Wilson P, Meyers DER, Kunze WA, Snow PJ (1986a). Synaptic action of single hair follicle afferent fibers on spinocervical tract cells with overlapping and non-overlapping receptive fields. Proc XXX Congr IUPS.

Wilson P, Meyers DER, Snow PJ (1986b). The detailed somatotopic organization of the dorsal horn in the lumbosacral enlargement of the cat. J Neurophysiol 55: 604-617.

Wilson P, Snow PJ (1987). Reorganization of the receptive fields of spinocervical tract neurons following denervation of a single digit in the cat. J Neurophysiol In the Press.

Woolf CJ, Wall PD (1982). Chronic peripheral nerve section diminishes the primary afferent A-fibre mediated inhibition of rat dorsal horn neurones. Brain Res 242: 77-85.

Effects of Injury on Trigeminal and Spinal Somatosensory Systems, pages 239–248

PERIPHERAL NERVE LESIONS CAUSE EXPANSION OF NEIGHBOURING INPUTS TO SPINAL CORD, CUNEATE NUCLEUS AND CORTEX

Bruce Pomeranz

Departments of Zoology and Physiology
University of Toronto
Toronto, Ontario M5S 1A1, Canada

INTRODUCTION

In 1975 when we began our studies on the central effects of peripheral nerve lesions, there was no literature on the subject. All previous lesions had been on more central structures such as dorsal columns (Wall and Egger, 1971) or dorsal roots (Liu and Chambers, 1958) and these lesions had produced expansion of the somatotopic maps of surviving neighbouring inputs. As central lesions (proximal to the dorsal root ganglion - DRG) would cause terminal degeneration in the central nervous system we reasoned that degeneration products might be the stimulus for "spreading" of neighbouring inputs. In contrast, peripheral nerve section, we reasoned, would leave the DRG intact with no degeneration of central terminals. If we were also to see "spreading" this might imply an active competition for territory, rather than a passive response to degenerating terminals (i.e. a dynamic physiological phenomenon rather than a pathological response).

As we were worried about obtaining negative results in an untried paradigm we optimized our chances of seeing a "plastic" change. To do so we chose to study somatosensory cortex (rather than the less plastic spinal cord) and we chose to study young kittens as they might show more plasticity than adults. When we began to see enormous expansions after peripheral lesions we became brave and studied cuneate nucleus, and adult cats where we also saw similar expansions.

As this was done by a Ph.D. student, John Kalaska it

was 4 to 7 years before we published this work (Kalaska and Pomeranz, 1979, 1982) and by that time we were scooped by Devor and Wall (1978) who showed that peripheral nerve lesions in the adult cat caused expansions of neighbouring inputs in the spinal cord from lateral cord into denervated medial cord. However, their results were not robust as others had difficulties reproducing it (Brown et al., 1984; Pubols, 1984; but see Lisney, 1983). When we switched our attention to spinal cord of adult rats in 1982 we sought a more robust phenomenon and tried cutting the sciatic while sparing the saphenous nerve (others had cut both sciatic and saphenous nerves). This was a fortunate decision, as rostrocaudal expansion in the cord seems to be more vigorous than medio-lateral spreading (Snow and Wilson, 1985).

In the course of all this work many speculations were made on the possible mechanisms of this expansion of neighbouring inputs into denervated zones of the CNS. Two major hypotheses emerged: either there was collateral sprouting of the spared neighbours, or else there was strengthening of weak ineffective (latent) synapses (Wall, 1977). The former hypothesis would be tested by anatomists, the latter by physiologists. We studied the weak synapse hypothesis in the spinal cord of adult rats in which the saphenous nerve had been spared after sciatic lesion (Markus et al., 1984; Markus and Pomeranz, in preparation).

In the following pages we will summarize the research in two parts: (A) the cat cuneate-cortex work and (B) the rat spinal cord work.

A. Cat Cuneate and Cortex Experiments

Methods: Kittens (1.5 to 3 wk old) and adult cats (>6 mo) had the right front paw partially denervated by ligating and transecting the right superficial radial, median and ulnar nerves at the wrist at a level just proximal to the carpal pad. Recordings were made in the left S1 cortex 8-10 weeks after surgery under either Nembutal or Dial anesthesia (no paralyzing agents were used, allowing us to maintain light anesthesia by keeping hindpaw pinch withdrawal reflexes intact). Electrodes for single unit extracellular recordings consisted of glass microelectrodes filled with 1.25 M Na citrate - 5% pontamine blue and bevelled to 5 MΩ resistance (this allowed us to mark electrode paths by injecting dye). Receptive fields for each cell in a track were determined using natural stimulation and cell responses were obtained to electrical stimuli applied at 4 times threshold to each of two nerves: the medial cutaneous which served the spared forearm region, and the ulnar which served the denervated paw. In the S1 cortex study data were obtained in 28 kittens (14 control, 14 operated) and in 14 adult cats (6 control, 8 operated). In the cuneate study 9 kittens were used (5 controls and 4 operated).

Results: Figure 1 shows the results obtained in kittens, while recording from paw cortex (PC), 8-10 weeks after denervating the paw. As can be seen there was a marked expansion of forearm RFs into PC. Only 19% of cells in PC had no detectable RFs. In two kittens in which the neuroma at the wrist was resected just prior to recording, the wrist RFs dropped from 24% to 13%, suggesting only some of the wrist responses were due to neuroma artifacts.

There was a complete loss of somatotopic pattern in the paw cortex of denervated kittens. Forearm and wrist RFs were all intermingled, even within single electrode tracks. All the paw cortex showed the novel forearm and wrist RFs, and hence there was not just a partial encroachment of forearm projections into paw cortex. There was no change in forearm cortex (FC).

When denervation was made in adult cats similar expansion was seen, but not as marked (Fig. 2). Only 7% of neurons in PC had forearm RFs (compared to 52% in kittens). 54% of cells in PC had wrist RFs (compared to 24% in kittens) perhaps suggested a more sensitive neuroma; 37% of cells in PC had no RFs (compared to 19% in kittens). This latter finding suggested that adult "plasticity" was less successful than in kittens. In 2 adult cats, in which the cortex was studied 6-7 months after lesion of the paw (and in which the neuroma was removed just prior to recording), the results were essentially the same as in the 8-10 week adult denervation study shown in Figure 2.

Results obtained with electrical stimulation of the peripheral nerves confirmed these RF studies: the medial cutaneous nerve, which innervates the forearm, drove cells in the PC of kittens and adult cats only after chronic denervation of the paw.

Results in the cuneate nucleus of kittens (adult cats

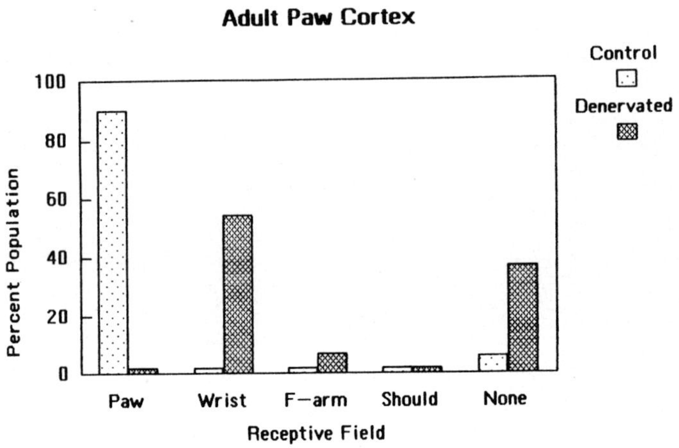

Figure 1. Receptive field locations in paw cortex of 14 control unoperated kittens (white bars), and 14 paw denervated kittens (dark bars). Denervated kittens showed a marked increase in wrist and forearm RF's in paw cortex.

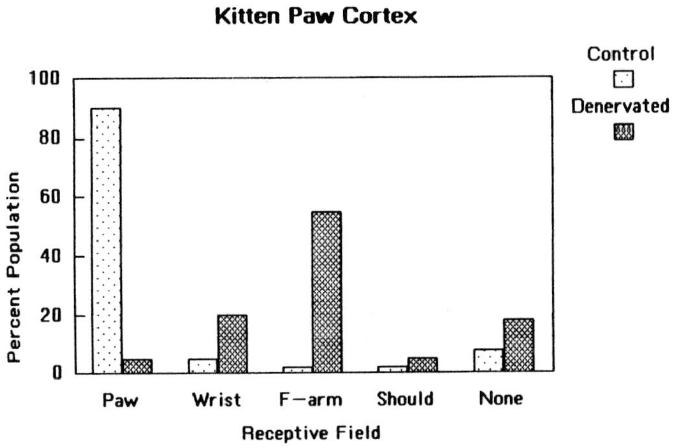

Figure 2. Receptive field locations in paw cortex of 6 control unoperated adult cats (white bars) and 8 paw denervated cats (dark bars). Denervated adults showed less expansion than kittens and more cells with no RF's.

were not studied) showed a spread of forearm RFs from the forearm-cuneate in medial tracks into the paw-cuneate in lateral tracks previously containing RFs in the paw. Thus forearm inputs had expanded into paw-cuneate zones. Moreover, most cells in the paw-cuneate responded to electrical stimulation of medial cutaneous nerve in the lesioned kittens, but not in the unoperated controls.

Discussion: There are four possible hypotheses to explain the expansions which we observed. In hypothesis 1 the expansion could be entirely in the dorsal column to cuneate projection, in hypothesis 2 in the dorsal column to cuneate and cuneate to thalamus projections, in hypothesis 3 in the dorsal column to cuneate and thalamus to cortex projections, and finally, in hypothesis 4 in projections at several levels. As it is almost impossible to determine at what level the expansion occurs by physiological mapping techniques we decided to focus our attention on the first central synapse. However, because of the compact nature of the cuneate nucleus making for small expansions (from medial to lateral), we decided to switch our study to the spinal cord following the reports of expansions by Devor and Hall (1978). We were especially interested in testing the alternative mechanisms to explain the expansion: collateral sprouting versus strengthening of "latent" weak synapses. In addition we concentrated our efforts on adult animals in order to avoid confusing developmental with adult plasticity phenomena.

B. Rat Spinal Cord Experiments

Methods: For all these studies in adult Wistar rats (350-450 g) major surgery was done under halothane anesthesia, which was gradually withdrawn and chloralose substituted to produce a light anesthesia for recording purposes. Gallamine was also used. Touch up doses of chloralose were given every few hours based on anesthetic depth determinations made when gallamine wore off. Somatotopic maps were made with 3 Mohm glass microelectrodes filled with 3 M NaCl for extracellular recording from neurons in dorsal horn of the cord from Lumbar 2 to Sacral 2. Electrode tracks were marked by cutting off the micropipette in situ and clearing the cord post mortem to directly observe the electrode in thick sections of the cord.

Because we spared the saphenous nerve while cutting the sciatic (unlike Devor and Wall (1978) who cut both sciatic and saphenous) we confined our maps to the rostrocaudal direction of the medial cord (where the distal hindleg is mapped), making 6 tracks between L3 and S1 at about 0.5 mm intervals on each side of the cord. Natural stimuli were applied to the hindleg to map RFs, while electrical stimuli were applied to the saphenous nerve in the calf.

Two different experiments were run using the above methods. In the first study, the left sciatic nerve was ligated and cut in the midthigh region (saphenous was spared). On various days post lesion (5, 10, 15, 18 or 21 days) the right sciatic nerve was cut to permit comparisons of left cord (chronically denervated many days before), and right cord (acutely denervated on the day of recording). In the second study no nerves were cut prior to the day of recording, and on the day of the study the sciatic nerve was cut bilaterally (acute denervation), in order to observe the effect of drugs on presumptive weak synapses in the sciatic territory. For this purpose two drugs were used (both by intravenous and direct application onto the cord surface): picrotoxin to block GABA inhibition, and 4 aminopyridine (4AP) to block K channels. The latter potentiates spike invasion into synaptic terminals which should strengthen weak (latent) synapses.

Results: In our initial paper on the rat paradigm (Markus et al., 1984) we established in 15 rats that, at 21 days after chronic sciatic denervation, the saphenous nerve had expanded in a caudal direction in excess of 2 mm to invade, and completely cover sciatic territory. Figure 3A and 3D illustrate the results of this first paper. Figure 3A was obtained from the right side of the spinal cord and 3D from the left side of the cord, on day 21 after chronic denervation of the left sciatic nerve. As shown in Figure 3A, the acute denervation of the right sciatic produced a silent zone (white) in which no RFs could be mapped using natural stimulation. This zone was labelled "sciatic" territory in the figure and extends from the caudal part of lumbar 3 cord segment, to the rostral part of lumbar 6. In the same diagram can be seen the "saphenous" territory rostral to lumbar 3 where RFs from the medial foot could be mapped due to the spared saphenous nerve (cross hatched thick lines). Caudal to lumbar 6 were RFs in thigh and hip area carried by intact thigh nerves (dotted zone). As all tracks were made in the medial cord, thigh inputs were not seen rostral to L6 as these are located in the lateral cord rostrally. The scale in the upper right hand corner is 1 mm long.

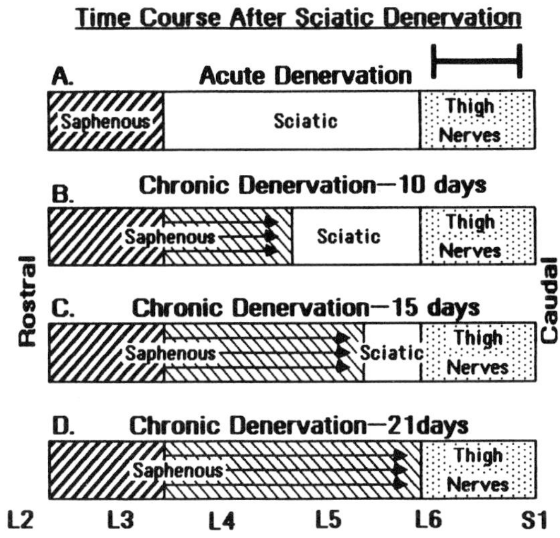

Figure 3. Time course of saphenous expansion after sciatic lesion. Cross hatch=saphenous RF, dots=thigh RFs, white=no RFs in sciatic territory. 3A is control; 3B,C and D show expansion of saphenous caudal boundary from L3 into L4, 5 and 6. Expansion is complete at 21 days. Scale is 1 mm.

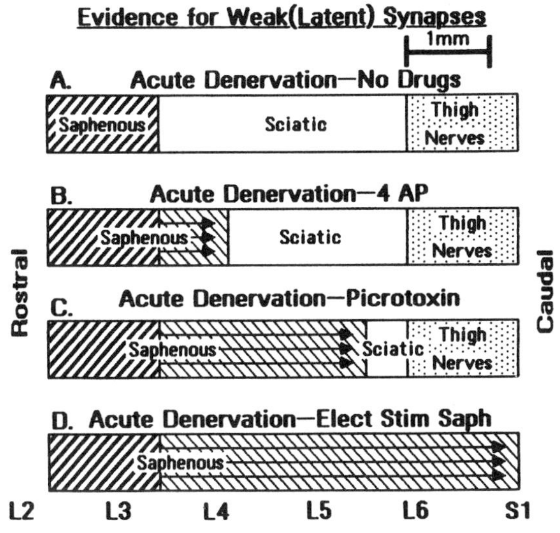

Figure 4. 4B and C show expansion of saphenous RFs into sciatic territory after drugs. 4D shows responses in sciatic territory from electrical stimuli of saphenous.

Figure 3D illustrates the expansion of saphenous RFs into lumbar 4 and 5 (cross hatched thin lines and arrows). In addition to expansion of saphenous inputs into sciatic territory, we also observed enlarged RF sizes; whereas normal saphenous RFs were limited to one toe, after chronic sciatic denervation this enlarged to two or more toes.

Figures 3B and 3C show some of the results of the time course study. Saphenous expansion began at 5 days, reached half way across sciatic territory by 10 days (Fig. 3B), further at 15 days (Fig. 3C), was not complete at 18 days, and only reached completion in the 21 day rats (Fig. 3D).

Figure 4 summarizes the results of the studies to test the possibility that the expansions described above were due to expression of weak (latent) synapses which were present prior to chronic sciatic denervation. In all 4 cases illustrated, the results were obtained in acutely denervated cords (sciatic was cut on the day of recording). The drug 4 aminopyridine (4AP) caused the appearance of saphenous RFs in lumbar 4 cord (Fig. 4B) but only close to the original untreated caudal boundary of the saphenous input in lumbar 3. The rest of the sciatic territory remained unresponsive to natural stimulation of the hindleg. In Figure 4C it can be seen that picrotoxin had much bigger effects causing the expression of saphenous RFs as far caudally as lumbar 5. Only a small zone remained unresponsive. However in both drug experiments we were puzzled by the fact that only a portion of the rats showed this "expansion". For 4AP only four out of 10 rats showed the expression of weak saphenous inputs after drug application, for picrotoxin only five out of 18 rats showed the effect. The remainder of the rats showed no drug effects whether the drugs were given by intravenous or by direct application to the cord surface.

Figure 4D illustrates another test of the weak synapse hypothesis. In acutely sciatic denervated cords, single unit responses were recorded from electrical stimulation of the saphenous nerve not only in sciatic territory (where no RFs were detectable), but also as far caudally as S1 and S2. Post stimulus histograms comparing responses to electrical stimulation of saphenous in acute or chronically sciatic denervated cords showed no significant differences in these ectopic caudal segments (L4 to S2). Because we were using extracellular recording techniques it was impossible to determine whether these ectopic unit responses evoked by electrical stimulation of the saphenous were mono- or polysynaptic in nature.

Discussion: The expansions we observed of saphenous RFs into sciatic territory 21 days after sciatic denervation were very marked and robust. The expansions covered several segments, were in excess of 2 mm away from the usual saphenous boundary, and were observed in all 15 rats studied. Moreover, we did not see thigh inputs spread into sciatic territory even though their boundaries were often closer than the saphenous boundaries. There has been considerable controversy over the Devor and Wall (1978) observations that thigh inputs spread from lateral cord into medial cord after cutting both sciatic and saphenous nerves, some labs replicating (Lisney, 1983), others failing to find any changes (Brown et al., 1984; Pubols, 1984). Devor attributes some of the failures to depressed spinal cords attributed to anesthesia (M. Devor, pers. commun.). On the other hand Snow and Wilson (1985) claim that rostro-caudal expansions are more likely to occur than latero-medial ones as his group has been able to denervate the 3rd toe and find expansion of 2nd and 4th toe inputs in a rostro-caudal direction. Our expansions are also in a caudal direction which is consistent with this latter view, but our results do not directly test the Devor and Wall phenomenon and hence cannot speak to that issue. In addition the time course of the changes we observed was much slower than that of Devor and Wall: in their rat experiments expansion occurred within 5 days, in ours it took 21 days for completion.

Perhaps more important were the studies to determine whether weak saphenous synapses exist which could ultimately explain the expansion if they became stronger over the 21 day period of sciatic denervation. Both 4AP and picrotoxin showed expansion of saphenous RFs in the acutely denervated animal, but we could not explain why the expansions were not seen in every animal. Also electrically evoked responses from saphenous stimulation were consistent with weak synapses being activated by synchronous volleys giving spatial summation.

In the absence of any evidence for long distance collateral sprouting after chronic denervation, it is tempting to speculate that these pre-existing weak synapses become strengthened over the 21 days. How they became stronger is not known. Indeed local collateral sprouting is a definite possibility as M. Murray (pers. commun.) has found electron-microscopic evidence that this can occur in the spinal cord.

ACKNOWLEDGEMENT

This work was supported by grants from NSERC of Canada.

REFERENCES

Brown AG, Fyffe REW, Noble R, Rowe MJ (1984). Effect of hind limb nerve section on lumbosacral dorsal horn neurons in the cat. J Physiol Lond 354:375-394.

Devor M, Wall PD (1978). Reorganization of spinal cord sensory map after peripheral nerve injury. Nature (Lond) 275:75-76.

Kalaska J, Pomeranz B (1979). Chronic paw denervation causes an age-dependent appearance of novel responses from forearm in "paw cortex" of kittens and adult cats. J Neurophysiol 42:618-633.

Kalaska J, Pomeranz B (1982). Chronic peripheral nerve injuries alter the somatotopic organization of the cuneate nucleus in kittens. Brain Res 236:35-47.

Lisney SJW (1983). Changes in the somatotopic organization of the cat lumbar cord following peripheral nerve transection and regeneration. Brain Res 259:31-39.

Liu CM, Chambers WW (1958). Intraspinal sprouting of dorsal root axons. Arch Neurol Psychol 79:48-61.

Markus H, Pomeranz B, Krushelnycky D (1984). Spread of saphenous somatotopic projection map in spinal cord and hypersensitivity of foot after chronic sciatic denervation in adult rat. Brain Res 296:27-39.

Pubols L (1984). The boundary of proximal hindlimb representation in the dorsal horn following peripheral nerve lesions in cats. A reevaluation of plasticity in the somatotopic map. Somatosen Res 2:19-32.

Snow PJ, Wilson P (1985). Plasticity of somatosensory maps in the adult mammalian spinal cord. Soc Neurosci Abs 11: 965.

Wall PD (1977). The presence of ineffective synapses and the circumstances which unmask them. Phil Trans Roy Soc Lond B 278:361-372.

Effects of Injury on Trigeminal and Spinal Somatosensory Systems,
pages 249–259

THE SPARED ROOT PREPARATION: EVIDENCE FOR SELECTIVE CHANGES OF PROJECTIONS FROM SURVIVING FIBERS

Lorne M. Mendell, H. Richard Koerber and Richard J. Traub.

Department of Neurobiology and Behavior, SUNY, Stony Brook, NY 11794.

INTRODUCTION

The spinal cord has been the site of numerous investigations of plasticity of neuronal connections (Mendell, 1984). A potentially attractive feature of this region is its somatotopic organization, from which deviations could provide evidence for plasticity. One potential complicating factor is that the somatotopy is overlaid by a dermatomal organization. Each segment exhibits a medial to lateral somatotopy which represents a distal to proximal "strip" of skin on the dermatome. However, since the dermatomes of adjacent dorsal roots overlap, there is potentially more than a single representation of a given patch of skin in the dorsal horn. Recording the receptive fields of postsynaptic cells in the lumbar dorsal horn suggests that this is not the case (Brown and Fuchs, 1975); however, it is clear that afferent fibers can send terminals beyond zones that are responsive to stimulation of their receptive field (Wall and Werman, 1976; Meyers and Snow, 1984). Such relatively ineffective projections could be a substrate for changes occurring after lesions which partially deafferent the spinal cord (Wall, 1977).

Chronic dorsal rhizotomy has been shown to result in rearrangement in functional central projections of surviving fibers analyzed in terms of receptive fields of the spinal neurons and the distribution of secure short latency projections from the periphery. Such changes have been noted by some (Basbaum and Wall, 1976; Mendell et al., 1978) but not all (Brown et al., 1983) investigators. Possible mechanisms to account for such alterations include sprouting from terminals of surviving afferent fibers and "derepression" of previously present but non-functional connections. Some evidence for sprouting has been reported in the "spared root" preparation (Liu and Chambers, 1958; Goldberger and Murray, 1982) but there is presently considerable debate concerning the operation of this mechanism under these conditions (Rodin et al., 1983).

A further complication is the recent finding that the small primary afferents responsive to noxious stimulation may participate disproportionately in the central adjustments which accompany deafferentation (Sedivec et al., 1983; Pubols and Brenowitz, 1982). Indeed, it is noteworthy that in the periphery, small fibers (nociceptors) seem more able to sprout into neighbouring denervated skin than large fibers (Devor et al., 1979 Nixon et al., 1984; Horch, 1981).

Recently, we demonstrated that spinocervical tract cells in the segment adjacent to a spared root in acutely deafferented cats lost much of their ability to respond to nociceptive and pressure stimuli (Sedivec et al., 1983). This ability was regained beginning 6 weeks after rhizotomy. The implication drawn from these findings was that small diameter afferents in the (spared) L7 dorsal root normally had a weak projection into the tested (deafferented) L6 segment, and that these were strengthened following the chronic deafferentation.

Rostral Extent of Small Afferents

We have investigated these issues by establishing the rostral extent of the small fiber projection in the lumbar enlargement of the cat. Afferent fibers whose peripheral axons are in the A-delta and C fiber groups are known to have a rostral projection although the distance they project is not well established. Anatomically it has been estimated to be as little as 1 (Lamotte, 1977) and as much as 3-4 segments (Culberson and Brown, 1984). These fibers are generally thought to run in Lissauer's Tract separated from the large fibers running in the dorsal columns (Chung and Coggeshall, 1979).

We have used tungsten micro electrodes to stimulate Lissauer's Tract at different levels while recording primary afferent fibers either as volleys in dorsal roots or peripheral nerves, or as single fibers in Lissauer's Tract or intracellularly in dorsal root ganglion (DRG) cells. Control studies revealed that such stimulation using currents up to 100 uA can be highly selective for small fibers in Lissauer's Tract (Traub et al., 1985). By recording from rootlets at various segmental levels combined with stimulation at sites rostral to such rootlets, it was established that at least some A-delta afferents project rostrally as far as 4-5 segments although the decrease in the magnitude of the compound volley measured at a given site indicates that many fibers fail to project more than 1 segment. Simultaneous recordings from a peripheral nerve at 2 sites confirmed that the volleys were generated by A-delta afferent fibers rather than being dorsal root reflexes in large fibers. C fibers were found to project rostrally in Lissauer's Tract but to a much lesser extent than A-delta fibers.

Since A-delta fibers can supply either D-Hair or high threshold mechanoreceptors (HTMR) (Burgess, Petit and Warren, 1968), it was of interest in the present context to establish to what extent each of these populations of afferent fibers projects rostrally. Recordings from primary axons in Lissauer's Tract in the vicinity of their root entry zone revealed the presence of both D-Hair and HTMR axons. About half the axons of each type were found to project rostrally at least 1 segment. Many axons recorded in Lissauer's Tract near their entry zone could be activated antidromically from the dorsal columns and not Lissauer's Tract although many did run in the latter pathway. These physiological findings confirm previous anatomical results (Light and Perl, 1979) that some small fibers pass <u>through</u> Lissauer's Tract to run rostrally in the dorsal columns. In this study such dorsal column fibers, when characterized, were exclusively from D-Hairs. However, many could not be activated and may have innervated nociceptors or other types of receptors which were not found because of inadequate search or lack of an appropriate natural stimulus. All fully characterized fibers whose axons projected in Lissauer's Tract were found to be nociceptors. C fibers axons were too small to be sampled with these electrodes (3M KCl glass pipettes, 20-40 Mohm).

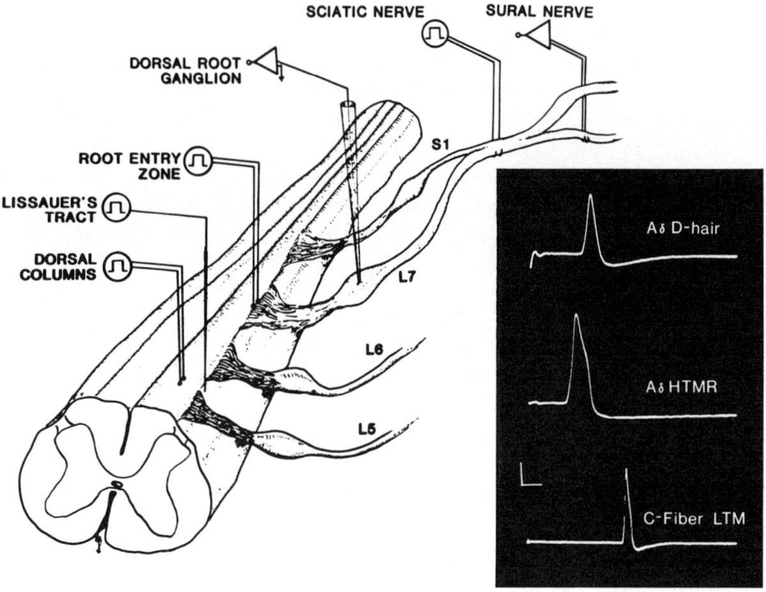

Figure 1. Electrode locations for DRG cell characterization and examples of three somal spikes. Search stimulus delivered to sciatic nerve and axonal projections determined by spinal stimulation. Calibration 2 ms (top trace), 10 ms (bottom trace) and 25 mV.

To circumvent our inability to characterize the adequate stimulus of some afferents and to record from C fibers, we carried out a further series of experiments recording from the DRG. Intracellular recordings from cell bodies with A-delta axons has revealed that HTMRs can be distinguished from D-Hairs based on action potential shape (Rose et al., 1986; Fig. 1); the former have much broader spikes with a characteristic inflection on the falling phase suggestive of a calcium component. It was thus useful to characterize the central projection of cells with these 2 different spike shapes even if peripheral receptors could not be established in each case. Furthermore, it was possible to record from C fibers in the DRG and to establish their projection in the spinal cord (Fig. 1).

These studies confirmed that both D-Hair (narrow spike) and HTMR (broad spike) afferents in the L7 ganglion could project rostrally to the L5 - L6 border in roughly the same proportions (50 - 70%). HTMRs could project either in the dorsal columns (Horch et al., 1976) or Lissauer's Tract. These findings largely replicate those obtained with Lissauer Tract recordings if one assumes that some of the afferents which could not be activated in that study were in fact nociceptors. Furthermore, it is clear from both studies that D-Hair afferents never project long distances in Lissauer's Tract even if they pass through this region close to their segment of entry. The DRG recordings also revealed that C-fibers, which all have broad spikes regardless of whether they innervate high or low threshold receptors, can project up Lissauer's Tract or the dorsal columns for 1 segment although in smaller proportions than A-delta fibers.

Functional Projection of Small Afferents

We then tried to establish whether small afferent fibers could activate postsynaptic neurons in segments distant from the segment of entry. Initial attempts involved recording in the L6 segment with the L5 and L6 dorsal roots cut and stimulating the sciatic nerve in 2 locations. Superficial cells in L6 dorsal horn responded with mean latency differences to stimulation at the 2 peripheral electrode sites indicative of A-delta fiber activation (i.e. distance between sciatic electrode sites (mm)/mean latency difference (ms) $<$ 36 mm/ms). However, it could not be established whether such responses were monosynaptic. A similar problem arose in the interpretation of the responses of such cells to Lissauer Tract stimulation - i.e. were the responses monosynaptic, and in addition, were they responding to primary afferents in this tract or to the axons of interneurons which are also known to project in Lissauer's Tract (see Chung and Coggeshall, 1979)?

To resolve these problems we have carried out a series of studies utilizing intracellular stimulation of single

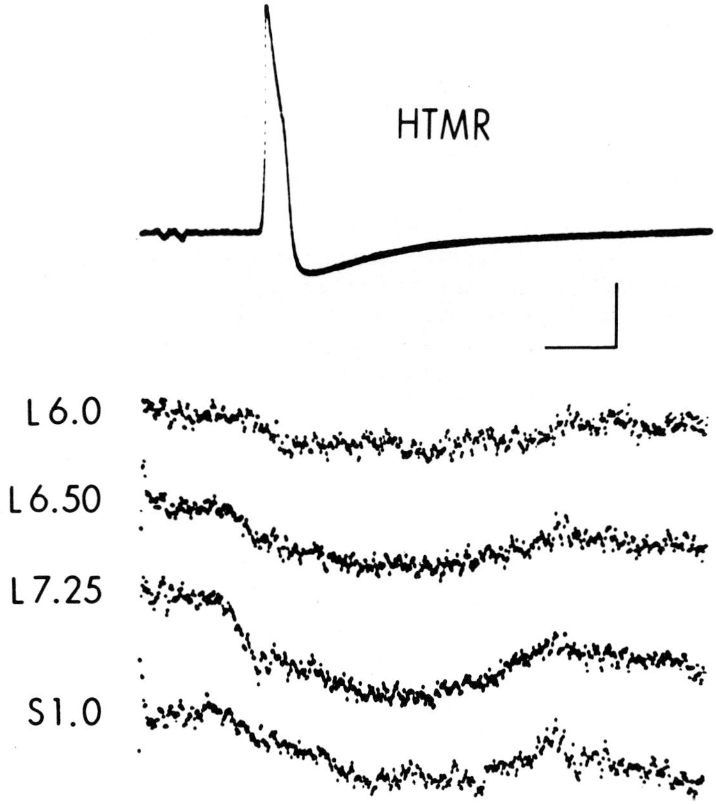

Figure 2. Cord dorsum potentials (CDP) averaged simultaneously at 4 positions ranging from L5/L6 segmental border (L6.0) to L7/S1 border (S1.0). Orthodromic somal spike of activated HTMR in L7 DRG displayed above. Note increased latency of CDP at more rostral positions from L7.25 to L6.0. Latency of CDP suggests monosynaptic delay. Calibrations 30 mV, 5 ms (spike); 2.5uV, 5 ms (CDP).

identified L7 DRG cells while simultaneously recording averaged cord dorsum potentials at 4 sites ranging from rostral S1 to the L5/L6 border (Fig. 2). Stimulation of identified HTMRs evoked short latency components at L5/L6 border which were likely to be monosynaptic. Even with the possible overestimate of the spatial extent of postsynaptic cell activation inherent in the field potential method (i.e. compared to current source density mapping - see Brown and Ritz, 1986), cells in the L6 segment are likely to be activated monosynaptically by HTMRs arriving over the L7 dorsal root.

Taken together, our studies indicate that small primary afferent fibers can travel several segments rostral from their entry zone and can activate postsynaptic cells monosynaptically in at least the neighbouring segment. Thus it seems clear that the enhanced responses in the segment neighbouring the spared root in chronically deafferented preparations, which we have attributed to the action of small fibers, could involve the strengthening of pathways which are already present in the normal animal. This then raises the question of why such responses are so weakened after acute deafferentation. One possibility is that postsynaptic cells cannot be driven by natural stimulation of small fibers in the neighbouring root because so few of them project as far as the neighbouring segment. The central action of these fibers would be strengthened after chronic rhizotomy, perhaps as a result of local sprouting, and would then be able to drive postsynaptic cells when activated with natural stimulation.

What factors might give small afferent fibers an advantage in responding to denervation peripherally or centrally? Previous authors (Yoshida and Matsuda, 1979; also see Fulton, 1986) have suggested that afferents with broad somatic spikes might be less differentiated than those with narrow somatic spikes. Our studies indicate that these neurons persist in the adult and in the case of those with myelinated fibers, are associated with a particular class of sensory receptor (Rose et al., 1986). Since these fibers (A-delta fibers supplying nociceptors) are the only myelinated ones which sprout in the periphery (and possibly centrally), we suggest that this advantage is conferred by their relative immaturity. Whether this ability is related to the particular ion exchanges mediated by channels responsible for the broad spike is at present not known.

Although certain small fibers may play an important role in these adjustments, we have also studied the alteration in functional projections of a more complete spectrum of afferent fibers in a spared root. Studies were carried out for over 150 single afferents in the L7 DRG in seven intact animals and over 50 afferents in two animals surviving 2 months after cutting the L5, L6 and S1 dorsal roots. In intact animals averaged cord dorsum potentials recorded in response to intracellular stimulation of large diameter cutaneous afferents at 18 Hz consisted of a fiber spike followed at monosynaptic latency (0.4 - 0.8 ms) by a potential which rose smoothly to a peak within 0.4 to 0.9 ms. This short latency response was followed by a slow wave of much longer duration. The longer latency wave was present only if preceded by a short latency wave. The amplitude of the short latency response was maximal at one recording location and fell monotonically at adjacent positions (Fig. 3-dashed). The segmental location of the maximum response varied among afferents in strict accordance with receptive field location.

Preliminary results indicate that most afferents in spared-root animals evoked cord dorsum field potentials in response to 18 Hz stimulation similar to those observed in intact animals. There were, however, exceptions: (1) In a few cases the short latency component recorded at the focus of the functional response did not rise smoothly to a peak. Instead there was a break in the slope at 0.5 - 0.8 ms following the onset which was followed by a second potential reaching a peak at a latency indicative of a disynaptic or delayed monosynaptic response; (2) In two instances the response recorded at adjacent locations had central latency longer (1.3 - 1.5 ms) than that elicited at 18 Hz in intact animals; (3) In three different instances (two in one animal) short latency responses were recorded at two different foci, separated by areas at which we could record the fiber spike but no response (Fig. 3). The afferents which gave these unusual responses had receptive fields in the periphery of the L7 dermatome (as determined in each animal by examining the receptive fields of all the sampled afferents) and therefore were probably projecting into areas of more severely deafferented dorsal horn.

The results of these preliminary studies indicate that polysynaptic propriospinal projections from the spared root are strengthened such that they are now

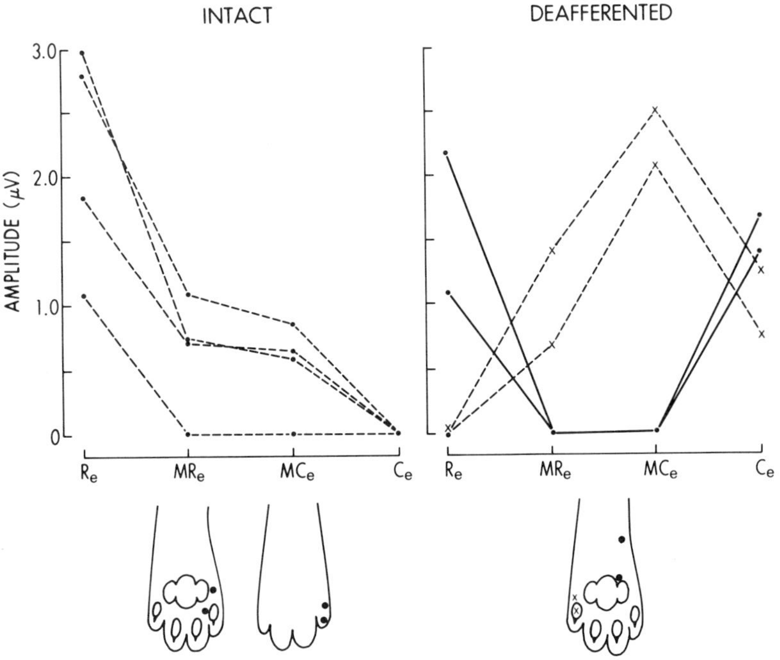

Figure 3. Examples of "profiles" of monosynaptic response amplitudes evoked by single afferents at 4 recording sites (Re, MRe, MCe, Ce). In intact cats profiles always exhibit a single peak. In deafferented cats examples of double peaks were noted in some (solid lines) but not all (dashed lines) cases. R - rostral, C - caudal, M - mid.

capable of following the stimulation at 18 Hz. The finding of 2 discrete monosynaptic response zones in some cases indicates changes in functional projections from afferents in the spared root although the underlying mechanisms cannot be specified at present. Thus changes in functional projections from fibers in the chronically spared root may involve the action of several mechanisms.

Supported by NS 14899, NS 16996 and Harry and Helen Aibinder Scholarship to Richard J. Traub.

REFERENCES

Basbaum AI, Wall PD (1976). Chronic changes in the response of cells in adult cat dorsal horn following partial deafferentation: the appearance of responding cells in a previously non-responsive region. Brain Res 116:181-204.

Brown AG, Brown PB, Fyffe REW, Pubols LM (1983). Effects of dorsal root section on spinocervical tract neurones in the cat. J Physiol London 337:589-608.

Brown PB, Fuchs J (1975). Somatotopic representation of hindlimb skin in cat dorsal horn. J Neurophysiol 38:1-9.

Brown, PB and Ritz, LA (1986). Dorsal horn potentials and current source densities evoked by single action potentials in single slowly adapting type I axons. J Neurophysiol. 55:1104-1113.

Burgess PR, Petit D, Warren RM (1968). Receptor types in cat hairy skin supplied by myelinated fibers. J Neurophysiol 31:833-848.

Culberson JL, Brown PB (1984). Projections of hindlimb dorsal roots to lumbosacral spinal cord of cat. J Neurophysiol 51:516-528.

Chung K, Coggeshall RE (1979). Primary afferent axons in the tract of Lissauer in the cat. J Comp Neurol 186:451-464.

Devor M, Schonfeld D, Seltzer Z, Wall PD (1979). Two modes of cutaneous reinnervation following peripheral nerve injury. J Comp Neurol. 185:211-220.

Fulton, BP (1986). Postnatal changes in active membrane properties of rat dorsal root ganglion neurones. J Physiol Proc (in press).

Goldberger ME, Murray M (1982). Lack of sprouting and its presence after lesions of the cat spinal cord. Brain Res 241:227-239.

Horch KW (1981). Absence of functional collateral sprouting of mechanoreceptor axons into denervated areas of mammalian skin. Exp Neurol 74:313-317.

Horch KW, Burgess PR, Whitehorn D (1976) Ascending collaterals of cutaneous neurones in the fasciculus gracilis of the cat. Brain Res 117: 1-17.

Lamotte C (1977). Distribution of the tract of Lissauer and the dorsal root fibers in the primate spinal cord. J Comp Neurol 172:529-562.

Light AR, Perl ER (1979). Spinal termination of functionally identified primary afferent neurons in the marginal zone and substantia gelatinosa of the spinal dorsal horn. J Comp Neurol 186:151-172.

Liu CM, Chambers WW (1958). Interspinal sprouting of dorsal root axons. Arch Neurol 79:46-61.

Mendell LM (1984). Modifiability of spinal synapses. Physiol Rev 64:260-324.

Mendell LM, Sassoon EM, Wall PD (1978). Properties of synaptic linkage from long ranging afferents onto dorsal horn neurones in normal and deafferented cats. J Physiol (London) 285:299-310.

Meyers DER, Snow PJ (1984). Somatotopically inappropriate projections of single hair follicle afferent fibers to the cat spinal cord. J Physiol 347:59-73.

Nixon, BJ, Doucette, R, Jackson, PC and Diamond, J (1984). Impulse activity evokes precocious sprouting of nociceptive nerves into denervated skin.. Somatosen Res 2:97-126.

Pubols LM, Brenowitz GL (1982). Maintenance of dorsal horn somatotopic organization and increased high-threshold response after single-root or spared-root deafferentation in cats. J Neurophysiol 47:103-112.

Rose RD, Koerber HR, Sedivec MJ, and Mendell LM (1986). Somal action potential duration differs in identified primary afferents. Neuroscience Letters. 63:259-263.

Rodin BE, Sampogna S, Kruger L (1983). An evaluation of intraspinal sprouting in dorsal root axons with the tracer horseradish peroxidase. J Comp Neurol 215:187-198.

Sedivec MJ, Ovelmen-Levitt J, Karp R, Mendell LM (1983). Increase in nociceptive input to spinocervical tract neurons following chronic partial deafferentation.J Neurosci 3:1511-1519.

Traub RJ, Sedivec MJ, Mendell LM (1985). Extent of the rostral projection of small diameter (A & C) primary afferent fibers in Lissauer's Tract. Soc Neurosci Abstr 11.

Wall PD, Werman R (1976). The physiology and anatomy of long ranging afferent fibers within the spinal cord. J Physiol London 255:321-334.

Wall PD (1977). The presence of ineffective synapses and the circumstances which unmask them. Phil Trans R Soc Ser B 278:361-372.

Yoshida, S, Matsuda, Y (1979). Studies on sensory neurons of the mouse with intracellular-recording and horseradish peroxidase-injection techniques. J. Neurophysiol. 42:1134-1145.

Effects of Injury on Trigeminal and Spinal Somatosensory Systems, pages 261–271

SPARED ROOT DEAFFERENTATION OF CAT SPINAL CORD: ANATOMICAL RECOVERY

Marion Murray, Liang-Fang Wu, and Michael E. Goldberger.
Department of Anatomy, Medical College of Pennsylvania, Philadelphia,Pennsylvania and West China Med. Col. Chengdu, PRC

INTRODUCTION

There is now considerable evidence for lesion induced axonal sprouting in the mammalian CNS (reviewed in Cotman, et al.1981). Sprouting remains of continued interest since it is one mechanism which may underlie recovery of function after brain damage and also because sprouting leading to reactive reinnervation implies that the synaptogenesis that occurs in the adult CNS may not obey the strict laws of specificity which obtain during development. Sprouting in the spinal cord, however, is controversial. Most of the evidence for sprouting in the spinal cord is based on light microscopic methods which demonstrate an increased projection of intact pathways after loss of other pathways (Liu and Chambers, 1958, reviewed in Goldberger and Murray, 1978, 1982, 1985). It must be shown, however, that the lesion-induced increase in a projection, which is taken as evidence for sprouting when light microscopic methods are used, is in fact associated with formation of new synaptic contacts by the spared axonal systems. Furthermore, while most of the evidence for sprouting in the CNS has been obtained from rat models, most of the evidence supporting sprouting in the spinal cord has been obtained from the cat. In the rat spinal cord, experiments comparable in some respects to those carried out in the cat have not produced results consistent with axonal sprouting; some authors have interpreted these findings as indicating that sprouting does not occur in the spinal cord (Rodin et al.,1983 , Rodin and Kruger, 1984). Thus, there is the possibility that sprouting described in the cat is artefactual or that the conditions necessary for eliciting or demonstrating sprouting in rat and cat spinal cord differ in ways which may reveal some of the properties regulating sprouting. There are two ways to resolve these issues. One approach is to repeat in the rat the experiments done in the cat to determine to what extent the contradictory results represent species differences which may reflect underlying anatomical differences and to what extent they represent methodological differences. A second approach is to compare, at the EM level, the synaptic population in regions in which sprouting has been described. An absence of sprouting should be reflected in a permanent denervation; a recovery of synaptic number should indicate sprouting. In this paper, we will describe results concerning the second of these two approaches: changes in the synaptic population in a target zone implicated in the sprouting response. We chose to study two preparations in which sprouting has been described in the adult cat: the complete lumbosacral deafferentation model in which propriospinal or descending systems sprout to replace dorsal roots (Goldberger and Murray, 1974, Tessler et al., 1980, 1981, 1984), and the spared root preparation in which all lumbosacral roots except L6 have been sectioned and in which the spared dorsal root sprouts (Liu and Chambers, 1958, Goldberger and Murray, 1982). We have focussed on the synaptic population in lamina II at the L6 level in these two preparations.

METHODS

We sectioned lumbosacral dorsal roots extradurally (or removed the ganglia) unilaterally in adult cats according to methods described in detail elsewhere (Goldberger and Murray, 1974, 1982). Animals were allowed to survive for 2 days to 2 years and then sacrificed by intracardiac perfusion. The spinal cords were dissected out and blocks of tissue were prepared for EM. On semithin sections, stained with toluidine blue, lamina II was identified, using cytoatchitectural criteria, and the area measured planimetrically to estimate shrinkage due to the deafferentation. Thin sections were then cut to include the entire cross section of lamina II. At the electron microscope, lamina II was outlined and systematically photographed.

Synaptic terminals were counted and the size, vesicle content, number of postsynaptic contacts, the length of the postsynaptic contact and the identity of the postsynaptic structure were measured or classified. The photographs from lumbosacral deafferented animals were further analyzed stereologically to determine changes in composition of the neuropil (Murray and Goldberger, 1986). All results were analyzed statistically.

RESULTS

1. Lamina II. Lamina II contains densely packed small neurons. These cells receive a dense projection from the unmyelinated population of dorsal root axons as well as descending projections and projections from local interneurons. The laminar boundaries are rather easily recognized owing to the paucity of myelinated fibers in lamina II compared to laminae I and III. The synaptic population includes central (or scalloped or glomerular) terminals, those large terminals which contain spherical vesicles and make more than one synaptic contact upon different postsynaptic profiles. There are at least 3 morphologically distinguishable subtypes of central terminals (Wu et al., 1986a) but all appear to arise from dorsal root axons and some may be peptidergic (deLanerolle and Lamotte, 1983). These central terminals make up approximately 20% of the population of terminals in lamina II and account for about 40% of the area occupied by terminals. For ease of classification we refer to all terminals which make 2 or more contacts per profile as "complex terminals"; in control animals virtually all complex terminals are clearly recognizable as central terminals described by other authors (Ralston and Ralston, 1979, Coimbra, et al., 1974). Most of the remaining terminals are small, about 1/4 the size of central terminals, contain spherical vesicles and make only one synaptic contact per profile; we refer to these as simple terminals. A small percentage of terminals contain pleomorphic vesicles and also make only one synaptic contact per profile. Most terminals make axodendritic contacts (fig. 1).

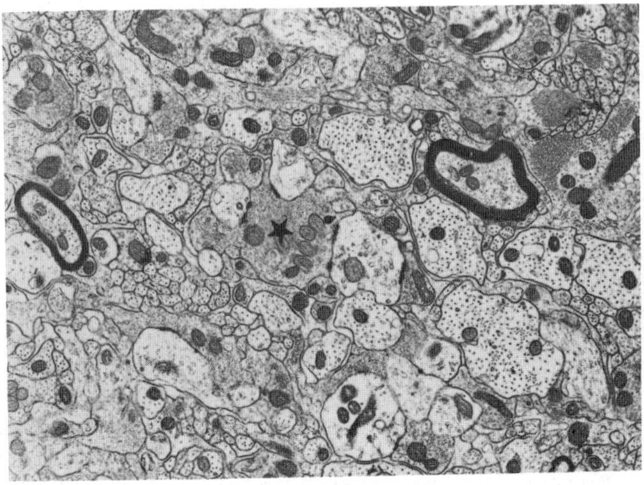

Fig. 1. Electron micrograph of lamina II neuropil showing Complex central terminals (star) and simple terminals.

2. Lumbosacral deafferentation. This lesion elicits a significant increase in glial cytoplasm, recognized by stereological analysis, that persists indefinitely. The lesion also produces a loss in area occupied by axons; the loss of axonal cytoplasm is comparable to the increase in glial cytoplasm and as a result, the deafferentation does not produce measurable shrinkage in lamina II. At early postoperative periods, some examples of degenerating complex and simple terminals can be seen. At later times, conventional central terminals are completely eliminated.

We calculated the number of terminals in lamina II, taking into account the area of the lamina, the total area occuppied by terminals and the mean area of terminals. Interestingly, deafferentation does not produce a loss in the calculated number of synaptic terminals in lamina II, at either acute or chronic survivals, despite the loss of the central terminals. We have suggested that this conservation of terminal number is achieved by a rapid formation of new terminals by spared descending and intraspinal axons (Murray and Goldberger, 1986). Furthermore, our morphometric study of the remaining terminals in the dorsal horn reveals the presence of an unusual type of terminal not found in normal lamina II (fig. 2). This aberrant terminal is small, the size of simple terminals, but makes more than one contact per profile (and thus by our criteria has become a complex terminal) and the active zone is unusual in being convex in contour (Wu et al., 1986b). We suggest that this terminal type may represent another form of lesion induced plasticity expressed by simple terminals.

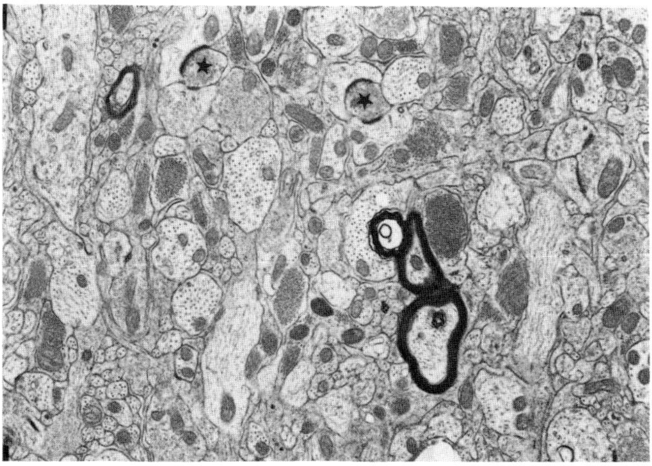

Fig. 2. Electron micrograph of lamina II after lumbosacral deafferentation showing examples of aberrant, small complex terminals (stars).

3. Spared Root Preparation. We examined central terminals in lamina II in several segments. All 3 types of central terminals were found but in reduced numbers on the deafferented side (fig. 3). Since, after complete deafferentation, normal terminal number is maintained and the reduction of synapse number is very slight, we assumed that the smaller lesion (spared root) would not result in a larger reduction in terminals. At the L5 level central terminal profiles were 10% larger, made more contacts and the mean contact length was greater than for terminals on the control side (fig. 4). These results suggest that the remaining central terminals, supplied by the spared L6 root, may undergo morphological changes in response to partial denervation of a shared target and that these altered terminals may compensate for some of the synaptic contacts lost as a result of partial dorsal rhizotomy. The aberrant terminals seen after complete deafferentation were not seen in spared root animals.

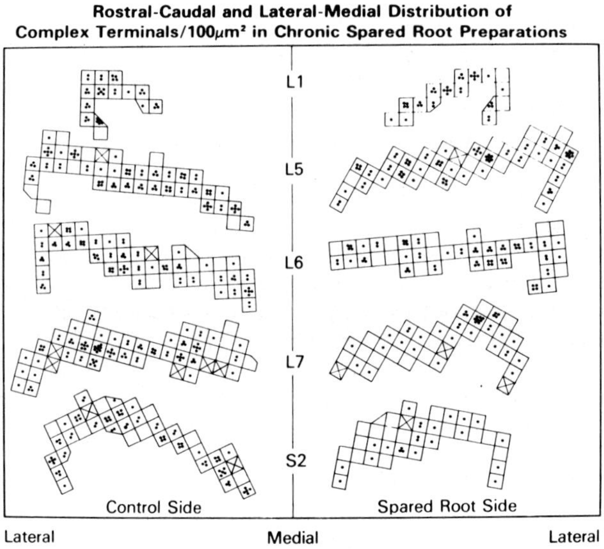

Fig. 3. Distribution of complex terminals and lamina II on spared root preparation on control and operated side. Each square indicates one grid square. Each dot indicates the complex terminals/100 μm^2.

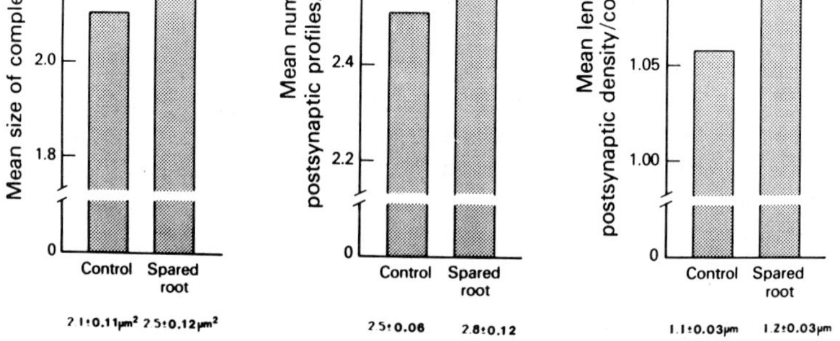

Fig. 4. Comparison of mean cross sectional area, number of postsynaptic contacts, and length of postsynaptic contacts at L5 level on control and operated side in chronic spared root animal.

DISCUSSION

Our results suggest several forms of lesion induced plasticity of synaptic terminals elicited by partial or complete lumbosacral deafferentation in lamina II of the cat spinal cord. These changes include 1) proliferation of simple synaptic terminals from intact systems in response to loss of dorsal root afferents, 2) formation of an aberrant form of simple terminal arising from intact axons in which the number and shape of contacts is changed, and 3) increase in size, number of synaptic contacts and length of postsynaptic density of scalloped dorsal root terminals . Similar changes in synaptic terminals have been described in other systems. Proliferation of synaptic terminals by intact systems has been described in several regions of the CNS (McWilliams and Lynch, 1979 ;Murray et al., 1979, reviewed in Cotman, et al., 1981; reviewed in Raisman, 1985). Formation of additional synaptic contacts by a simple terminal was first described by Raisman in the septum (1969) and has more recently been described for supraoptic neurons under conditions of chronic dehydration stress (Perlmutter et al., 1985). Changes in size and in length of postsynaptic density have been described in the cerebellum (Chen and Hillman ,1982, reviewed in Hillman and Chen, 1985)and changes in the shape of the postsynaptic density have been described in cortex afer several manipulations (Devon and Jones, 1979). Synaptic terminals in the spinal cord therefore seems to share characteristics of morphological plasticity with other synaptic terminals in the CNS of mammals. Important questions remain to be answered, however, before we can predict the functional consequences of these changes: how complete is the replacement and what are the sources of the replacement terminals.

After complete deafferentations, all of the central terminals and some of the simple terminals are lost, but they are replaced rapidly by an equal number of simple terminals from descending and intraspinal sources. It should be emphasized that while the terminal number is conserved, the number of synaptic contacts is decreased since central terminals, making several contacts, are replaced by simple terminals, making fewer contacts. We cannot determine to what extent the replacement is achieved by the formation of new synaptic terminals and to what extent it is achieved by the development of aberrent complexes in which simple terminals make additional synaptic contacts. We have also not identified the source of the replacement terminals, but we can suggest two candidates, the substance P (SP) and serotonergic systems, both of which show postdeafferentation increases in density. Lumbosacral deafferentation in the cat eliminates 75% of the SP from the dorsal horn. The amount of SP partially recovers; the source of this recovered SP appears to be local SP containing interneurons (Tessler et al., 1980, 1981, 1984). These SP interneurons may therefore contribute to the replacement of those dorsal root terminals which contain SP and the replacement may therefore represent a form of homotypic collateral sprouting. A second candidate is the descending serotonergic system, arising from the raphe nuclei, which supplies both lamina I and II. After unilateral deafferentation the density of the serotonin projection in lamina II, as measured stereologically from immunocytochemical preparations, increases significantly (Goldberger et al. 1985, Goldberger and Paige, 1986). These results are consistent with a lesion induced sprouting by serotonergic axons, but in this case the sprouting is apparently heterotypic in nature. The functional significance of sprouting by either of these systems is difficult to predict at present.

Our results in the spared root preparation suggest a form of synaptic plasticity attributable to dorsal root terminals. We know that dorsal roots are capable of considerable plasticity. In the rat, the number of unmyelinated axons in the roots increases following several procedures, including partial deafferentation (Hulsebosch and Coggeshall, 1981). We also know that intracentral dorsal root terminals undergo degenerative and regenerative changes when their peripheral processes are sectioned and that some of these changes are reflected in marked morphological alterations in the central terminals (Knyihar and Csillik, 1985). In our study we were able to provide preliminary evidence that some of these central terminals increase their cross sectional area, the number of contacts and the length of their postsynaptic contact. These changes could be expected to increase the sphere of influence of these terminals coming from axons in the spared root which could sompensate in part for the loss of adjacent dorsal root axons. Since the compensatory reactions occur in neurons similar to those lost, the recovery mediated by these compensatory changes might be expected to be greater than recovery mediated by dissimilar systems after a complete deafferentation.

REFERENCES

Chen S, Hillman DE (1982). Plasticity of the parallel fiber-Purkinje cell synapse by spine takeover and new synapse formation in the adult rat. Brain Res. 240:205-220.

Coimbra A, Sodre-Borges BP, Magalhaes MM (1974). The substantia gelatinosa Rolandi of the rat. Fine structure,cytochemistry and changes after dorsal root section. J. Neurocytol. 3:199-217.

Devon RM, Jones DG (1979). Synaptic terminal parameters in unanesthetized rat cerebral cortex. Cell Tissue Res. 203:189-200.

Goldberger ME, Murray M (1974). Restitution of function and collateral sprouting in the cat spinal cord: the deafferented animal. J. Comp. Neurol. 158:37-54.

Goldberger ME, Murray M (1978). Recovery of movement and axonal sprouting may obey some of the same laws. In Cotman, CW (ed.) "Neuronal plasticity" New York: Raven, Pp 73-96.

Goldberger ME, Murray M (1982). Lack of sprouting and its presence after lesions of the cat spinal cord. Brain Res. 241:227-239.

Goldberger ME, Murray M. (1985). Recovery of function and anatomical plasticity after damage to the adult and neonatal spinal cord. In Cotman, CW (ed.) "Synaptic Plasticity" New York, Guilford Press. Pp. 77-110.

Goldberger ME, Coleman E, Segal S. (1985). Plasticity in the serotonin system of the cat spinal cord. Anat Rec. 211:70A.

Goldberger ME, Paige E (1986). Anatomical plasticity of serotonin (5HT) projections after deafferentatiion of cat spinal cord. Neuroscience Abstracts. In press.

Hillman DE, Chen S. (1985). Plasticity in the size of presynaptic and postsynaptic membrane specializations. In Cotman, CW (ed.) "Synaptic Plasticity" New York: Guilford Press, Pp.39-76.

Hulsebosch CE, Coggeshall RE (1981). Sprouting of dorsal root axons. Brain Res. 224:170-174.

Knyihar E, Csillik B (1985). Fine structure of growth cones in upper dorsal horn of the adult primate spinal cord in the course of reactive synaptoneogenesis. Cell Tissue Res. 239:633-641.

deLanerrole NC, Lamotte CC (1983). Ultrastructure of chemically defined neuron systems in the dorsal horn of the monkey. I. Substance P immunoreactivity. Brain Res. 274:31-46.

Liu, CN, Chambers, WW (1958) Intraspinal sprouting of dorsal root axons. Arch. Neurol. Psychiat. 79:46-61.

Mc Williams R, Lynch G. (1979). Terminal proliferation in the partially deafferented dentate gyrus: time course for appearance and removal of degeneration and the replacement of lost terminals. J. Comp. Neurol. 187:191-198.

Murray M, Zimmer J, Raisman G (1979). Quantitative electron microscopic evidence for reinnervation in the adult rat interpeduncular nucleus after lesions of the fasciculus retroflexus. J. Comp. Neurol.187:447-468.

Murray M, Goldberger ME (1986). Replacement of synaptic terminals in lamina II and Clarke's nucleus after unilateral lumbosacral dorsal rhizotomy in adult cats. J. Neurosc. In press

Perlmutter LS, Tweedle CD, Hatton GI (1985) Neuronal/glial plasticity in the supraoptic dendritic zone in response to acute and chronic dehydratiion. Brain Res 261:225-232.

Raisman, G (1969). Neuronal plasticity in the septal nuclei of the adult rat. Brain Res. 14:25-48.

Raisman, G (1985). Synapse formation in the septal nuclei of adult rats. In Cotman, CW (ed.) " Synaptic Plasticity", New York Guilford Press Pp13-38.

Ralston HJ, Ralston DD (1979). The distribution of dorsal root axons in laminae I, II, and III of the macaque spinal cord. A quantitative electron microsocpic study. J. Comp. Neurol 184:643-684.

Rodin BE, Kruger L (1984). Absence of evidence for intraspinal sprouting in dorsal root axons caudal to a partial spinal hemisection: a horseradish peroxidase transport study. Somatosens. Res. 2:171-192,

Rodin BE, Sampogna S, Kruger L (1983). An examination of intraspinal sprouting in dorsal root axons with the tracer horseradish peroxidase. J. Comp. Neurol. 215:187-198.

Tessler A ,Glazer E, Artymyshyn R, Murray M, Goldberger ME (1980). Recovery of substance P in the cat spinal cord after unilateral lumbosacral deafferentation of cat spinal cord. Brain Res. 191:459-470.

Tessler A, Himes BT, Artymyshyn R, Murray M, Goldberger, ME (1981). Spinal neurons mediate return of substance P following deafferentation of cat spinal cord. Brain Res. 230:263-281.

Tessler A, Himes BT, Soper K, Murray M, Goldberger ME, Reichlin S. (1984). Recovery of substance P but not somatostatin in the cat spinal cord after unilateral lumbosacral dorsal rhizotomy: a quantitative study. Brain Res. 305:95-102.

Wu L-F, Goldberger ME, Murray M. (1986). Dorsal root terminals in lamina II of cat spinal cord: effects of partial deafferentation. Anat Rec. 214:147A.

Wu L-F, Petry-Battisti W, Goldberger ME, Murray M. (1986). Spared root deafferentation of cat spinal cord: anatomical recovery. Soc. Neurosc. Abst.

Effects of Injury on Trigeminal and Spinal Somatosensory Systems, pages 273–280

A REASSESSMENT OF EVIDENCE FOR PRIMARY AFFERENT SPROUTING IN THE DORSAL HORN

Paul B. Brown

Department of Physiology
West Virginia University Medical Center
Morgantown, West Virginia 26506
U.S.A.

INTRODUCTION

In 1958, Liu and Chambers published experimental results intended to demonstrate sprouting of primary afferent collaterals in the dorsal horn after partial deafferentation. Other workers have presented evidence for such sprouting (e.g., Goldberger and Murray, 1974, 1978, 1982; Murray and Goldberger, 1974). Although full unanimity does not exist among the laboratories which have addressed this question (viz., Kerr, 1972; Rodin et al., 1983; Rodin and Kruger, 1984), many describe primary afferent sprouting in the dorsal horn as well established. I suggest that the data are too ambiguous for this conclusion.

THE EVIDENCE FOR SPROUTING

We can exclude all studies of physiological and transmitter changes which occur after partial deafferentation, because all of these studies are amenable to interpretations other than sprouting. Physiological changes such as modifications of somatotopic organization, or of dorsal horn cell receptive fields or responsiveness to various types of afferent inputs, may result from the loss of afferent input and consequent modifications in local network properties (e.g., release from local and long-loop inhibition). Changes in regional densities of transmitters may be physiological responses to partial deafferentation (e.g., changes in synthesis and transport by primary afferents or postsynaptic neurons). Having excluded these types of data, we are left only with anatomical observations.

Liu and Chambers used a degeneration stain to examine the projection of a spared dorsal root, as compared with the projection of its homologue on the intact side. Since the original spared-root surgery would result in degeneration, they performed control experiments in which they produced lesions and examined the spinal cord at different survival times to determine when the degeneration from the lesions disappeared. Then, in chronic spared-root preparations, they severed the spared root and its contralateral homolog at intervals after the spared-root surgery when there was believed to be no residual degeneration from the first lesion. An increased distribution of degeneration stain or increased staining density within the normal distribution on the spared-root side was taken as evidence for collateral sprouting of the spared root.

Some subsequent degeneration studies have largely repeated these results (Goldberger and Murray, 1974; Murray and Goldberger, 1974) with variations on the original paradigm, although Kerr (1972) failed to find cervical afferent sprouting in the spinal trigeminal nucleus, and Goldberger and Murray (1982) found an increased density of degeneration stain in normal projection regions but no projections outside these regions.

Unfortunately, the controls in the Liu and Chambers experiments were inadequate for spared-root experiments. In the only two adult cats in which Liu and Chambers observed no residual degeneration, the lesion consisted of a dorsal quadrant section rather than a spared root. In one case, the only segment examined was 17 segments from the site of the lesion, and in the other case the description of the sections examined suggests a rather cursory sampling. No additional control data have ever been published. The fact that Goldberger and Murray (1982) saw no degeneration outside the normal projection of the test root suggests that there is no residual degeneration (because the initial lesion always involved inputs with other projections). However, their study involved 18 - 24 month survivals, and more modern degeneration stains, which may result in less staining of residual degeneration.

In these later studies, residual degeneration still

might cause the apparent increase in staining density on the previously operated side, but only in regions where the test root normally projects. This may occur in Clarke's nucleus, for example. Goldberger and Murray suggested that earlier reports of apparently novel staining in Clarke's nucleus after previous deafferentation were due to increased staining of a projection which is normally present. The normal projection is difficult to demonstrate because it stains poorly. However, the same argument can be made for old or scant residual degeneration: it may be present, and normally difficult to stain as well. In that case, it is conceivable that the increased stain in a normal projection region may be due to residual degeneration rather than sprouting. Also, as Micevych et al. (1986) have pointed out, there are good reasons to suspect possible staining of glial elements, degenerating dendrites, and degenerating neurons in the chronically denervated neuropil, as well as an increased tendency to impregnation of normal projections not normally seen with degeneration stains. No explanation has been offered for the increased extent of degeneration seen in early studies; if this was indeed an artifact, it seems possible that increased staining in normal areas of projection is an artifact as well.

Transneuronal atrophy and degeneration provide another important alternative explanation for fresh degeneration which is more concentrated or extensive on the previously deafferented side. On that side, the only remaining afferent input to the grey matter is provided by the one remaining dorsal root (except for ventral root afferents). Many neurons on the spared-root side may be sustained only by the one remaining root. When that root and its contralateral homologue are severed, the last remaining sensory input is removed on the previously lesioned side and many dorsal horn cells could die or atrophy. This is transneuronal degeneration or atrophy, which had already been documented in other parts of the sensory nervous system (e.g., Cook et al., 1951) at the time of the Liu and Chambers experiments. However, it is unlikely that any cells on the previously intact side would lose all of their sensory input because most or all dorsal horn cells receive input from more than one dorsal root. This means that, if transneuronal degeneration or atrophy occurs, it will be far more extensive on the previously operated side. The dying cells or processes will contribute to the total distribution of degeneration seen.

Transneuronal degeneration or atrophy could also account for the patterns of degeneration, or the lack of degeneration, seen in these and other experiments. Thus, just as it can be argued that sprouting occurs preferentially in areas which are close to or which overlap the normal projection of the sprouted element (Goldberger and Murray, 1978), the same would be expected in the case of transneuronal effects. Neurons which die or atrophy must have their cell bodies and dendrites in the second denervation zone in order to be affected. These dying cells will often have cell bodies, dendrites, and axonal collaterals in adjacent zones. Therefore, there should be an increased staining density in the normal projection zone of the root, with possible degeneration in adjacent zones as well. The absence of increased degeneration stain in some zones also has a possible explanation: in these zones, the postsynaptic elements may be sustained by inputs from other sources, such as descending tracts.

No one has attempted to determine whether the spared-root preparation results in transneuronal degeneration after cutting the spared root. Cutting one or two roots does not result in loss of cell bodies in laminae IV - VI, but such a lesion may produce dendritic degeneration in these laminae (Brown et al., 1979). Murray and Goldberger (1986) have used stereological analysis of EM material to conclude that there was no detectable loss of postsynaptic neuropil in the substantia gelatinosa after partial deafferentation. It is unclear whether this is a sufficiently sensitive technique to rule out material which would be picked up by a degeneration stain and which might constitute only a fraction of a percent of the total volume. It must be pointed out, however, that transneuronal degeneration occurs mostly in infants; and transneuronal atrophy need not lead to increased argyrophilia (Goldberger, personal communication).

The other methods used to test for primary afferent sprouting include transport methods and electron microscopic counting of synapses. The first studies using axonal transport used the intraganglionic injection of radiolabeled amino acids, and grain counting in different regions of the grey matter (Goldberger and Murray, 1974; Murray and Goldberger, 1974). Goldberger and Murray (1982) have subsequently decided that this method is unreliable, because of asymmetrical uptake. Another axonal transport experiment involved the use of transganglionic transport of horseradish peroxidase (HRP) in peripheral nerves; here no difference was seen in the intraspinal distribution of HRP in experimental and control rats (Rodin et al., 1983; Rodin and Kruger, 1984). The sum of evidence from transport studies is not supportive of afferent sprouting.

In their EM stereological study, Murray and Goldberger (1986) counted the number of synapses in lamina II and Clarke's nucleus after partial deafferentation. They concluded that lost terminals were rapidly replaced by small axodendritic terminals with spherical vesicles. Although these experiments may indicate that something is sprouting, there is no evidence that the sprouted elements are primary afferent fibers. Re-disappearance of the new synapses after cutting remaining roots would provide indirect evidence that they belong to primary afferent fibers, unless they belong to postsynaptic cells and are lost due to transneuronal effects.

In summary, although collateral sprouting of primary afferents may occur in the partially deafferented dorsal horn, and degeneration stain results may reflect such sprouting, other phenomena such as residual degeneration or transneuronal effects may contribute to the positive results obtained with degeneration methods. EM methods show promise of providing the conclusive evidence needed, but such a method would be very tedious for a full description of the distribution of sprouted terminals. I suggest another approach which may be less prone to artifact than degeneration stains.

AN ALTERNATIVE METHOD USING AXONAL TRANSPORT

The main advantage of using axonal transport to study sprouting is that residual degeneration debris and transneuronal degeneration will not affect the results, because we are not looking at degeneration. The method I propose uses transganglionic transport of HRP, as was done by Rodin and Kruger (1984) in the rat, with several built-in controls.

In the <u>control</u> animals, the same root, say L6, is

spared on both sides. This is done on the same day that a peripheral nerve (say, the saphenous nerve) which passes through the spared root is loaded with HRP bilaterally. Thus, the control animals have a bilateral acutely spared root. In the experimental animals, the same procedure is used except that on one side, the experimental side, the spared-root condition is chronic: that is, of longer duration than the acute spared root on the control side.

Both the level of entry through the dorsal roots and the projections of the cutaneous nerves have a high degree of bilateral symmetry in the normal animal (Koerber and Brown, 1981). Crossed projections can be avoided by using hindlimb, tail, or trunk nerves which do not contain axons with receptive fields near the dorsal or ventral midline of the tail or trunk (Ritz et al., 1985). By using bilaterally symmetric lesions of the roots, the nerves have a symmetrical limitation in their access to the spinal cord. There is no experimental asymmetry in the control animals, so they can be used to control for natural asymmetries of projections, levels of entry of the loaded nerves, and uptake of HRP by fibers in the loaded nerves. The only added experimental asymmetry in the experimental animals is in the length of time the fibers have to sprout: on the acute side only a few days are allowed, whereas on the chronic side any longer period can be allowed.

Quantitative methods can be applied to the analysis of projections on the two sides. For each section, a normalized variable is measured, e.g., the fractional mediolateral width of the dorsal horn occupied by stained terminal arbors of sensory axons. The symmetry index for each section is computed from a simple formula:

$$i = \frac{(x_E - x_C)}{(x_E + x_C)},$$

where i is the index of symmetry, and x_E and x_C are the measured values of the variable on experimental and control sides. The symmetry index can vary from −1 (skewed entirely to the control side), through 0 (perfectly symmetrical), to +1 (skewed entirely to the experimental side). This symmetry index can be averaged over adjacent sections to smoothe random variation within an animal, and corresponding rostrocaudal zones from different animals can be compared to assess interanimal variation.

In our application, we would assess populations of symmetry indices for a given rostrocaudal zone, comparing the distribution for control animals against that for experimental animals. A significant difference in populations would reflect a significant change in the regional distribution of stained elements. With an adequate sample size, this approach could compensate for random variations in HRP loading, so that density measurements could be compared.

Naturally, there are possible sources of artifact even after having taken the precautions outlined above. The most obvious is the possibility that sprouted elements may not transport HRP. There is no *a priori* reason to expect this -- if anything, the opposite is to be expected during the sprouting phase, because axonal transport is presumably essential to sprouting. However, altered specificity of transport could affect results. Also, it is necessary to examine such material for transneuronal transport of HRP, to exclude the mis-identification of stained dorsal horn cells and their processes as stained terminal arbors of primary sensory axons. Finally, some method must be developed to compensate for shrinkage.

REFERENCES

Brown PB, Busch GR, Whittington, J (1979). Anatomical changes in cat dorsal horn cells after transection of a single dorsal root. Exp Neurol 64: 453-468.

Cook WH, Walter JH, Barr ML (1951). A cytological study of transneuronal atrophy in the cat and the rabbit. J Comp Neurol 94: 267-292.

Goldberger ME, Murray M (1974). Restitution of function and collateral sprouting in the cat spinal cord: the deafferented animal. J Comp Neurol 158: 37-54.

Goldberger ME, Murray M (1978). Recovery of movement and axonal sprouting may obey some of the same laws. In Cotman CW (ed): "Neuronal Plasticity," New York: Raven, pp 73-96.

Goldberger ME, Murray M (1982). Lack of sprouting and its

presence after lesions of the cat spinal cord. Brain Res 241: 227-239.

Kerr FWL (1972). The potential of cervical primary afferents to sprout in the spinal nucleus of V following long term trigeminal denervation. Brain Res 43: 547-560.

Koerber HR, Brown PB (1982). Somatotopic organization of cutaneous nerve projections to cat dorsal horn. J Neurophysiol 48: 481-489.

Liu C-N, Chambers, WW (1958). Intraspinal sprouting of dorsal root axons. Arch Neurol Psychiat 79: 46-61.

Micevych P, Rodin B, Kruger L (1986). The controversial nature of the evidence for neuroplasticity of afferent axons in the spinal cord. In Yaksh TL (ed): "Spinal Afferent Processing," New York: Plenum, pp 417-443.

Murray M, Goldberger ME (1974). Restitution of function and collateral sprouting in the cat spinal cord: the partially hemisected animal. J Comp Neurol 158: 19-36.

Murray M, Goldberger ME (1986). Replacement of synaptic terminals in lamina II and Clarke's nucleus after unilateral lumbosacral dorsal rhizotomy in adult cats. J Neurosci (in press).

Ritz LA, Culberson JL, Brown PB (1985). Somatotopic organization in cat spinal cord segments with fused dorsal horns: caudal and thoracic levels. J. Neurophysiol 54: 1167-1177.

Rodin BE, Kruger L (1984). Absence of evidence for intraspinal sprouting in dorsal root axons caudal to a partial spinal hemisection: a horseradish peroxidase transport study. Somatosens Res 2: 171-192.

Rodin BE, Sampogna S, Kruger L (1983). An examination of intraspinal sprouting in dorsal root axons with the tracer horseradish peroxidase. J Comp Neurol 215: 187-198.

ACKNOWLEDGEMENTS

This paper was greatly improved thanks to the suggestions of ME Goldberger, BH Pubols, LM Pubols, and PJ Reier.

Effects of Injury on Trigeminal and Spinal Somatosensory Systems, pages 281–288

EFFECTS OF DORSAL COLUMN CUTS ON VARIOUS PAIN TESTING METHODS IN AWAKE AND ACUTE DECEREBRATE RATS

Suhayl J. Jabbur, Nayef E. Saadé and Samir F. Atweh

Dept. of Physiology (S.J.J.) and Div. of Neurology (S.F.A.), Faculty of Medicine, Amer. Univ. of Beirut and Dept. Natural Sci, Faculty of Sciences, Lebanese University, Beirut, Lebanon

INTRODUCTION

Traditional views on pain pathways maintain that spinal nociceptive-carrying systems lie in the ventral half of the spinal cord and are collectively referred to as the ventrolateral tracts. The somatic sensory systems which lie in the dorsal half of the spinal cord including the dorsal column (DC) and the spinocervical tracts are thought not to play a direct role in pain sensation (reviewed in Kerr, 1975). Enough experimental evidence accumulated during the past two decades, however, either modifies or does not readily fit with the traditional views.

The new findings can be briefly categorized as follows: first, pain experience has several dimensions including tonic (or chronic) vs phasic (or acute) aspects and also sensory-discriminative, affective-motivational and cognitive-evaluative aspects with corresponding neural substrates (reviewed in Melzack, 1984); second, descending systems from various areas in the brain can readily influence information along the various ascending nociceptive pathways (reviewed in Fields and Basbaum, 1984); third, reciprocal interconnections have been shown to link the neural stations that define the spinal somatic sensory systems including the spinal dorsal horn, the lateral cervical nucleus and the dorsal column nuclei (reviewed in Jabbur and Saadé, 1985); fourth, the dorsal spinal pathways may play a more direct role, than traditionally assumed, in pain perception (reviewed in Dennis and Melzack, 1977).

Two possible roles in pain mechanisms, either nociceptive-carrying or nociceptive-inhibiting, have been separately proposed for the DC system. Dennis and Melzack (1977) have reviewed the electrophysiological and behavioural evidence from experiments on anesthetized and freely moving animals or man and suggested a nociceptive-carrying role of the DCs, particularly involving the postsynaptic fibers which originate from neurons in the spinal gray. On the other hand, the better-documented pain-inhibiting role of the DC system led to the use of DC stimulation for the alleviation of pain in humans (Shealy et al., 1970). The analgesic effects of DC stimulation were assumed to be due to the activation of 'gating' mechanisms at spinal and/or supraspinal levels. The importance of a DC-brainstem-spinal loop in analgesia has been recently documented in our laboratory in decerebrate decerebellate cats (Saadé et al., 1984, 1985a,b) and in awake rats (Saadé et al., 1986).

The purpose of the present study is to examine further the possible role of the DC system in nociception by observing the effects of DC cuts on tests for phasic and tonic pain in awake rats and the effects of DC stimulation rostral to DC cuts on a phasic pain test in acute decerebrate rats.

MATERIALS AND METHODS

Experiments were carried out on 26 male Sprague-Dawley rats (150-200 g), which underwent surgery under ketamine anesthesia with 7 serving as sham controls and 19 having DC cuts. Through a posterior approach, the DC nuclei and the rostral part of the spinal cord were exposed and, with the aid of a dissecting microscope, a lesion was made at C_2 extending bilaterally from the midline to the entry of the dorsal roots. The completeness of the cuts was verified histologically after carrying out all the testing procedures. Sham-operated rats underwent similar surgery without the DC cuts. Rats were allowed at least one week to recover from the surgery before the start of the testing sessions.

The effects of DC cuts on baseline pain responsiveness were evaluated by employing the tail-immersion (TI) and hot-plate (HP) tests for phasic pain and the formalin (F) test for tonic pain. For the TI test (n=12) each rat was placed in a restraining cage and the distal 5 cm of the tail were dipped into hot water maintained at 50°C (±0.25°C) and the latency of the rat to curl its tail (or tail-flick) was measured and repeated at 5 min intervals during 30 min testing intervals. For the HP test (n=9), each rat was placed on a hot (55°C) copper plate and the latency of licking either forepaw was measured in one or two testing sessions per day (Saadé et al., 1986). For TI or HP test, two baseline latencies were determined and averaged for each rat in 3 testing sessions one week prior and one week after surgery. Each rat served as its own control.

For the F test (n=12), each rat received 0.03 ml of 5% F injected (s.c.) into the dorsal surface of a forepaw, and pain rating was started using the 4-step pain scale described by Dubuisson and Dennis (1977). Following the injection, data were continuously recorded for 60 min by manipulating a 4-position switch of a Grass Polygraph. A pain rating was then calculated for each 180 sec time interval using the formula $T_1+2T_2+3T_3/180$ sec (where T_1, T_2 or T_3 are the durations in sec spent in pain scale categories 1, 2 or 3 respectively). Each rat was used for one trial only because the inflammatory reaction produced by F requires one month for recovery (Dubuisson and Dennis, 1977). More details on the pain tests are described elsewhere (Vyklicky, 1984; Saadé et al., 1986).

The effects of stimulation of the DCs rostral to DC cuts were studied in 4 rats. Following decerebration, light anesthesia with Nembutal was given to insure a stable state of the animal for one hour during which the effects of DC stimulation on the TI test were observed.

RESULTS AND DISCUSSION

In agreement with previous studies using similar DC cuts, there was no evidence of gross behavioural deficits in sensory or motor functions in the recovered rats (Ganchrow et al., 1980; Hayes et al., 1978). This is important because virtually all pain tests rely on the display of motor behaviours. Anatomical verification showed that the lesions completely divided the DCs except for its ventralmost portion which contains the corticospinal tract.

Fig. 1-A and B show the effects of DC cuts on TI and HP tests, respectively; histograms of averages of individual scores (Fig. 1-A1 and B1) and of scores of all rats (Fig. 1-A2 and B2, left) in the respective tests are shown. DC cuts produced small but significant increases in the baseline TI latencies (P<0.01) and similar small increases in the baseline HP latencies which were not significant. No effects were observed on baseline TI and HP latencies in the respective sham-operated rats (Fig. 1-A2 and B2, right).

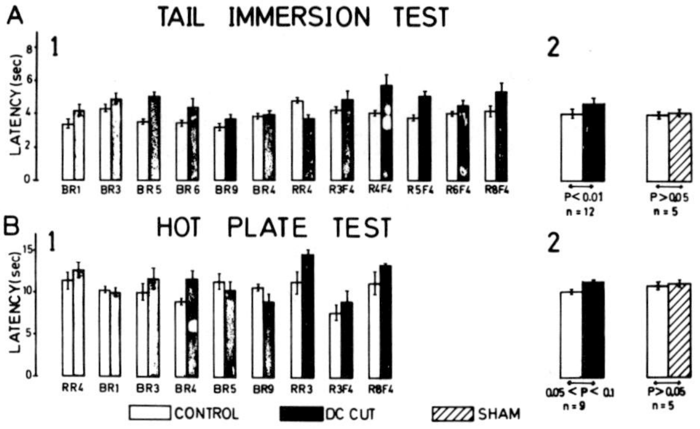

Figure 1. Histograms showing effects of DC cuts on latencies in TI (A) and HP (B) tests. Vertical lines indicate standard errors. 1: mean latencies for individual rats. 2: average for respective histograms in 1 (left) and for another group of sham rats (right). P: Student's t-test.

In monkeys, Vierck et al. (1971) had observed decreased pain reactivity, as evidenced by higher latencies and lower forces of escape responses to shock stimuli, following DC lesions. In rats, Hayes et al. (1978) also observed increase in baseline tail-flick latencies following DC lesions, but disregarded its significance in pain mechanisms because in the same animals shock- and morphine-produced analgesias were unchanged. In the present study, DC lesions produced significant increases in TI latencies while the changes in HP lick responses were not significant. This was not surprising because the two tests are not based on similar neural mechanisms; moreover, results with the two tests from other laboratories have not consistently yielded similar results under identical conditions (Kuraishi et al., 1985). This prompted us to use another kind of pain test.

In contrast to TI and HP tests, the F-test has been used for assessing moderate and continuous pain generated by injured tissues thus measuring tonic (or chronic) aspects of pain. The F-test, however, has two distinct phases: an immediate and short-lived increase in pain rating (the acute phase) followed by a slower and persistent increase in the rating (the tonic phase) that lasts 1.5-2 h in rats. Similar phases of intense burning pain lasting for 5 min followed by throbbing ache lasting 30-60 min have been reported in humans following injection of small amount of **F** into the index finger (Vyklicky, 1984). The tonic (or late) phase more clearly represents chronic pain due to inflammation but the acute (or early) phase is thought to be due to the direct action of F on sensory receptors and would thus be more analogous to the phasic pain produced by the TI and HP tests (Dubuisson and Dennis, 1977).

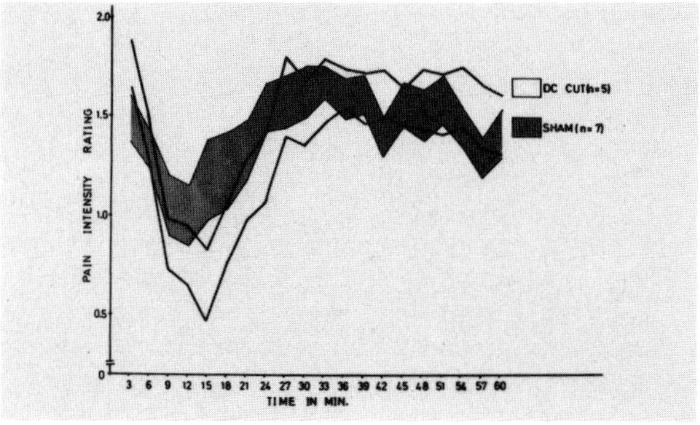

Figure 2. The effect of DC cuts on the time course of pain rating after F injection. Each curve represents a plot of the standard error of the mean (x2) within 3 min intervals.

A comparison of average F pain rating curves following F injection in rats with DC cuts (n=5) with sham-operated rats (n=7) revealed no significant differences in the tonic phase. DC cuts, however, produced a small but significant ($P<0.05$) changes in the acute phase of the pain rating curves including decreases in the 9-24 min interval (Fig. 2).

Thus, DC cuts produced small but significant changes in TI test and acute phase of F test both of which suggest a decrease in the phasic aspects of pain. This finding appears to contradict the better-documented analgesic effects from DC stimulation. We have previously shown that DC stimulation rostral to DC cuts in decerebrate-decerebellate cats produced primary afferent depolarization in lower spinal cord and inhibited flexor withdrawal reflexes and dorsal horn neuronal discharge evoked by various types of nociceptive stimuli (Saadé et al., 1984, 1985a,b). Furthermore, stimulation of the DC nuclei through chronically placed electrodes in awake rats with DC cuts produced clear inhibitory effects on TI test and both phases of the F test (Saadé et al., 1986).

The strong analgesic effect of DC stimulation has been assumed to be due to the antidromic and/or orthodromic activation of large and primary afferent fibers in the DCs (evidence reviewed by Saadé et al., 1984), while pain-signalling has been assumed to be mediated by non-primary high-threshold postsynaptic DC fibers which originate in the spinal cord. We compared the effects of high intensity vs low intensity DC conditioning stimulation rostral to DC cuts in 4 acute decerebrate rats on baseline latencies of the TI test. During high intensity conditioning DC stimulation (10 min, 100 Hz), TI latencies decreased during the first 5 min interval after the start of stimulation and returned to prestimulation values within 5 min after the termination of stimulation. Stimulation with lower intensity (0.05-0.5 mA peak current) shocks produced marked increases in TI latencies similar to what has been reported earlier in awake rats (Saadé et al., 1986). During DC stimulation (with either intensities), special precautions were taken to prevent spread of current to neighboring tracts.

The present results from DC cuts in awake rats and from DC stimulation in acute decerebrate rats are consistent with the notion that pain-signalling fibers are present in the DCs. In their review on pain-signalling tracts in the dorsal and ventral spinal cord, Dennis and Melzack (1977) characterized the post-synaptic DC with the spinocervicothalamic and neospinothalamic fibers as parts of a fast and direct system which mediates sensory discriminative dimensions of pain and triggers appropriate motor responses to minimize the damage done by the nociceptive stimuli in contrast to the paleospinothalamic, spinoreticular and propriospinal fibers which are parts of a slow, indirect and highly convergent system mediating affective-motivational aspects of pain. None of the fiber systems of either group are purely nociceptive and each fiber system has a significant population of multimodal neurons. In such a scheme, therefore, nociceptive and/or non-nociceptive somatic-sensory signalling in one or more pathways of either or both the fast or slow groups would depend on the behavioral state of the organism at the time of injury. In addition to the present study, data from our previous studies consistent with such a view include the demonstrations of analgesic effects via a DC-brainstem-spinal loop (Saadé et al., 1984, 1985a,b, 1986) and of modulatory interactions between DC and ventral tracts in various brain areas involved in nociception (reviewed in Jabbur and Saadé, 1985). These findings illustrate further the kind of complex balance that could exist between several systems carrying somatic sensory (including nociceptive) information and would account for the various dimensions of pain and the variability encountered in all forms of pain treatment.

CONCLUSIONS

First, DC cuts in awake rats caused small but significant decreases in tests for phasic pain as evidenced by increases in latencies of tail-immersion test and decreases in acute (but not tonic) phase of the formalin test.

Second, in acute decerebrate rats, DC stimulation rostral to DC cuts produced either increase or decrease in TI latencies dependent on intensity of electrical stimuli.

Third, the present and earlier findings from our laboratory are consistent with a role of the DCs in both pain-signalling and analgesia.

REFERENCES

Dennis SG, Melzack R (1977). Pain-signalling systems in the dorsal and ventral spinal cord. Pain 4:97-132.

Dubuisson D, Dennis SG (1977). The formalin test: a quantitative study of the analgesic effects of morphine, meperidine, and brain stem stimulation in rats and cats. Pain 4:161-174.

Fields HL, Basbaum AI (1984). Endogenous pain control mechanisms. In Wall PD, Melzack R (eds): "Textbook of Pain," Edinburgh: Churchill Livingstone, pp 142-152.

Ganchrow D, Margolin JK, Bernstein JJ (1980). Component analysis of hind limb behavioral alterations after damage to the rat dorsal funiculus. Exp Neurol 70:339-355.

Hayes RL, Price DD, Bennett GJ, Wilcox GL, Mayer DJ (1978). Differential effects of spinal cord lesions on narcotic and non-narcotic suppression of nociceptive reflexes: further evidence for the physiologic multiplicity of pain modulation. Brain Res 155:91-101.

Jabbur SJ, Saadé NE (1985). Interactions between dorsal column and ventral spinal inputs in somatosensory thalamo-cortical areas and in various brainstem nuclei in the cat. In Rowe M, Willis WD (eds): "Development, Organization, and Processing in Somatosensory Pathways," New York: Alan R. Liss, pp 223-229.

Kerr, FWL (1975). Neuroanatomical substrates of nociception in the spinal cord. Pain 1:325-356.

Kuraishi Y, Hirota N, Satoh M, Takagi H (1985). Antinociceptive effects of intrathecal opioids, noradrenaline and serotonin in rats: mechanical and thermal algesic tests. Brain Res 326:168-171.

Melzack R (1984). Neuropsychological basis of pain measurement. In Kruger L, Liebeskind JC (eds): "Advances in Pain Research and Therapy, Vol. 6," New York: Raven Press, pp 323-339.

Saade NE, Atweh SF, Tabet MS, Jabbur SJ (1985a). Inhibition of nociceptive withdrawal flexion reflexes through a dorsal column-brainstem-spinal loop. Brain Res 335:306-308.

Saadé NE, Tabet MS, Atweh SF, Jabbur SJ (1984). Modulation of segmental mechanisms by activation of a dorsal column brainstem spinal loop. Brain Res 310:180-184.

Saadé NE, Tabet MS, Banna NR, Atweh SF, Jabbur SJ (1985b). Inhibition of nociceptive evoked activity in spinal neurons through a dorsal column-brainstem-spinal loop. Brain Res 339:115-118.

Saadé NE, Tabet MS, Soueidan SA, Bitar M, Atweh SF, Jabbur SJ (1986). Supraspinal modulation of nociception in awake rats by stimulation of the dorsal column nuclei. Brain Res 369:307-310.

Shealy CN, Mortimer JT, Hagfors NR (1970). Dorsal column electroanalgesia. J Neursurg 32:560-564.

Vierck CJ, Hamilton DM, Thornby JI (1971). Pain reactivity of monkeys after lesions to the dorsal and lateral columns of the spinal cord. Exp Brain Res 13:140-158.

Vyklicky L (1984). Methods of testing pain mechanisms in animals. In Wall PD, Melzack R (eds): "Textbook of Pain," Edinburgh: Churchill Livingstone, pp 178-185.

Effects of Injury on Trigeminal and Spinal Somatosensory Systems,
pages 289–296

CHRONIC SPINAL CORD HEMISECTION INCREASES THE RESPONSE OF DORSAL HORN NEURONS TO NATURAL AND ELECTRICAL STIMULATION

Lillian M. Pubols, Harumitsu Hirata and Paul B. Brown
Neurological Sciences Institute (L.M.P.,H.H.) Good Samaritan Hospital & Medical Center, Portland, OR
Department of Physiology (P.B.B.), West Virginia University Medical Center, Morgantown, WV

INTRODUCTION

Early studies on the effects of injury to somatosensory systems were concerned primarily with documenting the behavioral, physiological, and anatomical changes brought about by such injuries. These studies generated hypotheses concerning the mechanisms underlying functional changes following lesions, with a strong emphasis on the mechanisms of reactive synaptogenesis (collateral sprouting) and/or the strengthening of already existing, but weak, projections (e.g., Goldberger & Murray, 1974; Murray & Goldberger, 1974; Wall, 1972). Much subsequent work dealt with evidence in favor of one or the other of these hypotheses. In most cases, however, this evidence was circumstantial. That is, collateral sprouting was shown to occur following injury, or weak projections were demonstrated in the normal animal, but no strong evidence linked these to the changes in function observed after lesions. One of the earliest studies attempting to forge such a link (Mendell et al., 1978) suggested that strengthening of projections which are subliminal in the normal animal is an insufficient explanation for changes seen following deafferentation. A much higher percentage of L7 dorsal horn neurons responded to electrical stimulation of flank skin following partial deafferentation than could be shown to have subliminal inputs from the flank in normal animals. Fortunately, as this volume attests, other investigators are now also attempting to design experiments which critically evaluate the relationship between sprouting and/or weak projections, and functional changes after lesions.

The present study was performed to correlate changes in the response properties of dorsal horn neurons following spinal cord hemisection with the extent and nature of weak projections of sural nerve afferent fibers in the normal animal. We chose this lesion paradigm because previous studies had shown an increase in both receptive field size and responsiveness to sural nerve stimulation following spinal cord hemisection (Brenowitz and Pubols, 1981a, 1981b).

METHODS

Subjects for these experiments were adult cats of either sex. All surgery and electrophysiological recording were carried out under sodium pentobarbital anesthesia. A recent publication (Pubols et al., 1986) describes in detail the methods used for dorsal horn recording.

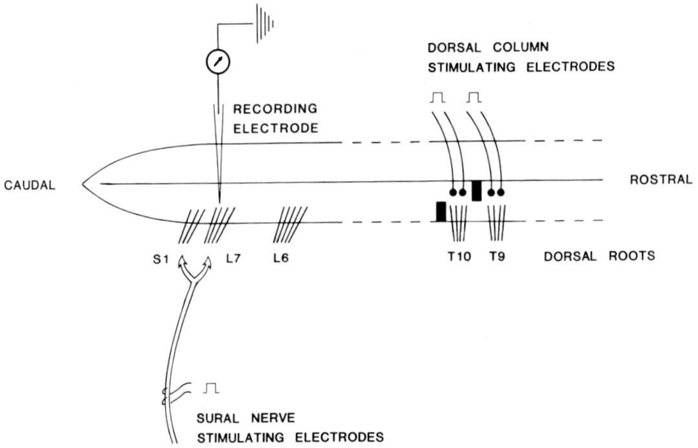

Figure 1. Diagram of recording and stimulating electrodes. Dorsal columns cut between the rostral and caudal thoracic electrodes. Dorsolateral column cut in normals.

In the experiments described in this communication we recorded from neurons in the dorsal horn of segments L6 and L7 (Figure 1). The region of skin supplied by the sural nerve (SN region) was identified in each cat by recording multiunit activity from the sural nerve electrodes while stimulating the skin mechanically. This region, while varying slightly from animal to animal, was generally on the lateral heel and lateral foot, and on the skin over the Achilles tendon and adjacent lateral leg. A dorsal column search stimulus was applied at the level of T9-10 as an aid in localizing dorsal horn neurons that were not spontaneously active. Neurons with well-isolated action potentials were evaluated with respect to their responses to low (1 g von Frey hair, movement of hairs), and high (pressure of up to 1-2 kg applied with hemostatic forceps) intensity mechanical stimuli applied to the skin, and the receptive field was drawn on a scale diagram of the cat's leg. Following this, the response of the cell to shocks to the sural nerve that were supramaximal for A fibers, but subthreshold for C fibers, was tested. Both extracellular and intracellular recording were carried out using unbevelled glass micropipettes filled with 2-3 M KCl and having tip resistances of 10-40 MΩ. Electrode tip potential and capacitance were neutralized by appropriate adjustment of the electrometer.

Spinal cord hemisections were performed in 12 of the animals, using aseptic technique. The lateral and ventral white matter was cut on the right side of the low thoracic spinal cord, sparing the dorsal columns. These animals showed hyperextension of the ipsilateral hindlimb, immediately following surgery. As reported by others (e.g., Murray and Golberger,1974), this symptom abated over a period of weeks, with good recovery of posture and locomotion. Survival times between hemisection and recording were <24 hr (2 cats), 2 weeks (2 cats), and 4 weeks or longer (8 cats).

RESULTS AND DISCUSSION

Evidence for Weak Sural Nerve Projections in Normal Cats

In a recent study (Pubols et al., 1986) we showed that approximately 30% of the cells in the L6 and L7 dorsal horn of the cat responded with impulses to sural nerve stimulation, and that about a third of these (10%) had natural receptive fields that lie outside the region of skin innervated by this nerve. We interpreted these data as supporting the concept of pre-existing, weak afferent projections. More recent experiments have shown that additional cells respond only with EPSPs to sural nerve stimulation (Pubols et al., 1985). An example of such a cell is shown in Figure 2. This cell responded to movement of hairs on the hip and back, well away from the skin region supplied by the sural nerve. It had no high threshold receptive field. Nevertheless, it responded with EPSPs to sural nerve stimulation. The latencies and wave forms of these responses were somewhat variable, suggesting that the projections which mediated them were not monosynaptic.

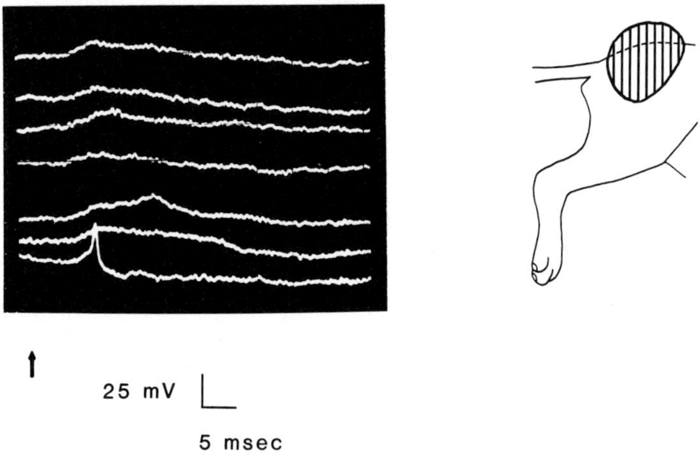

Figure 2. Intracellular recording of the responses to sural nerve stimulation (arrow). Seven successive trials are shown. Natural, low threshold RF of this cell at right.

A summary of the results from 42 cells recorded intracellularly is shown in Table 1. The data for impulse responses are in good agreement with those from a much larger extracellular sample (Pubols et al., 1986). For the subsample which gave no impulses to sural nerve stimulation, about a third (16.7 % of the total sample) nonetheless had a receptive field in the skin region supplied by the sural nerve. We have previously interpreted this to mean that the SN region may be supplied by other nerves. Intracellular recording revealed that one of these cells (2.4 % of the sample) did respond with EPSPs to sural nerve stimulation, but the others did not. For the cells which neither gave impulses to sural nerve stimulation, nor had a receptive field in the SN region, however, about a third gave EPSPs to nerve stimulation. Thus, approximately 19% of our intracellular sample responded only with EPSPs to sural nerve stimulation.

Table 1. Results of Normal Intracellular Sample (42 cells)

		% of Cells	
Response to Elect. Stim. of Sural N.		RF in SN Region	RF out of SN Region
Impulses		26.2	9.5
No Impulses		16.7	47.6
	EPSPs	2.4	16.7
	No EPSPs	14.3	30.9

Effect of Hemisection on Extracellular Responses to Sural Nerve Stimulation

Compared to normal animals, cats with with long term (> 4 weeks) spinal cord hemisections had significantly more cells responding to natural stimulation of the SN region (Table 2; $t = 2.53$, d.f. $= 22$, $p < 0.02$). This result suggests that, as the representation of other regions of skin are also likely to be increased following hemisection, the sizes of receptive fields in general should be increased. This was found to be the case for low threshold fields in the lateral dorsal horn in a previous study (Brenowitz & Pubols, 1981).

Cats with chronic hemisections also showed a moderate (16.8%), but significant, increase in the proportion of cells giving impulses to sural nerve stimulation (Table 3; $t = 2.53$, d.f. $= 20$, $p < 0.02$). This is numerically consistent with a strengthening of the subliminal projections observed in normal animals, where 19% of the intracellular sample responded only with EPSPs to sural nerve stimulation.

Table 2. Responses to Natural Stimulation

	Mean % of Cells with RF in SN Region	# of Animals
Hemisected	52.3	8
Normal	35.7	16
Difference	16.6	

Table 3. Responses to Electrical Stimulation

	Mean % of Cells Giving Impulses to Sural N. Stim.	# of Animals
Hemisected	50.6	7
Normal	33.8	15
Difference	16.8	

Examination of animals hemisected at shorter times prior to recording suggested that a period of several weeks is required for changes to become fully observable. Dorsal horns ipsilateral to acute hemisection appeared to be less excitable than in the normal animal. One of the two animals examined at a 2 week survival time resembled these acute animals, while the other was more similar to the long-term chronic animals.

SUMMARY AND CONCLUSIONS

In summary, then, (1) we have found evidence for weak sural nerve projections to dorsal horn neurons in normal animals, (2) we have observed a significant increase in the responsiveness to those projections following spinal cord hemisection, and (3) the magnitude of this change is consistent with the hypothesis that hemisection acts to strengthen the efficacy of existing afferent projections, rather than by creating new projections. Release of descending inhibition, known to be present in the intact spinal cord (e.g., Brown, 1971; Wall, 1967), is one obvious explanation for these findings. The fact that these changes take several weeks to appear, however, suggests that factors other than, or in addition to, simple release of descending inhibition are at work, as acute hemisection led to depression in responsiveness.

The present findings are not incompatible with an explanation based on very localized sprouting, but, as Brown points out in this volume, the spinal cord sprouting data are limited, and difficult to correlate directly with any current physiological findings. According to Murray et al. (this volume), sprouting may take place with a time course which is too rapid to relate to many slowly developing physiological changes. Studies attempting to correlate physiological changes temporally and spatially with anatomical sprouting of functionally identified projections are much needed.

As an alternative to sprouting, one should not overlook the possibility that denervation triggers changes in one or more types of transmitter receptors within the spinal cord. Receptors are known to be very plastic in terms of their numbers, affinity states, and biological efficacies (Hollenberg, 1985). Helke et al. (1985) have described increased substance P binding in the dorsal horn after destruction of primary afferent terminals by ricin. If denervation causes an increased response to a given amount of some transmitter, due to a change in receptor characteristics, this could explain the increased responsiveness we have observed following hemisection. The study of transmitter receptors appears to be a fruitful, and largely neglected, area of investigation for those interested in effects of injury on somatosensory systems.

ACKNOWLEDGMENT

The assistance of Sue Dawson, Joyce Gregory, Lynn Simmons, and Mark Foglesong is gratefully acknowledged. This work was supported by research grant NS19523 from the National Institutes of Health.

REFERENCES

Brenowitz GL, Pubols, LM (1981a). Increased response to sural nerve input in the dorsal horn following chronic spinal cord hemisection. Brain Research 208:421-425.
Brenowitz GL, Pubols, LM (1981b). Increased receptive field size of dorsal horn neurons following chronic spinal cord hemisection in cats. Brain Research 216:45-59.
Brown, AG (1971). Effects of descending impulses on transmission through the spinocervical tract. J Physiol (Lond) 219:103-125.
Goldberger ME, Murray M (1974). Restitution of function and collateral sprouting in the cat spinal cord: the deafferented animal. J Comp Neurol 158:37-54.
Helke, CJ, Charlton CG, Wiley RG (1985). Spinal cord substance P receptors are present on autonomic and somatic motor neurons: Studies with suicide transport, medullary lesions and neurotoxins. Soc Neurosci Abstr 11:903.
Hollenberg MD (1985). Receptor models and the action of neurotramsmitters and hormones: Some new perspectives. In Yamamura H.I, Enna SJ, Kuhar MJ (eds): "Neurotransmitter Receptor Binding," New York: Raven, pp 1-39.
Mendell LM, Sasson EM, Wall PD (1978). Properties of synaptic linkage from long ranging afferents onto dorsal horn neurones in normal and deafferented cats. J Physiol (Lond) 285:299-310.
Murray M, Goldberger ME (1974). Restitution of function and collateral sprouting in the cat spinal cord: The partially hemisected animal. J comp Neurol 158:19-36.
Pubols LM, Foglesong ME, Vahle-Hinz C (1986). Electrical stimulation reveals relatively ineffective sural nerve projections to dorsal horn neurons in the cat. Brain Research 371:109-122.
Pubols LM, Hirata H, Foglesong ME (1985). Evidence for the existence of relatively ineffective projections from the sural nerve to dorsal horn neurons using intracellular methods. Soc Neurosci Abstr 11:219.
Wall PD (1967). The laminar organization of the dorsal horn and the effects of descending impulses. J Physiol (Lond) 188:403-424.
Wall PD (1977). The presence of ineffective synapses and the circumstances which unmask them. Philos Trans R Soc London Ser B 278:361-372.

Effects of Injury on Trigeminal and Spinal Somatosensory Systems,
pages 297–302

SUMMARY AND CRITIQUE

E. R. Perl and L. Kruger

Dept. of Physiology 206H, University of North Carolina, Chapel Hill, N.C. 27514; and Dept. of Anatomy, Brain Research Institute, UCLA School of Medicine, Los Angeles, CA 90024

Recounting the discussion of the presentations on the effects of injury on dorsal root ganglion (DRG) neurons, primary afferent central terminations or the latter's target neurons is impractical because over 80 comments and questions were directed at the presenters by more than 30 different participants. The following, therefore, is an attempt to synthesize an overview of some issues that were touched upon and to provide some flavor of the concerns and reactions evoked by this set of reports.

The first session was concerned with degeneration or alterations in the central terminals of dorsal root ganglion (DRG) cells after injury or manipulation of the peripheral fibers of the same cells (i.e., transganglionic degeneration). One theme provided by this set of presentations was that almost any injury of the peripheral branches of primary afferent neurons can induce demonstrable changes in their central branches. Changes in central terminations can be provoked by selective removal of part of the afferent innervation to a sensory structure (e.g., vibrissae), or elimination of terminal tissue (e.g., teeth) by natural eruption or surgical removal. Such lesions and some specific cytotoxic agents generally mimic features associated with the more traditional crushing or cutting of peripheral nerve. In spite of general concurrence on the existence of central changes, it was valuable to have documented that even after the many years of study of neuronal injury there exists considerable disagreement about certain signs of degeneration and/or growth and the nature and extent of the various effects observed. The criteria used to evaluate changes in this first set of reports of the session were largely morphological and employed techniques for identifying degenerating or regenerating processes. There were differences in the way possible variations introduced by histological procedures were viewed or taken into account and the consideration given to the kind and significance of putative ultrastructural signs of degeneration. The discussion revealed our limited understanding of the range of morphological variation in normal animals and possible differences among species. Degeneration as evidenced by suppressive argyrophilic methods appears to have a different temporal course than certain presumed electron microscopic (EM) signs of degeneration. However, the timing of even accepted indicators is difficult to interpret because there is evidence for variation in the effects of peripheral injury on different subsets of DRG cells. It was argued by H.J. Ralston that the locus of injury to a DRG neuron determined the nature of the signs of "degeneration." It is not clear how recovery or reorganization might be related to variations in structure and to what extent it is a concomitant of degeneration. How growth, "sprouting" or any kind of extension of a neuronal terminal can be recognized from its fine structure was another point raised that needs to be adequately clarified. The effects of tissue preservation and the normal variants of the flocculent, fibrillary and dense osmiophilic forms of degeneration seen at the EM level diminish the reliability of these signs, an unreliability matched by the ambiguity in interpreting whorls of dilated endoplasmic reticulum and organelle displacement as reliable indicators of ′growth cones.′

Uncertainties in techniques for measuring degenerative changes and their magnitude diminish their value for quantitative analyses. This cautionary conclusion appears to apply to EM studies even when specific patterns of synaptic termination (e.g., the scalloped terminals and glomerular arrangements in the substantia gelatinosa) are utilized as markers to be counted or evaluated. The controls necessary to take into account distortions from fixation and tissue preparation or bias on the part of the observer (e.g., the blinded observer in M. Murray′s report) add to the complexity and the effort required. If, in addition, the temporal stages in the events are considered, appropriate and adequate sampling becomes a formidable task. In sum, the morphology of degeneration still awaits adequate tools.

M. Devor largely deviated from his announced topic and presented provocative data suggesting increases in the number of DRG neurons as a function of increasing age. In the course of studying the effects of section of sciatic nerve, an apparent bilateral increase in the number of DRG neurons was noted as the experimental population became progressively older. These findings sparked a lively discussion since the conclusions were contrary to those reached by Scandinavian workers (G. Grant and colleagues). These differing views evoked consideration of problems of adequately sampling cell numbers (e.g., is the presence of a nuclear profile sufficient for characterizing a cell?) and the methods for pulse labelling neurons so that the time of birth can be determined.

The general question of alterations in the central distribution of primary afferent fibers after some type of deafferentation or denervation was the central theme of a number of the remaining papers dealing with primary afferent neurons and their target central cells. It has become possible to use various combinations of morphological and electrophysiological techniques, but even combined approaches proved open to challenge. The discussion highlighted the equivocal nature of results or the ambiguity of experimental models even when the elegance of labeling single, functionally identified primary afferent fibers with established patterns of projection was employed (Hallas et al.). In the latter experiments no changes in distribution of branches proximal to an injured region were observed; however, the adequacy of the paradigm for testing the ability of primary afferent fibers to sprout in the adult nervous system is problematical. The uninjured processes of those neurons whose projections were evaluated may have been distributed only in areas in which available synaptic positions were occupied. The situation centrally may parallel that observed for peripheral innervation. Reorganization, sprouting or other effects dependent upon extension of cell processes may be possible only in regions where partial denervation of central cells has occurred. To properly test this idea, projections to denervated regions should be sampled, and soundly documented examples of proximal limb projection to spinal cord sites receiving distal limb input would be valuable.

The reorganization of projections to central neurons, as indicated in electrophysiological experiments by receptive field evaluations, was one of the more controversial topics. Given the complexity and heterogeneity of the dorsal horn of the spinal cord and its medullary equivalent, such experiments inherently are subject to doubts about the population studied. Heterogeneity in the population demands observations based upon single unit recordings. Even with systematic and careful efforts to characterize receptive fields of numerous neurons to provide an adequate sample, the general condition of the preparation, including anesthesia, the influence of descending modulation of afferent input and of responsiveness of the central neurons, all add factors difficult to control or evaluate. If these were not sufficient encumbrances to interpretation, there are the added factors of identification of the cell type, its location and the time elapsed following a denervation or modification of the afferent input. It is hardly surprising that there are differences of opinion on the type of effects produced on neuronal responsiveness by deafferentation. Most observers do seem to agree that changes probably take place. Those reported vary from the presence of inexcitable units or holes in a projection pattern from a given dorsal root to more subtle modifications of expected receptive field properties for neurons in given spinal gray loci. The latter include a slow invasion of projection from adjacent innervated tissue. There seems to be consensus that deafferentation in the presence of intact innervation by afferent fibers of nearby segments (e.g., the "spared root" preparation or in the lesser denervation produced by removal of the input from a single nerve) is associated with the appearance of unusual receptive fields or unusual proportions of certain responsive properties by neurons of the regions which had been the excitatory targets of the missing inputs. The new results presented indicate that extension of excitatory projections from innervated to denervated regions tend to occur rostro-caudally along the neuraxis. In most but not all instances, a temporal delay after denervation was required for such shifts in receptive field to become evident. Although the proximal shifts in receptive fields reported by Wilson et al. and Pomeranz et al. differ from the medio-lateral changes described previously by Devor and Wall ('78), the discussion concentrated on the underlying mechanisms rather than upon the receptive field changes.

Two mechanisms considered were "sprouting" or the physical establishment of new contacts and "unmasking" of sub-threshold synaptic connections, defined by Devor as "inappropriate." It is interesting to note that receptive field expansions are usually expressed along with a shift from low threshold to high threshold (nociceptor) mechanoreceptor representation.

In addition to changes in receptive field organization and distribution, the studies employing electro-physiological recordings also describe changes in the behavior of neurons, including enhanced responsiveness and changes in background activity as well as the more frequent appearance of neurons responding solely or principally to noxious stimulation. The change in responsiveness along with the equivocal evidence for sprouting, were probable reasons for the considerable attention paid to alterations of synaptic effectiveness. Some form of denervation supersensitivity to chemical synaptic mediators was postulated by Pubols et al. as possibly underlying certain alterations in neuronal behavior including receptive field modifications. In part, this idea was proposed to account for the delay in the observed alterations; however, supersensitivity as an explanation was challenged because of the absence of direct evidence that postsynaptic receptors had either modified in number or accessibility. The mechanism underlying the "unmasking" of synaptic connections, which is currently so much a part of the vernacular in the literature on denervation, may, in essence, constitute the subliminal fringe described in Sherrington's classical reflex studies. That is, connections made by presynaptic sources to a population of neurons include some effective enough to drive some neurons to discharge, but in others only produce subliminal effects. While this arrangement is generally discussed in terms of excitatory connections, it also applies to inhibitory interactions. Thus the uncovering of connections to neurons outside of the normal excitatory zone for a particular body region could be explained by the removal of the inhibitory connections that are associated with particular excitatory inputs. Such inhibitory arrangements underlie surround or adjacent region inhibition. Therefore, it is unnecessary for synapses to become more effective in order to unmask a subliminal projection; the weakness of the connection or its absence of expression in the intact organism could be the consequence of inhibitory suppression.

Several of the presentations and posters did offer evidence supporting structural reorganization of processes within the adult spinal cord as a consequence of CNS injury or peripheral denervation. The observation by Smith et al. that long processes capable of reinnervating skeletal muscle can grow through ventral roots implanted into the lateral spinal cord suggests that at least certain CNS neurons may possess the capacity for the kinds of growth or reconfiguration that once were widely denied as a possibility for the adult mammalian CNS.

These sessions made it evident that basic issues about changes produced by neuronal injury in the somatosensory system at the level of DRG neurons, in the spinal cord and in the trigeminal nuclei are far from solved. Structural and functional changes clearly do occur. Both the structural and functional changes alter with time after the injury. Do synapses change their capacity? Are new synapses formed? Are the apparent reorganizations in dendritic trees or terminal arrangements the result of growing processes possibly invading new territories? These all remain interesting and important possibilities. However, the evidence on many of these points remains ambiguous. It appears likely that the answers will not come easily and that the proper experiments are very difficult to design and to perform successfully. We have come a distance from the days of Ramon y Cajal, but we still have much to learn before there will be a firm understanding of how central terminations of primary afferent neurons could participate in recovery of function after injury. Resolution of questions concerning reorganization following injury may ultimately be achieved at a morphological level employing modern axon transport labels although the findings to date, including several studies reported at this meeting, have not described regrowth or sprouting of a sufficient magnitude to permit easy detection and measurement.

III
THALAMUS AND CORTEX

Effects of Injury on Trigeminal and Spinal Somatosensory Systems, pages 305–312

NOCICEPTIVE NEURONS IN THE SHELL REGION OF THE VENTROBASAL COMPLEX OF THE THALAMUS

Toshikatsu Yokota, Natsu Koyama and Yasuo Nishikawa

Department of Physiology,
Medical Collage of Shiga,
Seta, Otsu 520-21, Japan

INTRODUCTION

The ventrobasal (VB) complex of the thalamus is the somatosensory relay station. It has been well established that the VB complex receives mechanoreceptive and thermoreceptive inputs, but whether it also receives nociceptive input was uncertain. Recently several groups of investigators (Mitchell and Hellon, 1977; Kenshalo et al., 1980; Peschanski et al., 1980; Honda et al., 1983; Kniffki and Mizumura, 1983; Yokota and Matsumoto, 1983a,1983b; Yokota et al., 1985) have identified nociceptive neurons in the VB complex. The present paper will deal with these neurons.

RESULTS

1. Ventrobasal complex

Krieg (1948) divided the nucleus ventralis posterior into four parts: nucleus arcuatus lateralis, nucleus arcuatus medialis, nucleus posterior lateralis, and nucleus posterior inferior. In Olszewski's (1952) nomenclature, they are nucleus ventralis posterior medialis (VPM proper), nucleus ventralis posterior medialis parvocellularis (VPMpc), nucleus ventralis posterior lateralis (VPL), and nucleus ventralis posterior inferior (VPI), respectively. In higher primates, the VPL is further divided into pars oralis (VPLo) and pars caudalis (VPLc). J. E. Rose and Mountcastle (1952) reintroduced M. Rose's older term ventrobasal (VB) complex to include only somatosensory parts of the nucleus ventralis posterior. In most nonprimates, the VB complex is coextensive with the VPM proper and VPL. It excludes the VPMpc which is the taste relay nucleus. In primates, it also excludes the VPLo.

2. Trigeminal nociceptive neurons in cat VPM

The VPM proper is the thalamic somatosensory relay nucleus of the trigeminal system. The vast majority of neurons in this nucleus are low-threshold mechanoreceptive (LTM) neurons. They are maximally excited by gentle mechanical stimuli such as hair movements or light pressure, applied to the contralateral trigeminal integument. They are place-specific; that is, they have a circumscribed receptive field and show a somatotopic organization. They are also modality-specific; that is, a given neuron can be excited by one particular form of mechanical stimulation. Recently two classes of trigeminal nociceptive neurons have been found in the VPM proper of the cat (Yokota and Matsumoto, 1983a, 1983b; Yokota et al., 1985).

One class consists of nociceptive specific (NS) neurons. A great majority of them respond with a maintained discharge exclusively to noxious mechanical stimuli applied to a circumscribed, contralateral receptive field. Some of them respond to firm pressure, but discharge more vigorously when noxious stimuli are applied. Another class consists of wide dynamic range (WDR) neurons. They have a relatively large receptive field on the contralateral trigeminal integument, and have a graded response to touch, pressure and noxious mechanical stimuli in the center of the receptive field. In an area surrounding this central zone, they respond differentially to pressure and noxious stimuli. This area in turn is surrounded by another region in which only noxious stimuli can cause spike discharges.

NS neurons are located near the dorsal and/or ventral ends of a row of LTM neurons in perpendicular microelectrode penetrations across the caudal third of the VPM proper. They are not encountered in the VPMpc and in the ventrolateral region of the VPM proper bordering the VPL. Histologically it has been confirmed that they are located at or near the margin of the VPM proper. This marginal area is referred to as the shell region, and the shell region of the caudal third of the VPM proper in which NS neurons are located, is called the NS zone. WDR neurons are also located in the shell region of the VPM proper, but they are confined to a narrow band approximately 300 µm wide just rostral to the NS zone.

Both NS and WDR neurons are somatotopically organized. In general, ophthalmic NS neurons having a receptive field in the contralateral ophthalmic division and ophthalmic WDR neurons having a low threshold center in the same division are located dorsolaterally, maxillary NS and WDR neurons occur dorsomedially, and mandibular NS and WDR neurons are found ventromedially along the border between the VPM proper and the VPMpc. In the caudal part of the NS zone, only maxillary NS neurons are found in the dorsal shell region, whereas mandibular NS neurons are located ventromedially (Fig. 1).

3. Tooth pulp neurons in cat VPM

The role of the shell region of the VPM proper in trigeminal nociception has further been evaluated by utilizing electrical stimulation of tooth pulp in the cat (Yokota et al.,1986). Two classes of tooth pulp neurons have been identified. One class is only responsive to tooth pulp afferents. They are called tooth pulp specific (TPS) neurons. The other class of tooth pulp neurons is also responsive to mechanical stimulation of the trigeminal integument. They are WDR neurons responsive to tooth pulp afferents. Both classes of tooth pulp neurons are located in the shell region of the VPM proper; TPS neurons are coexistent with trigeminal NS neurons, and are found in the dorsomedial and ventromedial parts of the NS zone. WDR neurons responsive to tooth pulp afferents are located in the dorsomedial as well as ventromedial parts of the WDR zone. Tooth pulp neurons in the dorsomedial shell region respond to maxillary canine tooth afferents, whereas those in the ventromedial shell region respond to mandibular canine tooth pulp afferents. Some tooth pulp neurons in these two shell region respond to both maxillary and mandibular canine teeth. It has been demonstrated that these two classes of tooth pulp neurons are antidromically excited by electrical stimulation of the SI area of the somatosensory cortex.

4. Location of neurons relaying trigeminal nociceptive input to VPM

It has generally been held that the trigeminal subnucleus caudalis and its ventromedially adjacent bulbar lateral reticular formation are integral parts of the brainstem relaying trigeminal nociceptive input to the thalamus. It has been demonstrated that cooling of the caudal medulla oblongata reversibly supresses responses of NS, WDR and TPS neurons in the shell region of the caudal VPM proper. Responses of these neurons are irreversibly abolished after interruption of the spinal tract of the trigeminal nerve at a level just rostral to the obex, but electrical stimulation of the spinal tract at a level caudal to the incision still elicits excitation of these neurons (Yokota and Matsumoto,

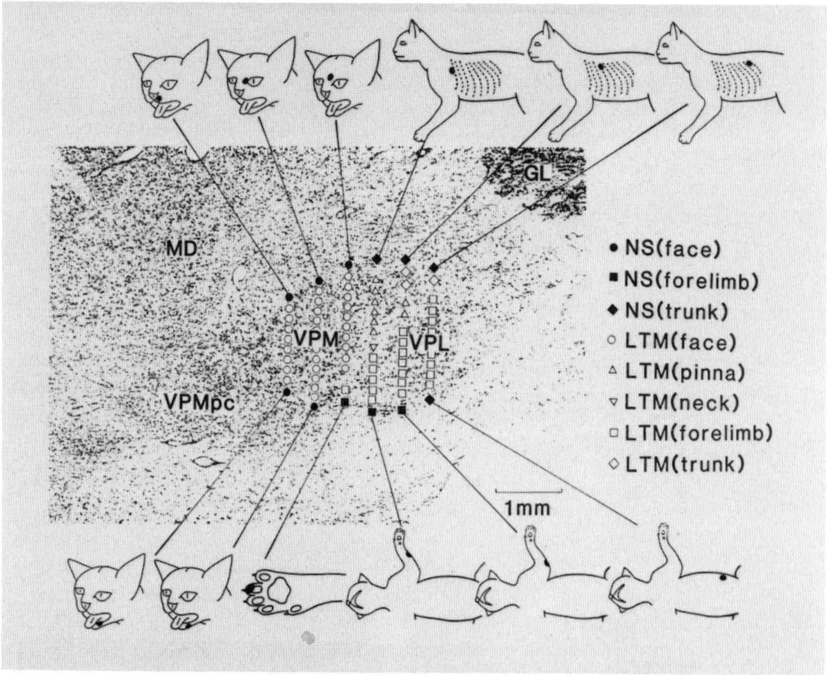

Fig. 1. A reconstruction of microelectrode penetrations through the VB complex, showing recording sites of NS and LTM units in one experiment. Individual figurines represent receptive fields of corresponding NS units which are located in the shell region of the VB complex. Abbreviations: GL, corpus geniculatum laterale; MD, nucleus medialis dorsalis; VPL; nucleus ventralis posterolateralis; VPM, nucleus ventralis posteromedialis; VPMpc, nucleus ventralis posteromedialis parvocellularis.

1983a; Yokota et al., 1986). Nociceptive responses of NS and WDR neurons and tooth pulp evoked responses of TPS and WDR neurons appear to depend on the integrity of the caudal medulla oblongata.

5. Nociceptive neurons in cat VPL

There have been reports of nociceptive responses of neurons in the marginal area of the VPL in the rat (Mitchell and Hellon, 1977), cat (Honda et al., 1983; Kniffki and Mizumura, 1983) and monkey (Kenshalo et al., 1980). It has been confirmed that trigeminal as well as spinal nociceptive neurons are located in a shell-like fashion around the VPL and VPM proper (Yokota et al., 1985). This marginal area is called the shell region of the VB complex (Fig.1).

Furthermore, it has been confirmed that NS and WDR neurons in the VPL are spatially segregated as in the case of the VPM proper. That is, NS neurons in the VPL are located at the level corresponding to the NS zone of the VPM proper, while WDR neurons are located in a narrow band just in front of the NS zone of the VPL. The border between the NS and WDR zones is slightly curved with its lateral end located more anteriorly, so that the WDR zone of the VPL tends to be located slightly more anterior to the WDR zone of the VPM proper. Nevertheless, the WDR zone of the VPL is continuous with the same zone of the VPM proper, and there is a belt around the whole VB complex, in which trigeminal and spinal WDR neurons are located.

6. Nociceptive neurons in VB complex of macaques

Nociceptive responses of neurons in the VPL of the monkey have already been reported (Kenshalo et al., 1980). They include NS and WDR neurons. We have explored the VB complex of the Japanese macaque (macaca fuscata), and confirmed the general distribution pattern as found in the cat. First of all, both NS and WDR neurons are located in the shell region of the caudal VB complex consisting of the VPM proper and VPLc. Secondly, NS and WDR neurons are spatially segregated, WDR neurons being located more anteriorly. However, there is a minor difference between cats and Japanese macaques. In the cat, nociceptive neurons are distributed over the whole surface of the caudal VB complex, so that there is no interruption in the location of nociceptive neurons around the VB complex in the transverse plane. In

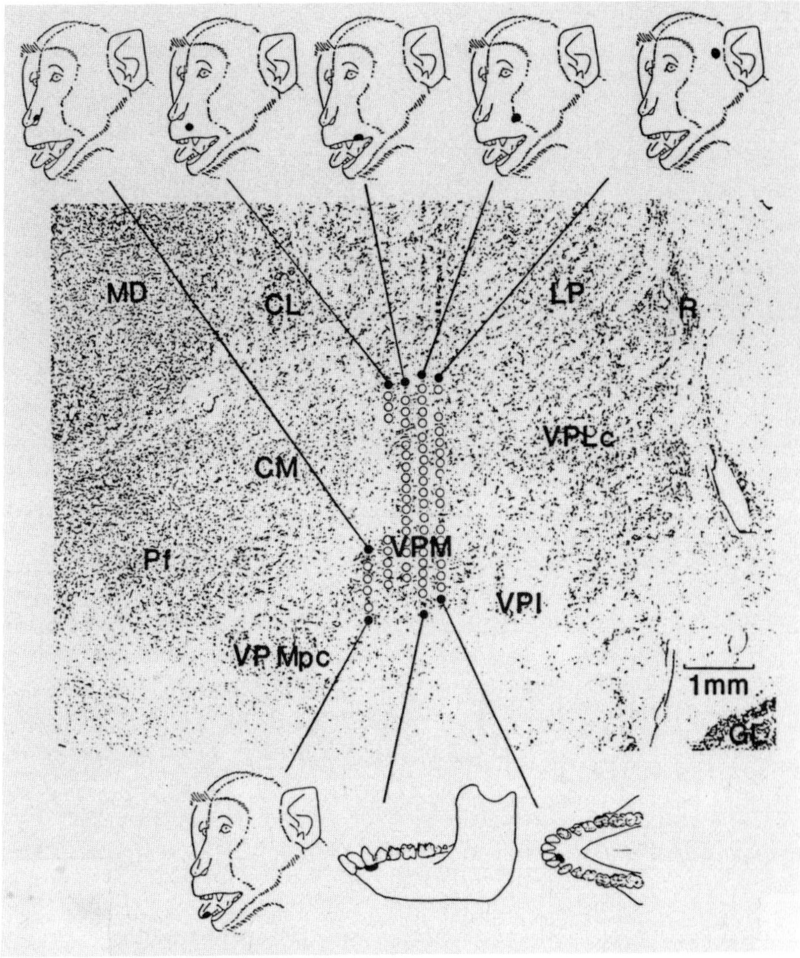

Fig. 2. A reconstruction of microelectrode penetrations showing recording sites of NS as well as LTM units and receptive fields of NS units. Filled circles and open circles in the photomicrograph indicate positions at which NS and LTM units were respectively encountered. Abbreviations; CL, nucleus centralis lateralis; CM, nucleus centrum medianum; LP, nucleus lateralis posterior; MD, nucleus medialis dorsalis; R, nucleus reticularis; VPI, nucleus ventralis inferior; VPLc, nucleus ventralis posterolateralis, pars caudalis; VPM, nucleus ventralis posteromedialis; VPMpc, nucleus ventralis posteromedialis parvocellularis.

the macaque, nociceptive neurons are missing along the medial edge of the VPM proper just dorsal and lateral to the nucleus centrum medianum (CM), although they are present just ventral to the CM (Fig.2).

SUMMARY

In both cats and Japanese macaques, there are nociceptive specific (NS) and wide dynamic range (WDR) neurons in the shell region of the caudal ventrobasal (VB) complex of the thalamus. They are spatially segregated, WDR neurons being located more anteriorly. There is a belt around the VB complex, in which WDR neurons are located. These two classes of nociceptive neurons constitute a thalamic link of the pain pathway between the spinal dorsal horn as well as trigeminal subnucleus caudalis and the primary somatosensory cortex.

REFERENCES

Honda CN, Mense S, Perl ED (1983). Neurons in ventrobasal region of cat thalamus selectively responsive to noxious mechanical stimulation. J Neurophysiol 49:662-673.

Kenshalo DRJr, Giesler GJJr, Leonard RB, Willis W (1980). Responses of neurons in primate ventral posterior lateral nucleus to noxious stimuli. J Neurophysiol 43:1594-1614.

Kniffki KD, Mizumura K (1983). Responses of neurons in VPL and VPL-VL region of the cat to algesic stimulation of muscle and tendon. J Neurophysiol 49:649-661.

Krieg WJS (1948). A reconstruction of the diencephalic nuclei of macacus rhesus. J Comp Neurol 88:1-51.

Mitchell D, Hellon RF (1977). Neuronal and behavioral responses in rats during noxious stimulation of the tail., Proc. Roy. Soc. London Ser. B. 197: 169-194.

Olszewski J(1952). The Thalamus of the Macaca Mulatta, Basel : Karger.

Peschanski M, Guilbaud G, Gautron M, Besson JM (1980). Encoding of noxious heat messages in neurons of the ventrobasal complex of the rat. Brain Res, 197: 401-413.

Rose M (1935). Das Zwischenhirn des Kaninchens. Mem Acad Pol Sci Lett Ser B: 81-108.

Rose JE, Mountcastle VB (1952). The thalamic tactile region in rabbit and cat. J Comp Neurol 97: 441-489.

Yokota T, Koyama N, Matsumoto N (1985) Somatotopic distribution of trigeminal nociceptive neurons in ventrobasal complex of cat thalamus. J Neurophysiol 53 :1387-1400.

Yokota T, Matsumoto N (1983a). Somatotopic distribution of trigeminal nociceptive specific neurons within the caudal somatosensory thalamus of the cat. Neurosci Lett 39: 125-130.

Yokota T, Matsumoto N (1983b). Location and functional organization of trigeminal wide dynamic range neurons within the nucleus ventralis posteromedialis of the cat. Neurosci Lett 39: 231-236.

Yokota T, Nishikawa Y, Koyama N (1986). Tooth pulp input to the shell region of nucleus ventralis posteromedialis of the cat thalamus. J Neurophysiol in press.

Effects of Injury on Trigeminal and Spinal Somatosensory Systems, pages 313–320

LATERAL THALAMIC NOCICEPTION: THE EFFECTS OF INTERRUPTION OF TRANSMISSION THROUGH THE VENTROLATERAL AND THE DORSOLATERAL SPINOTHALAMIC TRACTS

Charles J. Hodge, Jr., A. Vania Apkarian, Steven Martini and Robert J. Martin

Department of Neurosurgery, SUNY Health Science Center at Syracuse, Syracuse, New York 13210

The recurrence of clinical pain associated with the return of nociception that can occur following anterolateral spinal cord damage (White & Sweet, 1969) has prompted the hypothesis that alternate nociception signaling ascending spinal pathways exist outside the confines of the classical spinothalamic tract. Candidate alternate pain pathways considered include the spinocervical tract, the post synaptic dorsal column pathway and propriospinal pathways (Willis, 1985). Little attention has been given the possibility of a direct spinothalamic pathway existing outside the ventral quadrant. Recent evidence using retrograde transport of horseradish peroxidase (HRP) has, however, demonstrated the existence of a dorsolateral spinothalamic tract (DSTT) in cat and squirrel monkey (Jones et al., 1985a,b). The DSTT consists nearly exclusively of lamina I spinal neuron axons while the ventral spinothalamic tract (VSTT) consists of axons of spinal neurons located in laminae IV-X. Both pathways cross segmentally and have widespread thalamic terminations. Within the lateral thalamus, both pathways have terminals in the ventral posterior lateral nucleus (VPL) and the posterior nucleus (PO) (Apkarian et al., 1986b). This paper describes the changes in the response characteristics of nociceptive neurons of the cat lateral sensory thalamus following interruption of transmission through either the DSTT or the VSTT.

METHODS

Cats initially anesthetized with nembutal (35 mg/kg) and maintained with 2/3 nitrous oxide, 1/3 oxygen and supplemental halothane (0.1-0.2%) were used for these experiments. The thoracic spinal cord was exposed over two segments and a small craniectomy was done for thalamic access. Single unit recordings were made from the lateral sensory thalamus using parylene coated tungsten microelectrodes with impedances of 4-10 megohms. Only units responsive to noxious cutaneous inputs form the basis of this report. Following isolation, the response properties of the unit to innocuous and noxious (pinch and temperature >45 degrees C) stimuli were determined. Two methods of interrupting transmission through the thoracic ventral quadrant (VQ) or the dorsolateral funiculus (DLF) ipsilateral to the recording site were used. In some experiments, following characterization of the unit responses, microsurgical lesions of the DLF and/or the VQ were made. More commonly transmission through the DLF or the VQ was reversibly blocked by cooling the quadrant of interest to 1-3 degrees centigrade using 0.6 mm stainless steel tubing, in contact with the appropriate area of the thoracic spinal cord, through which cooled methanol was pumped. The contact temperature was monitored and could be set to any level by adjusting the methanol pump speed (Salsbury & Horel, 1983). The changes in the response properties of the thalamic units following interruption of transmission through the DLF or VQ were then determined. Each thalamic recording site was marked with an electrolytic lesion for later histologic localization.

RESULTS

Eighteen units responding to noxious cutaneous stimuli were studied. The receptive fields of all these units included the contralateral hindlimb. The locations of the units within the thalamus are shown in figure 1. Thirteen recording sites were in the shell region of the anterior lateral portion of the VPL nucleus, and two were located in PO. One of these units responded exclusively to noxious stimuli, while the remainder responded in a graded fashion to innocuous and noxious stimuli. Two units did not respond to noxious thermal stimulation, yet increased their ongoing activity when the receptive fields were

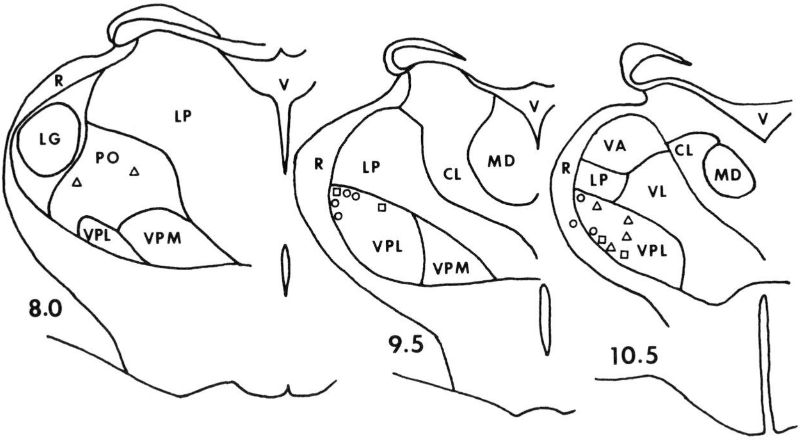

Figure 1. Locations of thalamic recording sites. The AP level of each thalamic section is indicated. The circles represent units unaffected by either DLF or VQ block. The triangles represent units whose responses were decreased by DLF block. The squares represent units whose responses were altered by VQ block.

pinched with serrated forceps. The activity of the units studied by thermal stimulation usually showed response saturation at receptive field temperatures above 50 degrees centigrade (figure 2). The nociceptive response properties of the units in PO were similar to those in VPL, though the receptive fields of the PO units were generally larger, at times consisting of the entire lower half of the body.

Six of eighteen units had their responses to noxious stimulation blocked by cooling or lesioning the DLF as shown in figure 2. The locations of these units are indicated in figure 1. When effective, DLF cooling or lesioning was able to completely abolish the thalamic response to noxious thermal cutaneous stimulation (figure 2). DLF blocking did not alter the responses or receptive field sizes of thalamic units elicited by innocuous skin stimulation, even when the responses to noxious stimuli were abolished. Two thalamic units showed an increase in responsiveness to noxious cutaneous stimulation during DLF cooling.

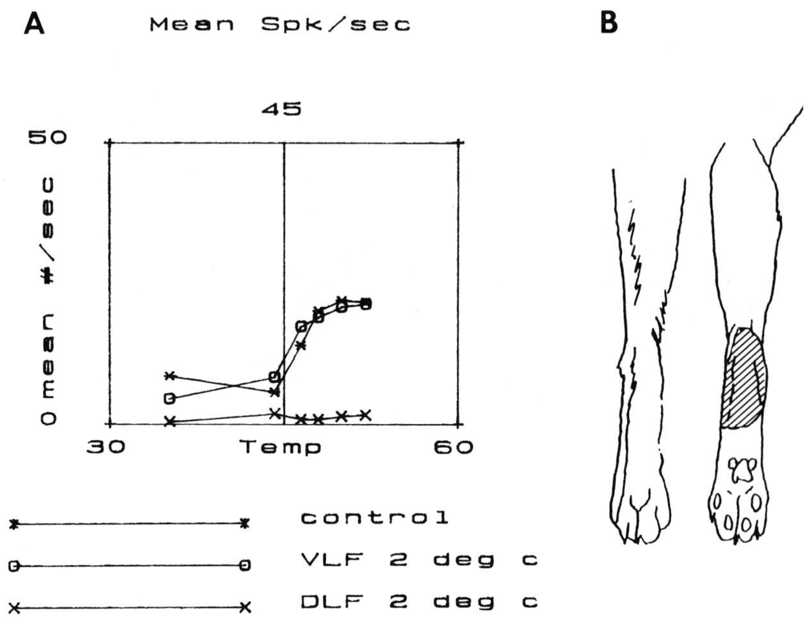

Figure 2. Effects of DLF and VLF blocks on a VPL unit responses to noxious cutaneous stimuli. A. Illustrates the mean number of spikes/second plotted against the cutaneous temperatures used to elicit the responses. In both the control state and when the VLF is cooled to 2 degrees C, the unit responds briskly to skin temperatures over 45 degrees C. When the DLF is cooled to 2 degrees C, the response to skin heating is lost. B. Shows the contralateral lower extremity receptive field to pinch of this unit. The heat stimulus was applied within this receptive field.

Four of sixteen units studied had their responses to nociceptive thermal cutaneous stimulation altered by cooling or lesioning the VQ. Of these, one showed a decrease (but not loss) to noxious cutaneous thermal stimulation, one showed an increased response to noxious thermal cutaneous stimulation, one showed an increase in background resting activity that masked any temperature response and one showed loss of response to pinch after VQ section which had been preceeded by an ineffective DLF

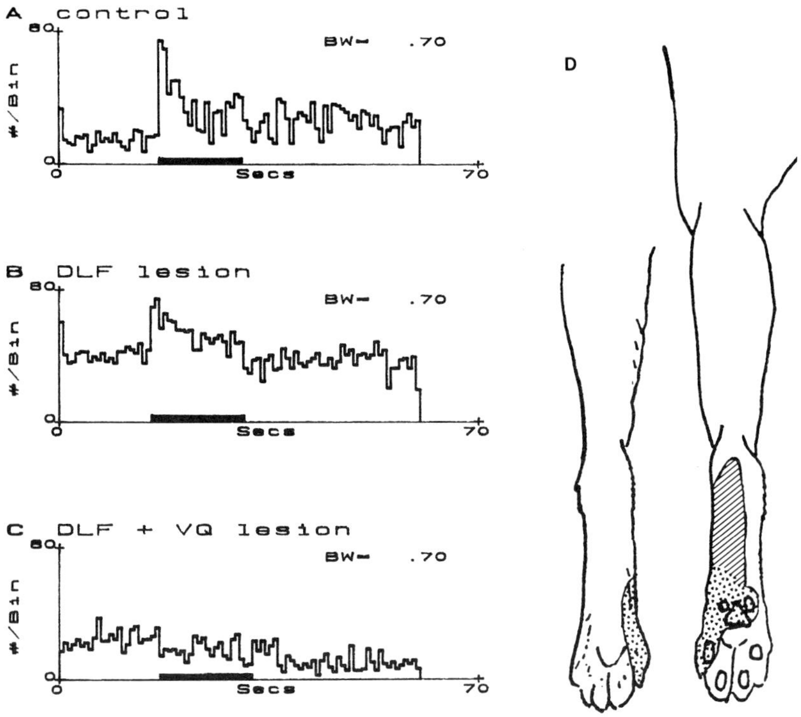

Figure 3. The effects of DLF and a combined DLF and VQ lesion on the responses of a VPL unit to pinch. A, B and C are peristimulus time histograms with binwidth of 0.7 seconds. The time of the occurence of the pinch is marked by the heavy black bar above the time axis. B. The effect of the DLF lesion ipsilateral to the recording site is to increase the spontaneous activity without altering the magnitude of the response to pinch. C. The response to pinch is abolished only when a VQ lesion ipsilateral to the recording site is added to the DLF lesion. D. The contralateral lower extremity receptive field to touch (stippled) and pinch (diagonal lines). Following the VQ lesion, the responses to both noxious and innocuous cutaneous stimuli are abolished.

lesion (figure 3).

In three units, where the response to noxious cutaneous stimulation could not be blocked by cooling either the VQ or the DLF, progressive surgical lesions of the spinal cord demonstrated that the input to these thalamic units traveled through multiple ascending pathways distributed bilaterally in the spinal cord.

DISCUSSION

These preliminary results indicate that information concerning the occurence of noxious peripheral stimulation ascends through the spinal cord in both the VQ and the DLF. It is impossible on the basis of this study to differentiate between the effects of interruption of direct spinothalamic pathways (DSTT, VSTT) and interruption of spinoreticulo-thalamic pathways or other multisynaptic pathways traveling in the VQ or DLF. The increase in responses to noxious peripheral stimulation that occurred with transmission block of either DLF or VQ were likely the result of loss of descending inhibition. The inability to block transmission to some of the units that were studied might indicate that the fibers traveling in the quadrant being cooled were too distant from the cold probe to be lowered to a blocking temperature, since when the contact probe is at 0 degrees centigrade, the effective blocking range is about 0.5 mm (Apkarian et al., 1986a). However, information concerning noxious peripheral events can also reach the thalamus through areas outside of the ipsilateral spinothalamic tracts.

Since the DSTT in the DLF is comprised almost entirely of lamina I cell axons (Jones et al., 1985a), it is clear that the nociceptive responses of some thalamic units is mediated by lamina I cell input. Based on the limited number of units in this study, it is uncertain whether there is a topographic preference in the lateral thalamus of units activated by lamina I cell input. Since there are essentially no lamina I cell axons traveling in the cat VSTT, it is apparent that lamina I cell input is not necessary for the nociceptive responses of all thalamic units.

This data is consistent with the work of Kennard (1954) who demonstrated the importance of the DLF for behavioral nociception in cats. Similarly, Vierck (1979) has shown that lesions of the DLF in macaque monkeys can, at least transiently, interfere with nociception. Interestingly, human pathologic specimens obtained following successful anterolateral cordotomy, indicate that some of the lesions were limited to the DLF (Sweet, 1973). It is possible, then, that the return of pain perception following anterolateral cordotomy or spinal trauma is a reflection, in part, of the spared lamina I cell input to the thalamus. The severe burning dysesthetic pain, typical of the post cordotomy syndrome, likewise is probably due in part to the activity in the thalamus elicited by lamina I cell nociceptive specific input. The role that the DSTT plays after long term denervation remains uninvestigated at present.

REFERENCES

Apkarian AV, Stevens RT, Martin RJ, Martini SM, Hodge CJ Jr (1986a). A spinal cord blocking technique which is reversible and localized. Soc Neurosci Abst Vol 12.

Apkarian AV, Hodge CJ Jr, Jones MW, Stevens RT (1986b). Thalamic terminations of the dorsolateral and the ventrolateral spinothalamic pathways. (This volume).

Jones MW, Apkarian AV, Stevens RT, Hodge CJ Jr (1985a). A dorsolateral spinothalamic pathway in squirrel monkey. Soc Neurosci Abst Vol 11 p. 577.

Jones MW, Hodge CJ Jr, Apkarian AV, Stevens RT (1985b). A dorsolateral spinothalamic pathway in cat. Brain Res 335:188-193.

Kennard MA (1954). The course of ascending fibers in spinal cord of the cat essential to the recognition of painful stimuli. J Comp Neurol 100:511-524.

Salsbury KG, Horel JA (1983). A cryogenic implant for producing reversible functional brain lesions. Behav Res Meth & Inst 15:433-436.

Sweet WH (1973). Craniospinal surgery for pain. Audio visual education in neurosurgery (AVENS), Lib Cong Cat No 73-701180, p.12.

Vierck CJ, Luck MM (1979). Loss and recovery of reactivity to noxious stimuli in monkeys with primary spinothalamic cordotomies, followed by secondary and tertiary lesions of other cord sectors. Brain 102:233-248.

White JC, Sweet WH (1969). "Pain and the Neurosurgeon." Springfield, Illinois: C. Thomas.

Willis WD (1985). "The Pain System" in Pain and Headache, vol 8, Basel: S. Karger.

Effects of Injury on Trigeminal and Spinal Somatosensory Systems, pages 321–330

EXPERIMENTALLY INDUCED DEGENERATION IN THE PRIMATE VENTROBASAL THALAMUS

Henry J. Ralston III and Diane D. Ralston

Department of Anatomy, University of California, San Francisco, CA 94143

INTRODUCTION

The ventrobasal complex of the thalamus (VB) is made up of complex neuronal networks which play a major and essential role in somatic sensation. In the primate, there is overlap within VB of three major systems conveying somatosensory stimuli from the body: the dorsal column projections-DCN (Boivie, 1978), the spinothalamic pathway-STT (Mehler et al., 1960; Boivie, 1979), and those from the lateral cervical nucleus-LCN (Boivie, 1980). This paper will be concerned with the DCN and STT pathways. The DCN projection is widely and densely distributed within that portion of VB representing the contralateral body, the ventroposterolateral nucleus (VPLC). The STT projections to VPLc overlap those of the DCN, but are patchy (Mehler et al., 1960; Ralston, 1984), being made up of rostrocaudally-running aggregations of fibers having a rod-like configuration (Jones et al., 1982)

This paper describes the normal fine structure of the primate VB, the types of degeneration undergone by terminals of DCN and STT fibers, and the long term consequences of chronic DCN ablation. Because of the fact that there is convergence of the DCN and STT pathway in primate VB, one can ask whether there is a reactive synaptogenesis of the STT pathway in the presence of chronic DCN lesions, as has been described in the rat somatosensory thalamus (Wells and Tripp, 1986) as well as in numerous other systems (Raisman, 1969; Cotman et al., 1981).

MATERIALS AND METHODS

This study is based upon the examination of tissues from the ventrobasal thalamus of Macaque monkeys, M. mulatta or M. fascicularis. Some of the monkeys were normal, others survived following various procedures to label projections to the thalamus, which have been described elsewhere (Ralston, 1985). These included lesions of either the dorsal column nuclei or the anterolateral cervical spinal cord, injections of tritiated amino acids into the DCN or the somatosensory cortex, the transport of wheat germ lectin conjugated to horseradish peroxidase (WGA-HRP) injected into one or two segments of the spinal cord dorsal horn, and immunocytochemical studies of GABAergic interneurons. In all cases, the animals were anesthetized at the time the experiments were performed and at the time the animals were sacrificed.

In experimentally induced lesions, most animals survived from one to ten days postoperatively, as it has been found that afferent fibers and terminals undergo their most prominent forms of degeneration during this time (Ralston, 1969). Two animals had longer survival periods: 42 and 66 days following a unilateral DCN lesion. It was in these animals that microinjections of WGA-HRP were made into the cervical spinal cord five days before sacrifice, in order to determine whether there is any evidence of expansion of the terminal field of STT fibers in the VB in which there had been chronic degeneration of DCN projections.

RESULTS

The normal fine structure of the monkey VB has been reported elsewhere (Ralston, 1985), and will only be briefly described here. There are four principal types of synaptic terminals; small profiles with round vesicles (SR) which constitute 80% of all synapses, and which arise in large part from the somatosensory cortex; profiles with pleomorphic or flattened vesicles (F) which are thought to be derived primarily from the thalamic reticular nucleus (Peschanski et al, 1983); large profiles with rounded vesicles (LR - figure 1) which have been shown to be the terminations of DCN, STT and LCN pathways (Ralston, 1983); and presynaptic dendrites (PSD) which are thought to be the

GABAergic branches of VB interneurons. PSDs receive synapses from SR, F and LR profiles. They have unique relationships with LR profiles in a complex arrangement known as a synaptic triad, in which LR is presynaptic to PSD and to a conventional dendrite, and the PSD is also presynaptic to a conventional dendrite.

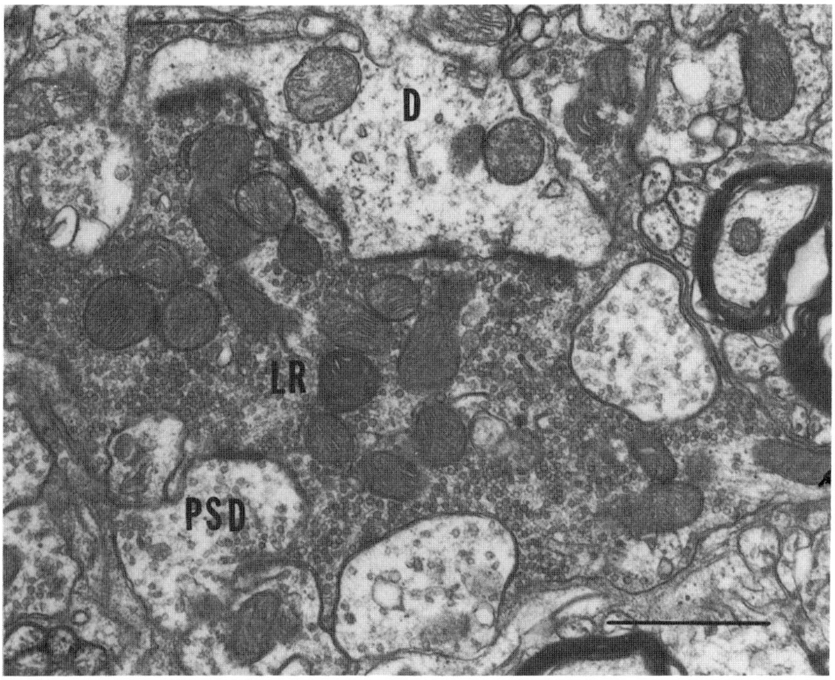

Figure 1. Electron micrograph of a normal LR synaptic profile in monkey VB, which makes synaptic contacts upon a conventional dendrite (D) and a presynaptic dendrite (PSD). scale bar - 1 um.

Following DCN, STT or LCN lesions, LR profiles are seen to undergo early neurofilamentous degeneration, in which synaptic vesicles disappear and there is a substantial neurofilamentous hyperplasia (figure 2). Subsequently, the terminals become electron-dense and within one week after the lesion have been phagocytosed and removed. LR profiles constitute only about 5% of the total synaptic population of VB, and of this number, more than 4/5 are of DCN origin, the remainder being principally derived from STT fibers and only a small percent from LCN.

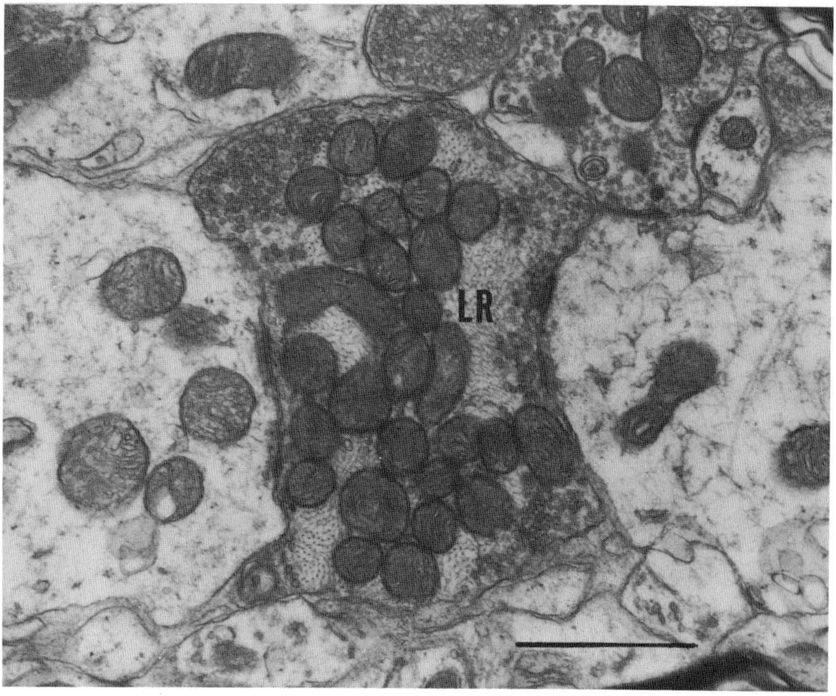

Figure 2. Neurofilamentous hyperplasia of an LR profile in monkey VB, 4 days after contralateral DCN lesions.

In the two animals having chronic DCN lesions, a careful study was made to determine whether or not there is any evidence of a reactive synaptogenesis, in which the terminal fields of the STT projection might expand to occupy the synaptic fields of the DCN projection. Light microscopy suggested that this might be the case, because the sizes of the patches of STT terminal fields in VB labeled by the orthorograde transport of WGA-HRP from the cervical spinal cord appeared to increase somewhat in size. A typical STT axonal arbor in normal VB measures approximately 0.3-0.5 um in diameter. In VB in which there was a chronic loss of DCN fibers, The STT projections measured about 0.5-0.7 um in diameter. These measurements pool the results of the diameters of 22 STT arbors in normal VB and 12 STT arbors in VB in which there had been a chronic lesion of DCN.

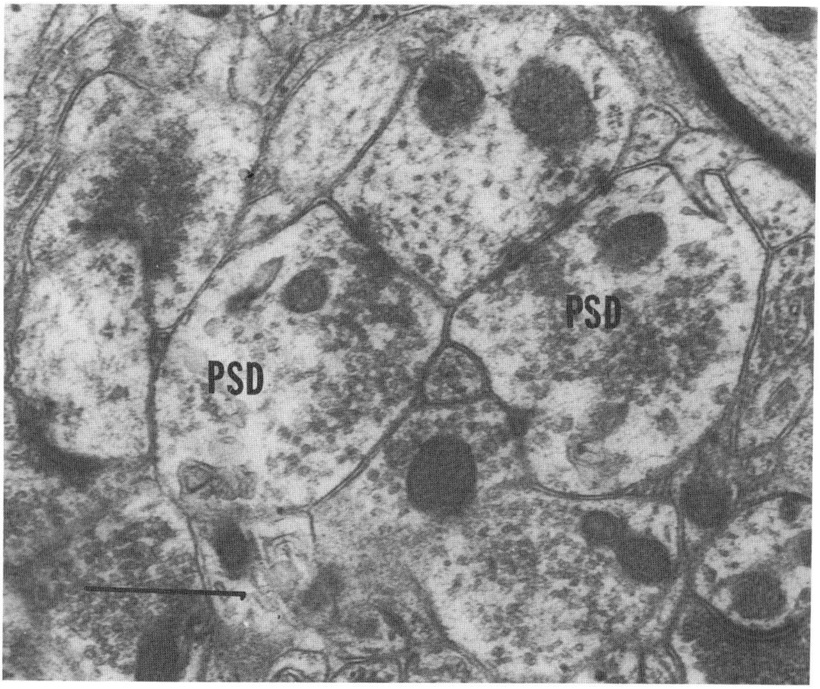

Figure 3. Several PSDs which normally have synaptic relationships with LR profiles form contacts with conventional dendrites but there is no LR profiles seen in this field or in numerous other similar fields. 42 days after contralateral DCN lesion.

Surprisingly, electron microscopic analysis of VB in the chronic cases did not reveal evidence of reactive synaptogenesis. As mentioned above, LR profiles typically form synaptic relationships with PSD profiles and conventional dendrites. The majority of the LR profiles degenerate in the first week following contralateral DCN lesions. In the chronic animals, it had been anticipated that there would be a reestablishment of LR profiles forming more or less normal synaptic relationships. However, this was not the case. Very few LR profiles were found in VB of the chronic animals despite extensive examination which would certainly have covered areas in which LR profiles of STT origin were present. Complex synaptic arrangements were found, in which multiple PSDs were found clustered together without LR profiles being present as in the normal case (Figure 3). Thus, in the two survival periods studied (42 and 66 days post DCN lesion), there was no evidence of reactive synaptogenesis in these two adult macaques.

DISCUSSION

The organization of the normal ventrobasal complex of the monkey shares many features in common with that of the cat (Ralston, 1969) and the degeneration undergone by the ascending afferent fibers to VB is similar in rat (Tripp and Wells, 1978), cat and monkey (Ralston, 1983). The principal features of the acute phase of Wallerian degeneration are an initial filamentous hyperplasia followed by markedly increased electron density of the profiles and rapid phagocytic removal of the degenerating axon terminals.

Reactive synaptogenesis in VB of rat and monkey might be expected to occur following removal of the DCN projections which form the dominant population of the ascending afferent projections to VB, because of the overlap of the DCN and STT projection into VB in these two species. Lund and Webster (1967a,b) demonstrated that STT and DCN projections occupy similar fields in rat VB. Ma et al (1986) demonstrated that these overlapping projections have a somatictopic organization in the rat. Furthermore, it has been recently been demonstrated that DCN and STT projections can terminate on the same neurons within rat VB (Ma et al, 1987). Similarly, there is extensive overlap of the STT and DCN projections in monkey VB (Boivie, 1978, 1979), and thus the STT projections might be expected to sprout to occupy synaptic sites previously occupied by DCN fibers. The cat, on the other hand, appears to have relatively nonoverlapping DCN and STT projections (Boivie, 1971a,b) and thus the opportunity for sprouting of one projection into the deafferentated zones previously occupied by the other is less likely to occur.

In studies of reactive synaptogenesis in rat VB, there is evidence that the number of LR profiles decreases significantly in the first week following DCN lesions, but then recovers to near normal levels 30-50 days postoperatively (Tripp and Wells, 1978; Wells and Tripp, 1986). In contrast to these results, the present study in the monkey demonstrates no recovery of LR profiles at survival times of 42 and 66 days following almost total lesions of the DCN. There are a number of possible explanations for this discrepancy, some of which relate to species differences. Although restoration of LR profiles in the rat VB begins by 30 days postlesion, this may be too short an interval in the primate. If so, our results suggest that survival times longer than 66 days will be required to demonstrate sprouting in primate VB. In addition, there may be species differences in the degree of overlap of STT and DCN projections. There is evidence for DCN and STT projections upon the same VB neurons in the rat (Ma et al., 1987), which means that a sprouting STT axon would have only a short distance to grow in order to take over the synaptic space previously occupied by a DCN profile. Although there is physiological evidence for convergence of DCN and STT projections to the same neurons in monkey VB (Willis, 1985), there is as yet no direct anatomical evidence that this is the case. Moreover, there is a fundamental difference in the organization of the rat VB compared to that of the primate. The rat lacks interneurons (Saporta and Kruger, 1977) which give rise to presynaptic dendrites (McAllister and Wells, 1981). These profiles are abundant in the monkey and there is a complex relationship between DCN or STT terminals and PSDs, which the rat does not have. A further difference between the present study and earlier studies in rats, unrelated to species differences, is the essentially complete lesions of the DCN which we performed in the monkey, in contrast to the partial lesions carried out in the rat. Thus, in the rat sprouting could have occurred from surviving DCN axons, as well as from STT projections.

CONCLUSION

The monkey ventrobasal thalamus demonstrates a complex synaptic organization which can be analyzed by a variety of experimental techniques used to label various constituent elements of this nucleus. Experimentally induced degeneration of major ascending projections to the nucleus results in a rapid neurofilamentous hyperplasia of axon terminals of DCN, STT or LCN projections, followed by increased electron density of the affected synapses and their rapid phagocytic removal. Following chronic lesions of DCN in the monkey, sprouting of surviving STT or LCN axons to occupy synaptic sites previously occupied by the DCN profiles did not occur at the 7 and 9 week survival times studied. Similar experiments in the rat VB by other investigators have indicated that such reactive synaptogenesis does take place in this species. We suggest that differences in the experimental approaches used, or fundamental differences in the organization of VB between the two species, may be responsible for these sharply differing results.

ACKNOWLEDGMENTS

We are indebted to Ms. Antonia Milroy for her skilled technical assistance in this project. Supported by grants NS21445 and NS23347 from the NIH.

REFERENCES

Boivie J (1971a). The termination in the thalamus and zona incerta of fibers from the dorsal column nuclei (DCN) in the cat: an experimental study with silver impregnation methods. Brain Res 28:459-490.

Boivie J (1971b). The termination of the spinothalamic tract in the cat: an experimental study with silver impregnation methods. Exp Brain Res 112:331-353.

Boivie J (1978). Anatomical observations on the dorsal column nuclei, the thalamic projection and the cytoarchitecture of some somatosensory thalamic nuclei in the monkey. J Comp Neurol 178:17-48.

Boivie J (1979). An anatomical reinvestigation of the termination of the spinothalamic tract in the monkey. J Comp Neurol 186:343-370.

Boivie J (1980). Thalamic projections from lateral cervical nucleus in monkey: a degeneration study. Brain Res 198:13-26.

Cotman CW, Nieto-Sampedro M, Harris EW (1981). Synapse replacement in the nervous system of adult vertebrates. Physiol Rev 61:684-784.

Jones EG, Friedman DP, Hendry SHC (1982). Thalamic basis of place and modality-specific columns in monkey somatosensory cortex: a correlative anatomical and physiological study. J Neurophysiol 48:545-568.

Lund RD, Webster KE (1967a). Thalamic afferents from the dorsal column nuclei: an experimental anatomical study in the rat. J Comp Neurol 130:301-312.

Lund RD, Webster KE (1967b). Thalamic afferents from the spinal cord and trigeminal nuclei: an experimental anatomical study in the rat. J Comp Neurol 130:313-328.

Ma W, Peschanski M, Besson JM (1986). The overlap of spinothalamic and dorsal column nuclei projection in the ventrobasal complex of the rat thalamus: a double anterograde labeling study using light microscopic analysis. J Comp Neurol 245:531-540.

Ma W, Peschanski M, Ralston HJ III (1987). The differential synaptic organization of the spinal and lemniscal projections to the ventrobasal complex of the rat thalamus. Evidence for convergence of the two systems upon single thalamic neurons. Neurosci (submitted).

McAllister JP, Wells J (1981). The structural organization of the ventral posterolateral nucleus in the rat. J Comp Neurol 197:271-301.

Mehler WR, Feferman ME, Nauta WJH (1960). Ascending axon degeneration following anterolateral cordotomy. An experimental study in the monkey. Brain 83:718-751.

Peschanski M, Ralston HJ III, Roudier F (1983). Reticularis thalami afferents to the ventrobasal complex of the rat thalamus: an electron microscope study. Brain Res 270:325-329.

Raisman G. (1969). Neuronal plasticity in the septal nuclei of the adult rat. Brain Res 14:25-48.

Ralston HJ III (1969). The synaptic organization of lemniscal projections to the ventrobasal thalamus of the cat. Brain Res 14:99-116.

Ralston HJ III (1983). The synaptic organization of the ventrobasal thalamus in the rat, cat and monkey. In: Macchi G, Rustioni A, Spreafico R (eds): "Somatosensory Integration in the Thalamus," Amsterdam: Elsevier, pp 241-250.

Ralston HJ III (1984). Synaptic organization of spinothalamic tract projections to the thalamus with special reference to pain. In: Kruger L, Liebeskind JC (eds): "Advance in Pain Research and Therapy," Vol. 6, New York: Raven Press, pp 183-195.

Ralston HJ III (1985). The fine structure of the ventrobasal thalamus of the monkey and cat. Brain Res Rev 9:228-242.

Saporta S, Kruger L (1977). The organization of the thalamocortical relay neurons in the rat ventrobasal complex studied by retrograde transport of horseradish peroxidase. J Comp Neurol 174:187-208.

Tripp LN, Wells J (1978). Formation of new synaptic terminals in the somatosensory thalamus of the rat after lesions of the dorsal column nuclei. Brain Res 155:362-367.

Wells J, Tripp LN (1986). Time course of a reactive synaptogenesis in the subcortical somatosensory system. J Comp Neurol (in press).

Willis WD (1985). Electrophysiological aspects of thalamic mechanisms of pain sensation. Brain Res Rev 9:242-259.

Effects of Injury on Trigeminal and Spinal Somatosensory Systems, pages 331–338

KAINIC ACID INDUCED NEURODEGENERATION IN VENTROBASAL COMPLEX OF THE RAT THALAMUS : GROWTH CONE-LIKE ENDINGS OF FUNCTIONAL AFFERENT FIBERS.

Marc Peschanski and Jean-Marie Besson

Unité de recherches de neurophysiologie pharmacologique, INSERM U 161, 2 rue d'Alésia, 75014 Paris, France.

For a decade, *in situ* injections of excitotoxic amino-acids into cerebral structures have been used to induce selective lesions of postsynaptic neurons. Excitotoxic lesions have been recognized in many cases as experimental models of neurodegenerative diseases (see refs in Coyle and Schwartz, 1983). Supporting this assumption, several anatomical and biochemical studies have provided substantial evidence that such injections had little, if any, acute effect on afferent fibers and axons of passage (see refs in Coyle and Schwartz, 1983). In contrast, little is known of the morphological and functional aspects of the long term afferent response to an excitotoxin induced degeneration of postsynaptic targets, although there is a general agreement that afferents retract over time. The question of the long term alteration of afferents to an area of neurodegeneration is, however, a question of importance if excitotoxic lesions are to be used as experimental models of chronic neurodegenerative diseases.

The present study was therefore undertaken to reconsider the fate of afferent fibers to an area of neurodegeneration. We decided to analyze this question in the ventrobasal complex of the rat thalamus (VB) because this structure possesses particularly simple and well described anatomical characteristics at the light and electron microscopic levels (Mc Allister and Wells, 1981 ; Peschanski et al., 1984). In addition, VB is one of the chief links involved in transmitting somatosensory information, which allowed us to easily identify the effects of a neurodegenerative lesion on afferent fibers using electrophysiological recordings in response to various somesthetic stimuli.

GENERAL PRESENTATION

The present data were obtained from male Sprague-Dawley rats weighing 200 g at the time of injection of kainic acid (KA). To obtain a large neuronal loss in VB without mechanical damage to afferent fibers, a slow pressure injection of 5 nmol of KA (in 0.2 µl of water, over 20 min) via a 1-µl Hamilton syringe was administered in anesthetized (400 mg/kg chloral hydrate) rats into the internal capsule at the level of the rostral part of the nucleus.
In preliminary studies (Kayser et al., 1985) it was observed that after a KA-induced lesion of VB, the threshold of the vocalization induced by pressure of the opposite paws was substantially increased. This observation demonstrated that the pathway necessary to produce an integrated behavioral response to noxious stimulation was profundly altered.
The results presented here were obtained from animals which survived for 30 days after the KA injection. After this survival time, shrinkage of the brain on the lesioned side was not evident. Preliminary experiments using Nissl-stained 100 µm-thick microtome sections or 16 µm-thick cryostat sections demonstrated that only small darkly stained glial cells were visible within an area of VB close to the injection site. There was not a gradual transition between lesioned and unlesioned tissue and the boundary of the normal tissue was easily demonstrated by the abrupt cessation of glial proliferation and the appearance of neurons. Within the area of lesion itself, the normal architecture of VB was completely lost. A particularly noteworthy observation was the lack of the regular arrays of large bundles of fibers which normally cross VB.

LIGHT MICROSCOPY

VB receives three types of afferents (see refs in Peschanski et al., 1984 ; Peschanski and Besson, 1984) which can be categorized in 1) point-to-point systems, including ascending somatosensory pathways and cortico-thalamic afferents ; 2) diffuse systems,of which the noradrenergic coerulear projection is by far the most significant ; 3) an inhibitory system originating from the thalamic reticular nucleus. Since this last system was completely eliminated by the KA injections in our experimental conditions, data will only be presented concerning the other two.

Point-to-point systems

Wheat-germ agglutinin conjugated to HRP (10% in water) was injected bilaterally into the dorsal column nuclei or the spinal cord, or ipsilaterally into the somatosensory cortex, 24 to 48 h before sacrifice of the animal and perfusion using aldehyde fixatives. Projections to the unlesioned VB from the ascending pathways could therefore serve as controls. Sixty µm-thick coronal sections were cut and treated for HRP histochemistry following the technique described by Mesulam (1978).

Gross observation of all three labeled pathways demonstrated that all three studied afferent systems were present within the area of neuronal loss. As expected from the observation that a complete neuronal loss ensued in VB following a lesion, cortical injections produced no retrogradely labeled neurons within the lesioned area. When the afferent inputs from the spinal cord to the lesioned VB were compared with the input to the normal side, no obvious re-routing of the spinal afferents toward unlesioned parts of VB was observed. A follow-up study of the spinothalamic projections failed to demonstrate any re-routing of these afferents as long as 9 months after KA injection. In contrast, it was possible to demonstrate a decrease in the number of fibers for all three point-to-point systems in the lesioned area as compared with the projections toward the normal side. The follow-up study of lemniscal projections demonstrated a progressive decrease in the number of labeled fibers although the disappearance was not yet complete up to 14 months after KA injection. This decrease, probably due to a progressive retrograde alteration of the cells of origin, was easily observed for lemniscal afferents originating from the dorsal column

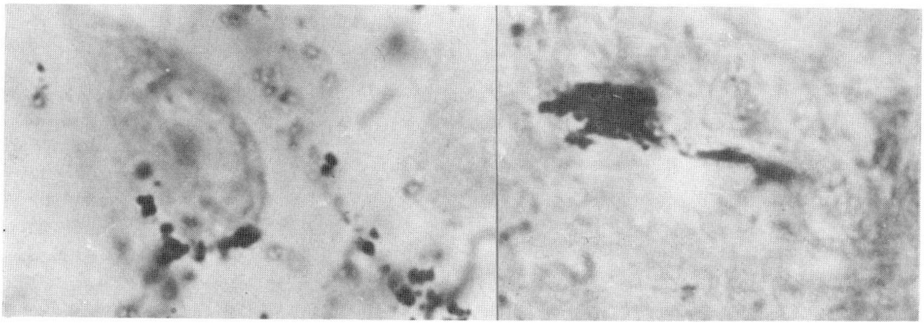

Figure 1 : High power photomicrographs showing anterogradely labeled lemniscal fiber terminals in the lesioned area (right) and in normal VB (left).

nuclei although the difference between sides was partly obscured by a swelling of terminal structures.
The major morphological change was the appearance of large terminal or preterminal swellings intermingled with apparently normal axons (fig. 1-right). These large structures, termed "varicosities" were densely filled by WGA-HRP and possessed diameters of more than 20 µm. The shapes were heterogeneous, the limits irregular, and protrusions were observed.

Catecholaminergic systems

Immunocytochemical studies of catecholaminergic systems were performed using an antibody raised against the enzyme tyrosine hydroxylase to analyze the noradrenergic projections from the locus coeruleus constituting one of the main diffuse systems to VB. In parallel, biochemical analysis of the aminergic content of VB was performed using high pressure liquid chromatography with electro detection.
TH-like immunoreactive fibers were present in the lesioned area one, two and four months after KA injection. This anatomical observation corresponded to the biochemical demonstration that the total amount of norepinephrine in VB was unchanged up to four months after KA injection. Additionally, there was no evident structural alteration of the TH-like immunoreactive fibers in the lesioned areas as compared to those observed in untreated animals.

As a whole, this first series of studies indicated that afferent fibers to an area of KA-induced neurodegeneration were still present one month or longer after the loss of their postsynaptic targets. The diffuse noradrenergic network was remarkably unaltered both morphologically at the light microscopic level and biochemically. In contrast, the fibers constituting point-to-point systems seemed to be relatively decreased in number and exhibited structural alterations of their terminal or preterminal portions. To characterize and further identify the "varicosities", an electron microscopic analysis of the lesioned tissue was carried out.

ELECTRON MICROSCOPY

The ultrastructure of the lesioned area one month after KA injection demonstrates substantial morphological differences from the normal VB. Large intercellular gaps occur so extensively that neural structures are only rarely in contact. As expected from the light microscopic analysis, there are numerous glial cells and a complete lack of neuronal somas, dendrites and observed synaptic contacts. The neural processes which do exist in the tissue are the varicosities - not observed at all in normal VB - and unmyelinated profiles. Both types of profiles were labeled anterogradely from the dorsal column nuclei or the somatosensory cortex.

Varicosities

Varicosities could be separated into two groups on the basis of morphological characteristics.

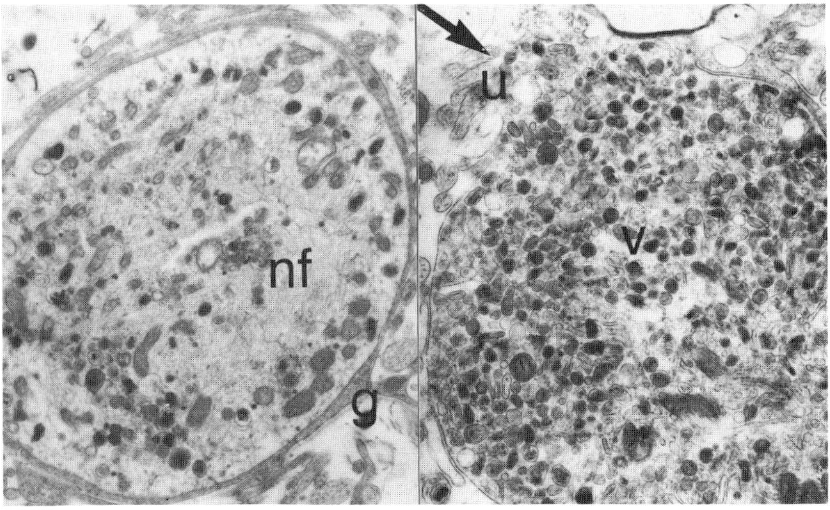

Figure 2 : Varicosities. left : varicosity ensheathed by a glial process (G) and filled with a neurofilamentous meshwork (nf); right : unensheathed varicosity (V) with thin excrescences (U, arrow).

Ensheathed varicosities (fig. 2 left) are axonal swellings completely ensheathed by glial processes. They demonstrate the morphological features of axonal degeneration, some exhibit a neurofilamentous meshwork occupying the center of the profile while the other organelles (including enlarged mitochondria) are pushed away along the external membranes. Other ensheathed varicosities are electron lucent and contain mostly smooth endoplasmic reticulum and enlarged mitochondria. Characteristically, these ensheathed,

presumably degenerating, varicosities are rounded in shape and no protrusions or thick expansions are observed. As a result, these ensheathed varicosities were considered to be morphological features of dying back axons.
Unensheathed varicosities (fig. 2) (i.e. not completely surrounded by glial processes) are, in contrast, quite variable in shape and size and rich in organelle content. The most predominent organelles in the unensheathed varicosities are arrays of microtubules observable in all portions of the swellings. Mitochondria are also particularly numerous in the central portion of the swelling; they are elongated, slender and relatively dense. Smooth endoplasmic reticulum is also widespread and organized in vesicles and tubules. Large structures containing electron dense material, which appeared comparable to lysosomes, are additionally present in these varicosities.
Three types of excrescences issue from the unensheathed varicosities : (i) thick "mound-like" expansions containing large vacuoles and dense-core vesicles (ii) thin protrusions containing only neurofilaments and resembling filopodia (iii) thin long excrescences resembling unmyelinated axons.

Unmyelinated axons

Numerous unmyelinated axons containing microtubules and occasional vesicles of smooth endoplasmic reticulum appear in bundles within the neuropil. The origin of some of these unmyelinated axons could be traced back either to unensheathed varicosities or to large unmyelinated or myelinated axons. The amount of unmyelinated axons within the neuropil was substantially increased compared to that observed in normal tissue.

As a whole, these results demonstrate that an area of KA-induced neurodegeneration contains axonal profiles undergoing two potentially opposing fates : presumptive "dying back" axons, characterized by ensheathed varicosities filled by a neurofilamentous meshwork, and probable "growing" elements including both proliferating unmyelinated axons and varicosities. The fine structure of these presumptive growing elements compares surprisingly well with that described for regenerating growth cones (Tennyson, 1970 ; Bunge, 1973), particularly their organelle content in terms of density and subcellular localization. Our interpretation of these changes is that in such an area of neuronal loss, the point-to-point afferent systems undergo morphological changes demonstrating both a progressive retrograde degeneration and the growth of processes taking the forms of growth-cone like structures and proliferating unmyelinated axons. If such a growing process exists, questions arise regarding the functional state of the afferent fibers undergoing these structural alterations.

ELECTROPHYSIOLOGICAL ANALYSIS

These data were obtained from 15 rats lesioned one or two months before recording. Fifty-six afferent fibers activated from an area of the body normally represented in the area of VB lesioned by KA were recorded extracellularly using glass micropipettes inserted into the lesioned area. Out of these 56 units, 38 responded to brushing, 14 to light pressure and 4 to both non-noxious and noxious mechanical stimulation of the skin. The conclusive element leading us to consider the recorded unit as a "targetless" fiber was a histologic control demonstrating that the location of the recorded fiber was in an area of VB devoid of neuronal cell bodies. All the response characteristics of these afferent fibers appeared consistant with the results obtained in unlesioned animals (see refs in Guilbaud et al., 1980) including a rough calculation of their conduction velocity.

CONCLUSIONS

The present data demonstrate that despite a complete neuronal loss in VB leading to an alteration of a noxious response in a behavioral test, there is an apparent preservation of the afferent circuitry as revealed by both anatomical and electrophysiological analyses. In addition, the ultrastructural analysis of the lesioned tissue reveals that despite terminal or preterminal processes undergoing an apparent degeneration, there exists both a proliferation of unmyelinated fibers and the appearance of axonal varicosities which can be compared to growth-cone like structures. Both latter types of axonal profiles might be interpreted as signs of a regenerative attempt. Since no unaltered afferent point-to-point fiber was observed anatomically, it can be inferred from electrophysiological results that structural alteration did not modify significantly the functional capacity of fibers. Further studies are needed to determine whether such apparently regenerative phenomena are present in other cases of neurodegeneration and in particular in neurodegenerative diseases. Experiments have been also undertaken to determine whether targetless afferent fibers belonging to point-to-point systems could make new functional contacts, with new postsynaptic elements introduced by intracerebral transplantation of embryonic neurons. We have now evidence that targetless fibers can form synaptic contacts with grafted embryonic neurons. Electrophysiological studies are in progress to determine whether these synaptic contacts are functional.

Bunge, M.B., Fine structure of nerve fibers and growth cones of isolated sympathetic neurons in culture. J. Cell Biol., 56, 1973, 702-712.

Coyle, J.T. and Schwarz, R., The use of excitatory amino acids as selective neurotoxins. In : Handbook of chemical neuroanatomy, A. Björklund and T. Hökfelt eds, Elsevier, Amsterdam, 1983, 508-527

Guilbaud, G., Peschanski, M., Gautron, M. and Binder, D., Neurones responding to noxious stimulation in VB complex and caudal adjacent regions in the thalamus of the rat. Pain, 8, 1980, 303-318.

Kayser, V., Peschanski, M. and Guilbaud, G., Neuronal loss in the ventrobasal complex of the rat thalamus alters behavioral responses to noxious stimulation. In : Adv. in Pain Res. and Ther., 1985, Raven Press, N.Y., 277-284.

Mc Allister, J.P. and Wells, J., The structural organization of the ventroposterolateral nucleus in the rat. J. Comp. Neurol., 197, 1981, 271-301.

Mesulam, M.M., Tetramethyl benzidine for horseradish peroxidase neurohistochemistry : a non carcinogenic blue reaction product with superior sensitivity for visualizing neural afferents and efferents. J. Histochem. Cytochem., 26, 1978, 106-117.

Peschanski, M. and Besson, J.M., Coerulear projections to the lateral diencephalon in the rat. Neurosci. Lett., 46, 1984, 329-334.

Peschanski, M., Lee, C.L. and Ralston, H.J. III, The structural organization of the ventrobasal complex of the rat as revealed by the analysis of physiologically characterized neurons injected intracellularly with horseradish peroxidase. Brain Res., 297, 1984, 63-74.

Tennyson, V.M., The fine structure of the axon and growth cone of the dorsal root neuroblast of the rabbit embryo. J. Cell Biol., 44, 1970, 62-79.

Acknowledgements : the authors whish to thank Drs G. Guilbaud, F. Godefroy, J. Weill-Fugazza and A. Basbaum for their participation to some of these experiments and Dr S.L. Juliano for her review of the manuscript.

Effects of Injury on Trigeminal and Spinal Somatosensory Systems, pages 339–346

NON-INVASIVE ASSESSMENT OF PERIPHERAL AND CENTRAL NEURAL INJURY BY CEREBRAL EVOKED POTENTIALS

Willie K. Dong, Yoriko Kawakami and Eric H. Chudler

Department of Anesthesiology (W.K.D., Y.K., E.H.C.), and Multidisciplinary Pain Center (W.K.D.), School of Medicine, University of Washington, Seattle, Washington 98195

INTRODUCTION

The clinical utility of trigeminal and spinal somatosensory evoked potentials in non-invasive assessment of peripheral and central neurological disorders has been demonstrated (Anziska and Cracco, 1980; Desmedt, 1980; Buettner et al., 1982; Leandri et al., 1985). The usefulness of this diagnostic tool has been increased by computers that permit resolution of both near-field (cortex) and far-field (brain stem, spinal cord, nerve) components of these potentials. Non-human primate studies using invasive stimulating and recording techniques and acute lesions or ablations have made important contributions to understanding the origins and biophysics of these potentials in man (Arezzo et al., 1979, 1981; Chudler et al., 1985, 1986). Evoked potentials, obtained non-invasively in a chronic animal model, may provide an important correlate to behavioral or neurological measurements that are often used in assessing peripheral or central neural injury. This paper presents findings from the cat that show 1) the effects of acute central injury on trigeminal and spinal somatosensory, far-field and early near-field evoked potentials and 2) the effects of chronic nerve injury on spinal somatosensory, early near-field potentials. The latter are preliminary observations intended to demonstrate the feasibility of non-invasive, long-term electrophysiological assessment of neural injury in the same animal.

MATERIALS AND METHODS

In acutely prepared, barbiturate-anesthetized cats, trigeminal and spinal somatosensory evoked potentials were

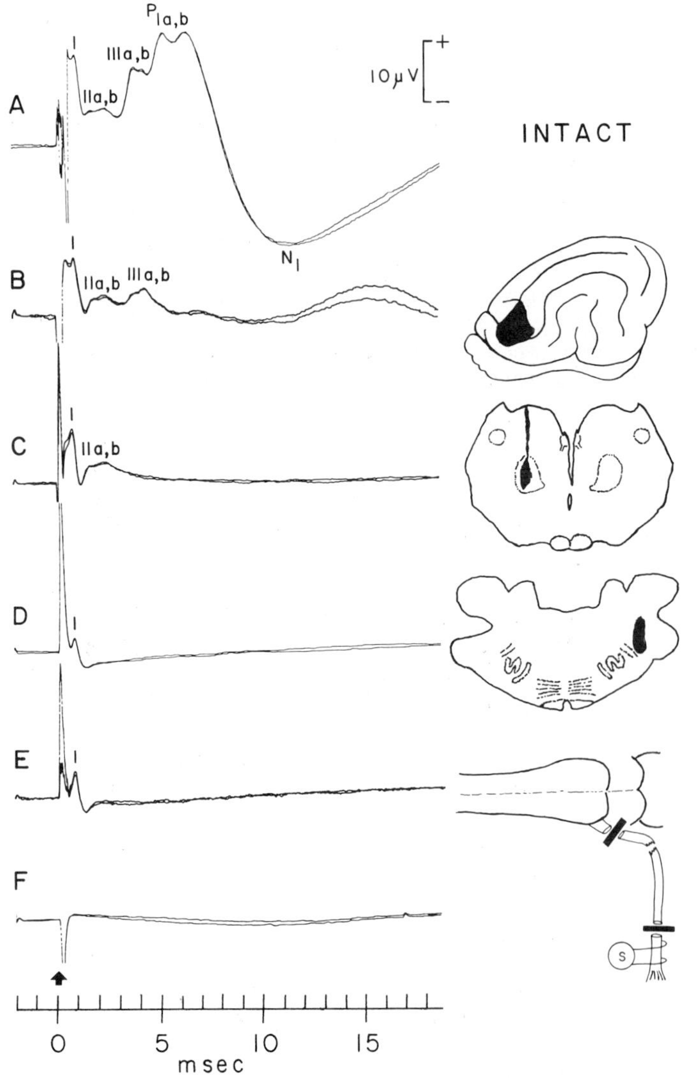

Figure 1. Effects of acute central injury on trigeminal evoked potentials. Each evoked potential in the pair of overlapping traces represents an average of 512 trials. A: nervous system intact. B: ablation of contralateral SI cortex and related white matter. C: lesion of contralateral VPM. D: lesion of ipsilateral PNV. E: dorsal rhizotomy of trigeminal nerve. F: transection of main mental nerve immediately proximal to stimulating electrodes (S). Reproduced with permission (Dong, 1982).

elicited by electrical bipolar stimulation of the main mental branch of the inferior alveloar (dental) nerve and superficial radial nerve (or dorsal columns), respectively. Evoked potentials were recorded from active electrodes implanted epidurally over the contralateral primary sensorimotor cortex (SI). Reference and ground electrodes were implanted in the nasal and occipital bones, respectively. Details of the animal preparation and of the stimulation and recording procedures are described in previous reports (see Dong, 1982; Dong et al., 1982). In chronically prepared, halothane-anesthetized cats, spinal somatosensory evoked potentials were elicited by electrical bipolar stimulation of the skin surface on the dorsal forepaw. Vitallium screw electrodes were implanted in the frontal bone for chronic epidural recordings over SI. All signals were led to preamplifiers with a frequency response of 30 Hz to 3 kHz (-3 dB cutoff points) and to a signal averager with a vertical resolution of 12 bits, maximum sweep length of 4096 points and maximum sampling rate of 1 µS/point.

RESULTS AND DISCUSSION

Short latency brain stem (far-field) and cortical (early near-field) potentials were evoked by activating large myelinated (Aβ) fibers in the main mental nerve (Fig. 1A). Barlow and Spangler (1985) recently reported far-field and early near-field components elicited by mechanical stimulation of the lip that are identical to those recorded in response to electrical stimulation of the mental nerve. As shown in Fig. 1B-1F, specific sets of response components are affected depending on the level of acute injury in the trigeminal lemniscal system. The generator sources were identified from these lesion/ablation results and from comparison of both latency and waveform of the epidurally-recorded components with those recorded at putative generator sites along the trigeminal lemniscal system (Dong, 1982). Far-field components I, II and III, respectively, originate from the inferior alveolar (dental) nerve/semilunar (gasserian) ganglion, trigeminal lemniscus (axons from principal sensory nucleus-PNV) and thalamocortical radiation (axons from VPM nucleus), whereas early near-field components P1 and N1 originate from the cell layers of cortical area 3. A recent study showed that tooth pulp-evoked far-field and early near-field potentials in the cat are also volume-conducted from the same generator sources (Dong and Chudler, 1984).

Activation of dorsal column fibers or large myelinated (Aβ) cutaneous nerve fibers in the spinal somatosensory system evokes

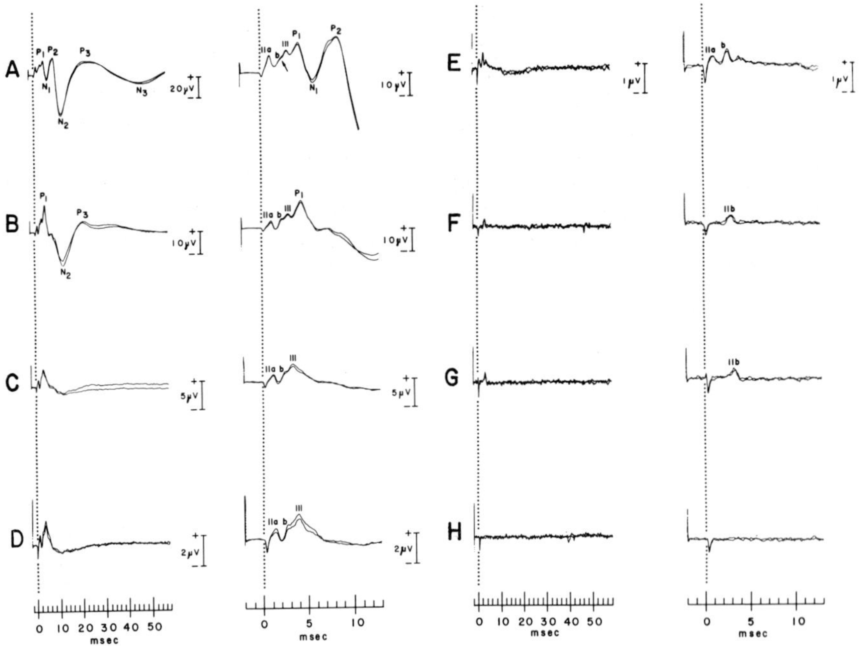

Figure 2. Effects of acute central injury on somatosensory evoked potentials. Each evoked potential in the pair of overlapping traces represents an average of 512 trials. All evoked potentials were evoked by stimulation of the contralateral dorsal columns between C6 and C7. A: nervous system intact. B: bilateral ablation of sensory (SI, SII) and motor (MI) cortices. C: bilateral posterior thalamotomy. D: transection of brain stem at medulla (within Horsley-Clarke frontal planes P9.0-10.0). E: bilateral lesion of dorsal columns between C1 and C2. F: bilateral lesion of dorsal columns at C6. G: bilateral rhizotomy of C5 to T1 dorsal roots, bilateral lesion of dorsolateral funiculi at C5 and spinal cord transection at C8. H: bilateral lesion of spinal cord ventrolateral quadrants (hemisection of ventral spinal cord) between C5 and C6. Reproduced with permission of publisher (Dong et al., 1982).

a complex pattern of far-field and early near-field components (Fig. 2A). As shown in Fig. 2B-H, acute injury at different levels of the lemniscal and extralemniscal systems affects specific sets of response components. The origins of these components were identified from the results of lesion/ablation and from comparison of latency and waveform of the epidurally-recorded components with those recorded at putative generator sources along the two spinal somatosensory projection systems (Dong et al., 1982). The following sites of origin are proposed: I - peripheral nerve; IIa - dorsal columns; IIb - spinothalamic tract; III - medial lemniscus (axons from DCN); P1 - thalamocortical projection (axons from VPL nucleus); N1, P2 - sensorimotor cortices; N2, P3 - association cortices.

A recent study was performed to determine the utility of evoked potentials in monitoring reinnervation of skin after crushing the superficial radial nerve (5mm proximal to radius styloid process). The following parameters were maintained constant across all recording sessions: inspired halothane (1.0-1.5%); impedance across skin stimulation electrodes (8 KΩ) and SI recording electrodes (3.0+1.0 KΩ); rate of stimulation (2/S); suprathreshold stimulation intensity (6mA). Shown in Fig. 3 are representative early near-field components evoked by stimulation of the radial (RN) and ulnar (UN) receptive fields before and after RN crush. In Fig. 4, the topographic amplitude distribution of the SI component (P2) is superimposed on the forepaw stimulation sites. Despite application of a constant stimulus intensity to RN or UN sites, the SI responses were not equipotential. The topographic amplitude distribution of the SI evoked potential underwent considerable alterations prior to complete reinnervation of the RN receptive field. An extensive overlap between UN and RN receptive fields is evident when the UN receptive field (after RN crush on day 4) is compared to the RN receptive field (after UN transection on day 85B). Our results in the cat suggest that functional expansion of the intact, neighboring UN fibers into the RN receptive fields does not occur after RN crush injury (see Devor et al., 1979).

CONCLUSION

The non-invasive measure of evoked potentials in chronically prepared animals is potentially useful in assessing the degree, extent and duration of peripheral or central neural injury.

Research supported by NIH grants DE05130 and NS16329.

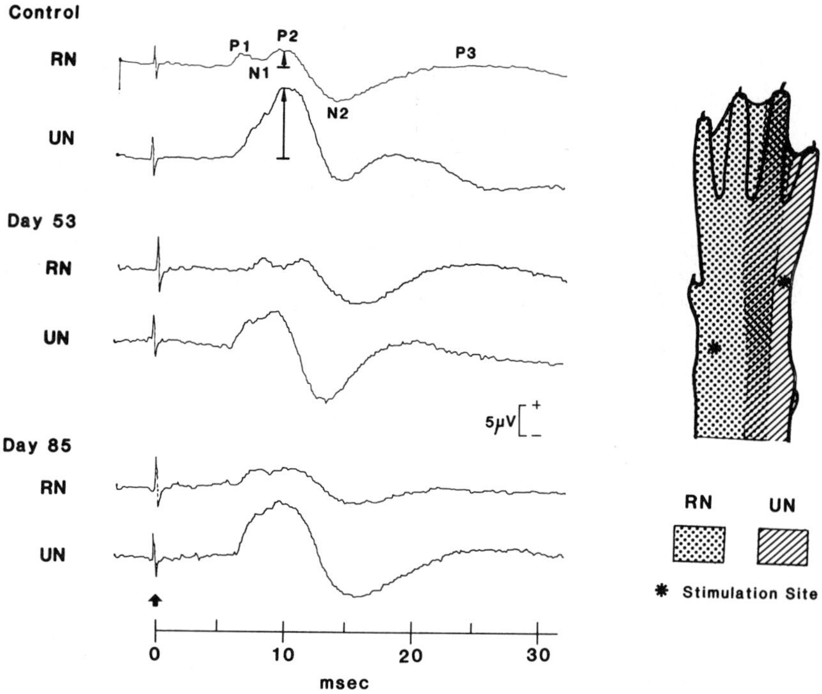

Figure 3. Somatosensory evoked potentials elicited by cutaneous stimulation. Each evoked potential, recorded from the same epidural electrode overlying the lateral sigmoid gyrus of the contralateral SI, represents an average of 64 trials. Electrical stimuli were applied at the same suprathreshold intensity (6mA) to an equally spaced, rectangular grid of loci on skin innervated by the radial nerve (RN) and/or ulnar nerve (UN). The bipolar platinum-ball stimulating electrodes, separated by 3mm, were oriented along the longitudinal axis of the forelimb with the anode and cathode located distal and proximal, respectively. Shown are representative potentials evoked by stimulation at two sites (*) on the RN and UN receptive fields before (control) and after (Days 53 and 85) RN crush. The amplitude of the first positive cortical potential, component P2, was measured from the prestimulus baseline activity to its peak (upward arrows in top traces). See Figure 4 for topographic representation of P2 amplitudes on the RN and UN receptive fields.

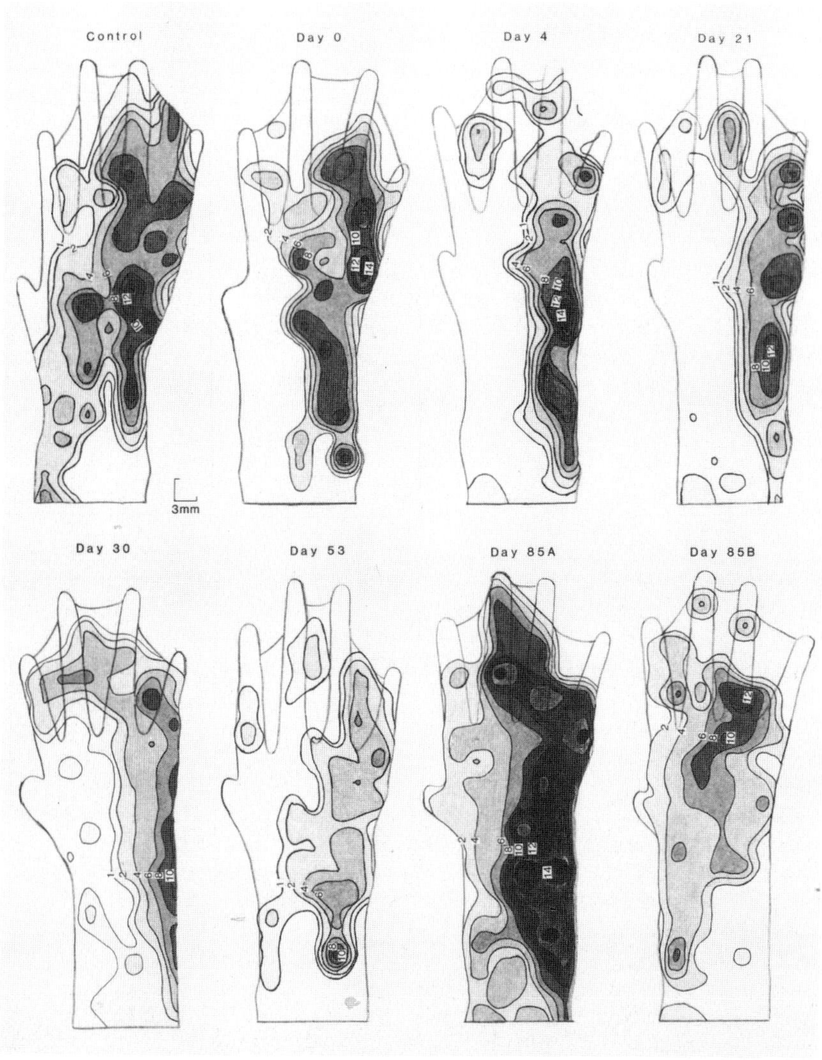

Figure 4. Topographic amplitude distribution of cortical component P2 on forepaw stimulation sites before and after radial nerve crush. Isopotential contour lines are displayed in incremental steps of 1 or 2 μV and superimposed on the stimulated forepaw (dorsal surface). On each day shown, suprathreshold stimuli (6mA) were applied to a grid of 121 ± 7 points that were equally spaced at 3mm intervals. The radial nerve was crushed on Day 0 and the ulnar nerve was transected on Day 85B.

REFERENCES

Anziska B, Cracco R (1980). Short latency somatosensory evoked potentials: Studies in patients with focal neurological disease. Electroencephalogr Clin Neurophysiol 49:227-239.

Arezzo JC, Vaughan HG, Legatt AD (1981). Topography and intracranial sources of somatosensory evoked potentials in the monkey. II. Cortical components. Electroencephalogr Clin Neurophysiol 51:1-18.

Arezzo J, Legatt AD, Vaughan HG (1979). Topography and intracranial sources of somatosensory evoked potentials in the monkey. I. Early components. Electroencephalogr Clin Neurophysiol 46:155-172.

Barlow SM, Spangler K (1985). Mechanically driven trigeminal evoked potentials in cat. Society for Neuroscience Abstracts 11:907.

Buettner UW, Petruch F, Scheglmann K, Stohr M (1982). Diagnostic significance of cortical somatosensory evoked potentials following trigeminal nerve stimulation. In Courjon J, Mauguiere F, Revol M (eds): "Clinical Applications of Evoked Potentials in Neurology," New York: Raven Press, pp. 339-345.

Chudler EH, Dong WK, Kawakami Y (1985). Tooth pulp-evoked potentials in the monkey: Cortical surface and intracortical distribution. Pain 22:221-223.

Chudler EH, Dong WK, Kawakami Y (1986). Cortical nociceptive responses and behavioral correlates in the monkey. Brain Res (in press).

Desmedt JE (1980). "Progress in Clinical Neurophysiology. Clinical Uses of Cerebral, Brainstem and Spinal Somatosensory Evoked Potentials." Basel: Karger, Vol. 7.

Devor M, Schonfeld D, Seltzer Z, Wall PD (1979). Two modes of cutaneous reinnervation following peripheral nerve injury. J Comp Neurol 185:211-220.

Dong WK (1982). Trigeminal evoked potentials: origins in the cat. Brain Res 223:205-210.

Dong WK, Harkins SW, Ashleman BT (1982). Origins of cat somatosensory far-field and early near-field evoked potentials. Electroencephalogr Clin Neurophysiol 53:143-165.

Dong WK, Chudler EH (1984). Origins of tooth pulp-evoked far-field and early near-field potentials in the cat. J Neurophysiol 51:859-889.

Leandri M, Parodi CI, Favale E (1985). Early evoked potentials detected from the scalp of man following infraorbital nerve stimulation. Electroencephalogr Clin Neurophysiol 62:99-107.

Effects of Injury on Trigeminal and Spinal Somatosensory Systems, pages 347–354

A "RECOVERY CYCLE" IN CENTRAL SOMATOSENSORY CIRCUITS OF PRIMATES AFTER DAMAGE AND REGENERATION OF NERVES: SYSTEM LEVEL REORGANIZATION DURING REGROWTH OF CONNECTIONS

J. T. Wall and J. H. Kaas

Department of Psychology, Vanderbilt University
Nashville, Tennessee 37240

Touch sensations are lost from skin regions that become denervated as a result of nerve injury, but can be recovered if these regions are subsequently reinnervated. This "sensory recovery cycle" is dependent on a relatively well understood cycle of peripheral degeneration and regeneration changes in the injured nerve. Although this "peripheral recovery cycle" is clearly necessary for restoring sensations, the key to understanding sensory recovery lies in a knowledge of the corresponding changes that occur in the central nervous system, since it is central activity that generates sensations. In an attempt to understand central changes, we have studied how topographical organization in the cortical area 3b representation of the hand skin of adult primates is affected when innervation patterns to the hand are changed as a result of damage and regeneration of nerves (Wall et al., 1983, 1986; Wall and Kaas, 1986). This paper briefly summarizes some of the findings and implications of these studies.

MATERIALS AND METHODS

The primate hand is innervated by the median, ulnar, and radial nerves. Cortical topography was studied with multiunit mapping procedures in owl or squirrel monkeys in which the innervation to the hand was manipulated in one of several ways. In studies of nerve damage, median nerves to glabrous skin on the radial palm and digits were injured so that cortical topography could be assessed under conditions where the hand was incompletely innervated. In studies of nerve regeneration, cortical organization was evaluated when regeneration followed crush injury of the median nerve and when regeneration followed end-to-end repair of a sectioned median nerve. Regeneration after crush injury allows cortical assessment under "optimal" reinnervation conditions where injury does not interrupt the continuity of extraaxonal tissue sheaths of the nerve; whereas, reinnervation after repair allows cortical study under more variable conditions where, due to the complete disruption of axons and tissue sheaths, the likelihood that regrowing fibers will reobtain their original target sites in the skin is lower than after crush and regeneration.

RESULTS

Two features of topographical organization will be considered: (1) overall topography of the hand representation and (2) the cortical representation of the glabrous index finger. Overall topography is useful for considering the extent of the cortical changes that are produced after nerve manipulation, whereas consideration of a finger representation illustrates how the location and spatial distribution of the cortical activation zone for a delimited skin region is transformed.

1. Overall Topography of the Hand Representation

Normal. The area 3b representation of the hand in normal owl and squirrel monkeys is topographically organized. Although the detailed patterns of organization vary somewhat in different monkeys, several features are consistently seen across individuals. (1) Neuronal clusters at all or most cortical recording sites in the hand cortex are responsive to cutaneous tactile stimuli and have a small, continuous receptive field. (2) Inputs from palmar pads primarily activate a mediolaterally oriented band of neurons along the caudal margin of the hand cortex (P's, Fig. 1A, B), whereas inputs from digits activate a similarly oriented but more rostrally located band (D's, Fig. 1A, B). (3) Within both these mediolateral bands there is an organized progression of inputs from the thumb (D1) to little finger (D5) side of the hand as cortical recording sites shift from lateral to medial in cortex. (4) Finally, glabrous skin areas on the hand are represented over larger cortical areas than hairy skin areas.

Damage. Crush or section of the median nerve results in a loss of inputs from the thumbward half of the palm and from glabrous digits 1, 2, and part of 3 (Fig. 1A stippled). Immediately after injury, much of the cortical zone that would normally represent this skin (e.g., stippled Fig. 1B)

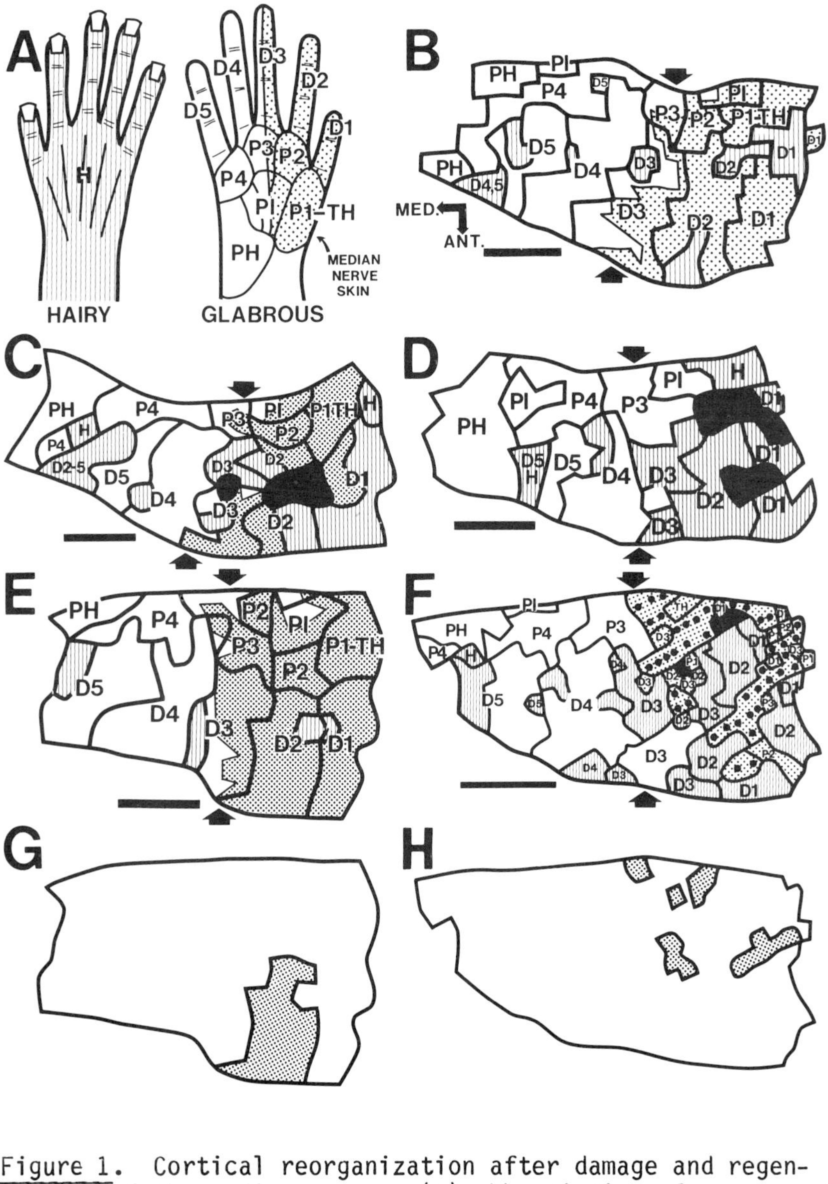

Figure 1. Cortical reorganization after damage and regeneration of the median nerve. (A) Abbreviations for parts of the hand: D1-5, digits 1-5; P2-4, pads 2-4; P1-TH, pad 1 and thenar pad; PI, insular pads; PH, hypothenar pad; H, hairy hand between wrist and knuckles. Glabrous hand parts

is unresponsive to cutaneous stimuli. Within a few days, however, this deprived zone of cortex begins to become responsive to cutaneous inputs from skin locations that adjoin the denervated skin (Merzenich et al., 1983). This "substitution" of intact inputs for injured, lost inputs results in an enlargement of the cortical representations of intact inputs (e.g., dorsal digits 1, 2, and 3, Figs. 1C, D). These changes in topographic patterns occur in the lateral 1/3-1/2 of the hand representation where median nerve inputs would normally be represented (e.g., to the right of arrows in Figs. 1B-D). In contrast, the topography in the more medial part of the hand representation appears to remain normal.

Regeneration after crush injury. The pattern of cortical topography that is seen after damage of the median nerve is

Figure 1 continued: indicated with stippling lose innervation after median nerve injury, whereas unshaded glabrous parts and hatched hairy parts remain innervated by the ulnar or radial nerves. Abbreviations and patterns of shading also apply to B-H. (B) Normal cortical topography. Note that the representation of the median nerve skin (stippling) is located laterally. The indicated spatial orientation also applies to C-H. Spatial calibration bar = 1 mm in all panels. (C) Topography 32 days after crush injury at a time when the hand was partially reinnervated. Note: relatively large representations of hairy digits 1-3, poorly responsive zones (blackened), and partial representation of the median nerve skin (stippling). (D) Topography 6 days after section injury and prior to any reinnervation. Note: relatively large representations of hairy digits 1-3, poorly responsive zones (blackened), and no representation of the median nerve skin (i.e., no stippling). (E) Topography following reinnervation of all parts of the hand after crush injury. Note: relatively normal representation of median nerve skin (stippling) and relatively small representations of hairy digits 1-3. (F) Topography following reinnervation of all parts of the hand after nerve section and repair. Note: large representations of hairy digits 1-3, poorly responsive zones (blackened), and a relatively small representation of the median nerve skin (stippling). (G-H) Comparison of the representation of glabrous D2 (stippling) following regeneration after (G) nerve crush and (H) nerve repair.

itself further changed when a crushed nerve regenerates back to the skin. Following regeneration, all regions of the hand, including the skin regions that were previously denervated, can again become represented in the hand cortex. Overall, the topographical features of the representation of the hand are often normal in major respects (Figs. 1B, E). For example, (1) neuronal clusters at all or most cortical recording sites have a delimited cutaneous receptive field, (2) normal topographical gradients are evident for proximal to distal hand locations in the caudorostral cortical direction, and for the thumb to little finger sides of the hand in the lateromedial direction, and (3) the representations of glabrous skin surfaces predominate. These normal features are seen in the lateral (e.g., to right of arrows Fig. 1E), as well as the medial part of the hand representation. These findings suggest that injury related cortical changes can be effectively reversed under optimal recovery conditions.

Regeneration after section and end-to-end repair. Regeneration after nerve repair can also result in the reestablishment of cortical representations of all regions of the hand. The topography in the hand representation, however, is often abnormal in several respects including the following: (1) neuronal clusters at some cortical sites have multiple receptive fields on discontinuous zones of skin (large dots, Fig. 1F), or are only poorly responsive to cutaneous stimuli, (2) the cortical area representing the reinnervated skin is often smaller than normal and commonly does not have normal topographical gradients for inputs from different locations on the hand, and (3) large representations of dorsal digits, similar to those seen after section injury, are often still apparent (Figs. 1D, F). These abnormalities occur in the lateral part of the hand cortex (e.g., to the right of arrows Fig. 1F); topography in the medial part of the hand cortex appears to remain normal. These findings suggest that the likelihood of recovering normal cortical topography is lower when regeneration follows nerve repair than when regeneration follows crush injury.

2. Cortical Representation of a Finger

Other features of cortical reorganization are best illustrated by considering the transformations that occur in the representation of a delimited skin region like a finger. Inputs from the glabrous index finger (D2) normally activate neuronal clusters in the rostrolateral part of the hand representation (Fig. 1B). Following injury of the median nerve, the cortical representation of this skin is lost (e.g., Fig. 1D). With subsequent regeneration of the median nerve, the representation of the index finger can be recovered; however, the spatial features of the newly established representation can vary widely. For example, following crush and regeneration, a representation that resembles that of normal animals in terms of size, location, and internal topographical order, is often reestablished (e.g., Figs. 1B, G). In contrast, following median nerve repair, the representation of the index finger is commonly abnormal in several respects, including the following (e.g., Figs. 1B, H). (1) Neuronal clusters that are activated by index finger inputs are frequently distributed in small "patches" of cortex. (2) These patches are often widely distributed across the lateral part of the hand cortex (e.g., Fig. 1H). This suggests there is an increased divergence in the flow of information from the skin to cortex. (3) As a result of abnormal multiple receptive field structure, neuronal clusters at some sites in these patches may be simultaneously activated by inputs from the index finger and by other widely separated parts of the hand. This suggests that there is an increased convergence of information from the skin to sites in cortex and that new patches are often not specific in representing the index finger.

DISCUSSION

Our findings suggest that both damage and regeneration of nerves cause central circuits up to the primary somatosensory (area 3b) cortex to undergo organizational changes which, considered together, constitute a "central recovery cycle." The following general features characterize this recovery cycle. (1) There are modifications in the functioning of cortical circuits that are at least 2-3 synapses removed from injured or regrown neurons. (2) At least 3 stages of modification occur: an early stage when cutaneous inputs are lost and cortical activation from the skin diminishes, a second stage when uninjured inputs may substitute for injured inputs, and a third stage when substitution changes may be reversed by reactivation from newly regenerated inputs. (3) Reorganizational changes appear restricted to zones of cortex that are normally activated by the damaged neurons. (4) There are changes in both the convergence and divergence of information transfer from skin receptors to cortical neurons. (5) There is a range of outcomes in how regenerated inputs are represented, which can vary from close replication of normal organization to highly abnormal organization.

There is little understanding of how organizational features of central circuits are transformed following nervous system damage and regrowth. In the past, most studies of nervous system injury have focussed on changes that result from the lesion or damage, itself (e.g., see Finger and Stein, 1982). In contrast, there are few studies of the cortical consequences of regeneration and, as a result, the concept of recovery, in the sense of an understanding of central modifications after injury and after actual replacement of injured circuits with regenerated circuits, has not been widely recognized. Although we took advantage of the natural regeneration capacities of peripheral neurons, the usefulness of understanding central recovery cycles is clearly not restricted to nerve regeneration. Recent studies on transplants of central or peripheral nervous tissue into different parts of the brain have shown that grafted tissues can survive, grow processes into neighboring structures, and support new axons from the host tissue (e.g., see Cotman, 1985, and Nottebohm, 1985). In demonstrating that damaged central connections can regrow, these findings have changed traditional views on the regenerative capacities of the brain. It seems likely that features of central recovery defined in the present experiments will also be apparent in the recovery cycles of other circuits. In particular, the present recovery cycle was determined in a system that is normally organized in a highly topographic fashion, and it is reasonable to propose that features of this cycle will hold for any system in which new circuits must integrate with spatially organized systems in the brain.

In a further attempt to determine central capacities for recovery, we have tried to build new, identifiable features into regenerating peripheral connections to specifically test whether these features become incorporated into cortical circuits (Wall and Kaas, 1986). In these studies, the innervation patterns to the hands of adult monkeys were changed by cross repair of the ulnar to the median nerve. As a result of this manipulation, the ulnar nerve regenerated into the skin territory normally innervated by the median nerve. This procedure allowed us to remodel the spatial relationship between an address on the skin, i.e., what skin territory the regenerated end of the ulnar nerve innervated, and the central activation zone of the ulnar nerve. The difference in the skin addresses of normal and cross regenerated ulnar nerves supplied a "tag" which could be used to identify whether this change in peripheral addressing became incorporated in cortical topographical organization. The results indicated (1) that area 3b cortical topography changed after cross reinnervation, (2) that many of these changes were tagged to peripheral readdressing, and (3) that these tagged cortical changes remained apparent for the longest period tested which was almost 3 years after peripheral readdressing. These results suggest that topographical organization in the polysynaptic system of connections up to cortex is strongly influenced by spatial addressing in the periphery. These findings are provocative from the viewpoint of central recovery because they demonstrate that it is possible to use regenerated nervous tissue and central recovery cycles to intentionally engineer long-lasting organizational changes in central circuits.

The above experiments provide useful insights into the "system" level consequences of injury and regrowth of circuits. We feel that further delineation of the factors that influence this central recovery cycle will increase our understanding of brain function after neural damage.

REFERENCES

Cotman CW (1985). "Synaptic Plasticity." New York: Guilford.

Finger S, Stein DG (1982). "Brain Damage and Recovery." New York: Academic.

Merzenich MM, Kaas JH, Wall JT, Sur M, Nelson RJ, Felleman DJ (1983). Progression of change following median nerve section in the cortical representation of the hand in areas 3b and 1 in adult owl and squirrel monkeys. Neuroscience 10:639-665.

Nottebohm F (1985). Hope for a new neurology. Ann NY Acad Sci 457:1-233.

Wall JT, Felleman DJ, Kaas JH (1983). Recovery of normal topography in the somatosensory cortex of monkeys after nerve crush and regeneration. Science 221:771-773.

Wall JT, Kaas JH (1986) Long-term cortical consequences of reinnervation errors after nerve regeneration in monkeys. Brain Res 372:400-404.

Wall JT, Kaas JH, Sur M, Nelson RJ, Felleman DJ, Merzenich MM (1986). Functional reorganization in somatosensory cortical areas 3b and 1 of adult monkeys after median nerve repair: possible relationships to sensory recovery in humans. J Neuroscience 6:218-233.

Effects of Injury on Trigeminal and Spinal Somatosensory Systems, pages 355–362

EFFECTS OF PYRAMIDAL TRACT LESIONS ON DEVELOPING LAYER 5 SENSORIMOTOR CORTICAL NEURONS

Katherine Kalil

Department of Anatomy and Neurosciences Training Program, University of Wisconsin, Madison, Wisconsin 53706

A number of recent studies have shown that interruption of afferent input from the periphery can have a profound effect on developing CNS neurons (Belford and Killackey, 1980; Killackey, this volume). In contrast, there is far less information about how the interaction of efferent axons with their targets affects the development of mammalian CNS axons. Further, although afferent and efferent connectivity are important, CNS neurons also have intrinsic programs for growth that proceed during certain phases of development in the absence of such connectivity. For example, in the mammalian visual system the growth of cells in the cat lateral geniculate nucleus continues relatively normally after early visual deafferentiation. Cells become arrested in their growth only at a stage when mature patterns of retinogeniculate terminations would normally develop (Kalil and Scott, 1979; Kalil, 1980).

The present chapter will describe how damage to their efferent axons in the pyramidal tract affects the growth and survival of neurons in layer 5B of the hamster sensorimotor cortex. Of particular interest are the differences related to the age at which the lesions are made and the developmental ages at which the effects of injury would manifest themselves. The hamster pyramidal tract is a good system for such studies since pyramidal tract axons arising from layer 5B of the sensorimotor cortex grow out almost entirely postnatally (Reh and Kalil, 1981, 1982). Cortical neurons in the lumbar representation were chosen for quantitative study (Ramirez and Kalil, 1985) since these are among the largest cells in the sensorimotor cortex.

Since their axons do not invade targets in the lumbar spinal cord until 10 days postnatal (Reh and Kalil, 1981) it is possible to measure the effects of axotomy on cortical neurons before the axons have reached their targets.

MATERIALS AND METHODS

Cell measurements of cortical neurons were made on celloidin-embedded 20 μm coronal sections stained with cresyl violet. Brain sections were obtained from 41 hamsters perfused with 10% formol saline at various stages of normal development or at various survival times following a unilateral lesion of the medullary pyramidal tract. Lesions of the tract in both infant and adult animals were made by a ventral approach through the basioccipital bone. One hundred cells from layer 5B were measured on a single coronal section from the normal or affected lumbar sensorimotor cortex. Landmarks, such as the hippocampus, as well as topographic maps obtained by retrograde HRP techniques (Kalil and Reh, 1981) were used to ensure that cell samples were taken from corresponding lumbar cortical areas regardless of age-related differences in cerebral size. Outlines of neurons from layer 5B containing nucleoli were traced at 1000X using a drawing tube. Cell areas were calculated with an electronic planimeter, and the data from each lumbar cortical area entered into a Harris 6024/5 computer for statistical analysis.

The possibility of cell loss was assessed by comparing normal cortical neuronal density with that of axotomized cortical neurons. Cell density measurements in layer 5B were taken from corresponding lumbar cortical areas by counting cells at 1000X, and computing the area of tissue examined as well as the section thickness.

RESULTS AND DISCUSSION

Normal Development

The rodent neocortex is extremely immature at birth. In the hamster, pyramidal tract neurons are migratory for several days after birth (Shimada and Langman, 1970). Not until days 3 and 4 can layer 5 be recognized in Nissl stained sections. Sublamination of this layer begins at the end of the postnatal week when some of the cells begin to enlarge at a rapid rate, thus differentiating 5B from 5A. Measurements of normal cell growth (Ramirez and Kalil, 1985) show that the mean cross sectional area of the population as a whole doubles between 7 and 14 days. The rate of growth declines after this and adult cell size is reached by about 7 weeks of age. If cell size is analyzed by histograms, the growth rate of the cell population projecting to the spinal cord is even more rapid than the population as a whole. Measurements of retrogradely HRP labeled lumbar corticospinal neurons in adult animals revealed that they comprise the upper 40% in size of the cells in this region of layer 5B. Thus, when histograms of cell size measurements were used to separate small cells (non-corticospinal) from large cells (corticospinal) it was found that the small cells have completed their growth by 11 days postnatal whereas the large cells almost triple in area between 7 and 14 days. During the second week after birth, injection of the cortex with anterograde tracers shows that axons from the lumbar projection area are approaching their targets in the spinal cord which they begin to innervate at about postnatal day 10; from 10-14 days fibers establish connections in the lumbar spinal cord (Reh and Kalil, 1981). Thus, an acceleration in cortical cell growth is accompanied by a period of rapid axonal growth and synaptogenesis.

There is no histologic evidence for cell death in layer 5B during normal development and this is confirmed by quantitative analysis of neuronal density (Ramirez and Kalil, 1985). This result is consistent with those of Finlay and Slattery (1983) who showed that cell death does occur in developing hamster neocortex but is confined largely to layers 2, 3 and 4, and is infrequent in layers 5 and 6. The lack of cell death among developing pyramidal tract neurons is of interest because in the hamster there is direct evidence for axon loss in the infant pyramidal tract (Reh and Kalil, 1982a). Electron microscopy revealed that between 3 and 10 days of age the population of pyramidal tract axons remains at about 200,000 fibers. Then, beginning at 10 days of age there is a large loss of axons resulting in an adult population of only half that of the infants. The largest percentage (65%) of fiber loss occurs between 10 and 14 days of age, followed by a more gradual decline over several weeks. Given the absence of

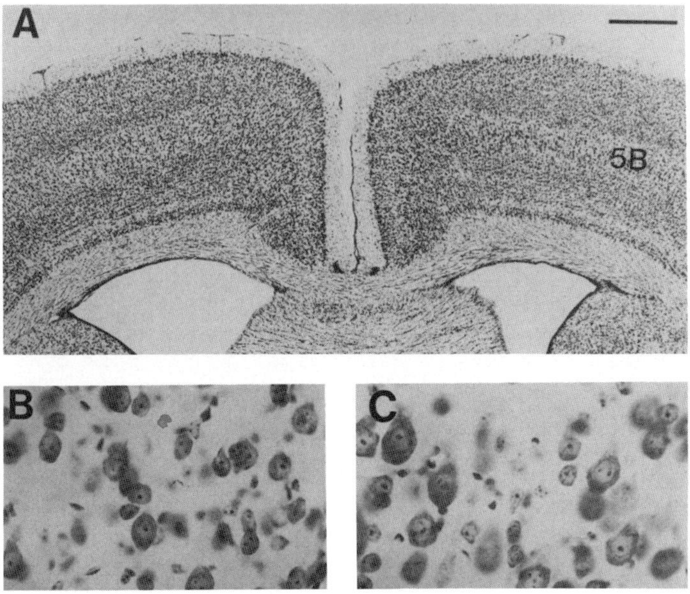

Figure 1. A. Photomicrograph of a Nissl-stained section through the lumbar sensorimotor cortex of an adult hamster with a lesion of the left pyramidal tract at 6 days of age. Note the band of large pyramidal cells in layer 5B of the unaffected (right) cortex and the smaller cells of the affected (left) cortex. B,C. Higher-power photomicrographs from the same section used in A showing large normal pyramidal tract cells (C) and smaller axotomized cells (B). Scale bar = 500 μm.

cortical cell death in layer 5B, it is likely that the lost axons represent transient collaterals whose cortical neurons survive to maturity.

Development After Pyramidotomy

Pyramidal tract lesions in animals at 4, 6 or 8 days of age have no effect on the normal cell growth of cortical neurons measured at 7 or 11 days of age. After 11 days, however, cell growth in layer 5B abruptly ceases. Thus, in the adult the overall distribution of cell size is virtu-

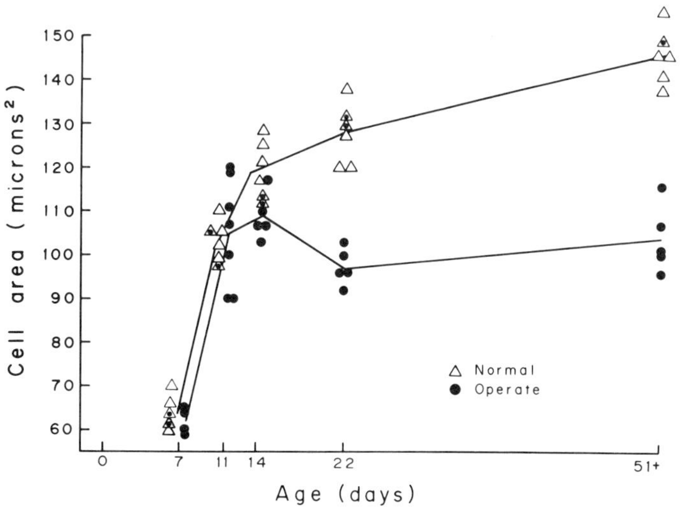

Figure 2. Mean cross-sectional area of cell bodies in layer 5B of lumbar sensorimotor cortex at various postnatal ages. Normal growth (triangles and triangles with central dots) is compared to growth after infant pyramidotomy (solid circles). Each data point represents the mean cross-sectional area of 100 cells.

ally the same as at 11 days. Analysis of cell size by histogram shows that it is the large cell population that is affected by the lesion; this is consistent with the finding that the large cells project their axons into the spinal cord such that lesions of the pyramidal tract in the medulla would sever them. Although the large cells are arrested in development and remain at 50% of normal adult size, small neurons are unaffected by the lesion, presumably because their axons terminate rostral to the lesion.

Large and small cells in layer 5B are also affected differently by adult pyramidotomy. In the adult, lesions of the pyramidal tract produce at least a 60% reduction in cross sectional area of the large cells. The result is that the shrunken neurons are indistinguishable from small cells. The effects of shrinkage are apparent as early as seven days after axotomy and are maximal by postoperative day 25. No additional shrinkage takes place after this.

In contrast, small cells are virtually unaffected by pyramidotomy, as suggested by the fact the lower limit of cell size is the same for normal and lesioned adults. As in normal development, there is no histologic evidence for cell death, nor do neuronal density measurements reveal evidence for any significant cell loss after pyramidal tract lesions in infants or adults.

There are often marked differences between the responses of neurons to axotomy in the CNS of young vs. adult animals. Previous studies have shown that damage to CNS axons early in development can result in either preservation of the cell body accompanied in some instances by collateral sprouting or else rapid and massive retrograde degeneration leading to cell death. A more likely outcome after axotomy in the adult CNS is a progressive cell shrinkage with some cell loss.

The results in hamster pyramidal tract neurons reveal major differences between infant and adult lesioned animals. Whereas adult lesions produce atrophy of corticospinal cells, infant lesions result in arrested growth of large cortical cells. In neither case does significant cell death occur. These results have significant consequences for the fate of the axon as well. In animals with lesions as adults, retrograde shrinkage of corticospinal cells is accompanied by a slowly progressing retrograde degeneration of the pyamidal tract (Kalil and Schneider, 1975). In animals with infant lesions, corticospinal cells, although they fail to achieve their full size, neither atrophy or die and are thus able to regrow their axons (Kalil and Reh, 1979, 1982). Regrowth of severed pyramidal tract axons is maximal if the lesion occurs between 4 and 8 days of age when rapid cell growth and axon elongation are taking place and before extensive corticospinal synaptogenesis occurs. After this period the ability of the severed axons to regrow declines, and no regrowth occurs if lesions are made in animals older than 3 weeks of age. Thus, an important consequence of the ability of immature cortical neurons to survive axotomy, is that the neurons can support regrowth of the severed axons which subsequently establish synapses in appropriate regions of the spinal cord (see Kalil, 1984 for a review). Regrowing fibers contribute to preservation of fine manipulatory movements of the forelimb digits, motor functions which are not restored if the lesion is made in adult animals (Reh and Kalil, 1982b). More recent studies of locomotion in hamsters with infant and adult lesions of the pyramidal tract show a similar difference in the ability of infant but not adult animals to recover motor function after injury to the pyramidal tract (see Keifer and Kalil, this volume).

CONCLUSIONS

Studies of corticospinal cell growth have revealed two distinct phases of cell growth. In the first phase the cells grow normally despite the lesion of their axons within the pyramidal tract. Suddenly at 11 days after birth the cells are arrested in development, regardless of whether the tract is cut at 4, 6 or 8 days postnatal. The cells do not die but remain at about 50% of the normal cross sectional area. The critical time at which growth of the cortical cell becomes dependent on its axon occurs at the beginning of corticospinal innervation of the lumbar cord. It is not known what features of synaptogenesis are important for continued cell growth, but it might be that the retrograde transport of trophic substances from the target and the initiation of synaptic activity are necessary for cortical neurons to achieve their full size. It is perhaps surprising that cortical cell growth is so severely affected because the pyramidal tract lesion cuts off corticospinal fibers but does not injure collaterals rostral to the medulla. Similarly, lesions of the tract in adult animals cause at least a 60% shrinkage of cortical neurons but not cell death. Apparently the remaining axon collaterals are not sufficient to ensure the full growth of the cell in infants or the maintenance of normal cell size in adults after the removal of corticospinal fibers.

The arrest in cortical cell development midway through the period of accelerated cell growth suggests that at early stages neurons may have programs of development regulated by intrinsic mechanisms but that after their axons begin to communicate with a target the further maturation of the cell body comes under environmental influences requiring the integrity of the axon. Since synaptogenesis also signals the end of regenerative growth for corticospinal axons after early injury, an understanding of the relationship between cellular and axonal development will be important in attempts to promote regeneration in the mammalian CNS.

REFERENCES

Belford GR, Killackey HP (1980) The sensitive period in the development of the trigeminal system of the neonatal rat. J Comp Neurol 193:335-350.
Finlay BL, Slattery M (1983) Local differences in the amount of early cell death in neocortex predict adult local specializations. Science 219:1349-1351.
Kalil K (1984) Development and regrowth of the rodent pyramidal tract. TINS 7:394-398.
Kalil K, Reh T (1979) Regrowth of severed axons in the neonatal central nervous system: Establishment of normal connections. Science 205:1158-1161.
Kalil K, Reh T (1981) Establishment of corticospinal topography in hamster pyramidal tract neurons during development. Soc Neurosci Abstr 7:177.
Kalil K, Reh T (1982) A light and electron microscopic study of regrowing pyramidal tract fibers. J Comp Neurol 211:265-275.
Kalil K, Schneider GE (1975) Retrograde cortical and axonal changes following lesions of the pyramidal tract. Brain Res 89:15-27.
Kalil R (1980) A quantitative study of the effects of monocular enucleation and deprivation on cell growth in the dorsal lateral geniculate nucleus of the cat. J Comp Neurol 189:483-524.
Kalil R, Scott G (1979) Development of retinogeniculate synapses in the dorsal lateral geniculate nucleus of the cat. Soc Neurosci Abstr 5:791.
Ramirez LF, Kalil K (1985) Critical stages for growth in the development of cortical neurons. J Comp Neurol 237:506-518.
Reh T, Kalil K (1981) Development of the pyramidal tract in the hamster. I. A light microscopic study. J Comp Neurol 200:55-67.
Reh T, Kalil K (1982a) Development of pyramidal tract in the hamster. II. An electron microscopic study. J Comp Neurol 205:77-88.
Reh T, Kalil K (1982b) Functional role of regrowing pyramidal tract fibers. J Comp Neurol 211:276-283.

Effects of Injury on Trigeminal and Spinal Somatosensory Systems, pages 363–370

THREE PHASES IN THE VULNERABILITY OF THE SOMATOSENSORY SYSTEM TO PERIPHERAL NERVE DAMAGE

Herbert P. Killackey

Departments of Psychobiology
and of Anatomy and Neurobiology,
University of California, Irvine
Irvine, CA 92717

In this short essay I would like to develop the thesis that there are at least three separate phases of somatosensory system vulnerability to peripheral nerve damage. Further, as a consequence of the changing morphological and functional state of the nervous system, each of these phases is characterized by a different response to peripheral injury. I will refer to these three phases rather arbitrarily as the early developmental phase, late developmental phase and the mature phase. In a similar arbitrary fashion, I will focus on the research of my laboratory on the somatosensory system of the rat and begin with a discussion of the late developmental phase as it has been most intensely studied.

LATE DEVELOPMENTAL PHASE

It was first demonstrated by Van der Loos and Woolsey (1973) that altering the somatosensory periphery (removal of a row of vibrissae) at about the time of birth affects the cytoarchitectonic organization of the fourth layer of primary somatosensory cortex. This intriguing finding was the starting point of my own laboratory's interest in the role of the periphery in the establishment of central patterns of neuronal connectivity. We have since utilized a variety of anatomical techniques, including anterograde and retrograde tracers, and most notably, a histochemical assay succinic dehydrogenase which marks the distribution of afferent terminals to study this problem. We first provided evidence that the initial distribution of thalamocortical afferents is altered by cautery of a row of vibrissae on the day of birth (Killackey and Belford, 1979). We also extended the analysis to subcortical stations of this pathway, the brainstem trigeminal complex and the ventral posterior nucleus of the dorsal thalamus, and demonstrated that peripheral injury has a similar effect on these structures (Belford and Killackey, 1980; Erzurumlu and Killackey, 1983).

In terms of normal development, we established that a vibrissae-related pattern is first formed in the periphery and then in the central nervous system in a sequential fashion from brainstem to cortex. In terms of altered development, we established that there is a "sensitive period" during which the periphery must be damaged in order to alter central morphology and that peripheral damage affects both the distribution of afferent terminals and cell bodies. We have also provided evidence that other portions of the somatosensory system besides the trigeminal representation respond to peripheral injury in a similar fashion (Dawson and Killackey, 1986a). Damage to the paws or their afferent innervation around the time of birth alters their associated central representations. Overall, we have interpreted these findings as suggesting that the periphery, acting through the brainstem, provides a template for the formation of central patterns of connectivity (Bates and Killackey, 1985).

Our operating hypothesis is that the main effect of peripheral damage is exerted at one of the central targets of the primary afferents and that the pattern "set up" in this target is replicated in more central stations. In terms of the trigeminal system, this central target is the principal sensory nucleus. This assertion is based on our recent finding that the formation of a vibrissae-related pattern in the ventral posterior nucleus is dependent on an intact principal sensory nucleus and not on other portions of the brainstem trigeminal complex to which primary trigeminal afferents project (Killackey and Fleming, 1985). Further, it is important to note that peripheral damage on the first five or six days following birth has the same effect on the principal sensory nucleus while the effect on more central stations is less severe on each successive day (Belford and Killackey, 1980; Bates and Killackey, 1985).

Our interpretation of these events is as follows. During the first few days of life (the "sensitive" period), the terminal arbors of the primary afferents are forming and their distribution pattern replicates the distribution of the vibrissae. The terminal arbors of the primary afferents in turn induce the vibrissae-related clustering of the thalamic projection neurons of the principal sensory nucleus. This pattern is then replicated in the thalamic terminations of these cells which in turn induce the clustering of thalamocortical relay cells. This same process is repeated still a third time at the cortical level. Cautery of a row of vibrissae in the neonatal animal results in the loss of the associated primary afferents, and hence, the related principal sensory nucleus relay neurons and their coupled central counterparts fail to cluster appropriately. It should be emphasized that there does not appear to be any loss of neuronal elements beyond the primary afferents. The gradation in the severity of the central effect is a result of the time available for interaction between the primary afferents and their target neurons. Cautery at the time of birth minimizes such interactions while damage at a later time allows interaction until the time of damage.

We have also examined aspects of this process at the level of individual thalamocortical afferent terminal arbors. At the time of birth, thalamocortical afferents have reached the white matter underneath the cortical layers and they are topographically organized but are not characterized by the detailed somatotopic organization which develops later (Dawson and Killackey, 1985). By the fourth day after birth, they are distributed in a discrete vibrissae related fashion. In the adult individual thalamocortical terminal arbors are the same size as the cluster with which they are associated (at all levels, cluster size is dependent on the particular vibrissae to which the cluster is related). Individual thalamocortical terminal arbors in adult rats in which the infraorbital nerve was severed on the day of birth differ dramatically from normal (Jensen and Killackey, 1986). They are two to three times as large as normal arbors, appear to have fewer branches and overlap more extensively than terminal arbors in normal animals. We interpret these findings as suggesting that the peripherally based somatotopy is a reflection of terminal arbor morphology.

In the foregoing interpretations major emphasis was placed on the loss of primary afferents following the cautery of a row of vibrissae. Our previous best evidence for this was based on horseradish peroxidase bulk labelling of primary afferents after cautery of a row of vibrissae which results in an unlabelled area in the brainstem

Table 1*

Age	Exp. Group	Synapse Number	Profile Number	Relative Profile Area
PND 3	Intact	6.33	33.64	9.09%
	Experimental	5.00	26.83	6.54%
PND 9	Intact	7.58	33.92	10.74%
	Experimental	4.92	26.67	5.94%

* Each entry is the average of data from 12 sections.

trigeminal complex corresponding to the damaged row (Bates and Killackey, 1985). We have recently followed up a previous study of the ultrastructural organization of the brainstem trigeminal complex (Ide and Killackey, 1985) and obtained evidence that cautery of a row of vibrissae at birth results in a decrease in synaptic density in the subnucleus interpolaris of the brainstem trigeminal complex. Figure 1 presents a low power photomicrograph of a plastic embedded section of the brainstem of the rat and illustrates how portions of the normal and altered subnucleus interpolaris are prepared for analysis and the presence of labelled primary afferent terminals in this nucleus at two days of age. Table 1 presents the results of a stereological analysis of synaptic density on two animals that had the middle row of vibrissae cauterized on the day of birth. There is a clear decrease in synaptic density in the experimental as compared to the intact side.

Developing primary sensory neurons are particularly dependent on nerve growth factor and other neurotrophic factors for survival (see Johnson et al., 1986 for recent review). These same authors also review evidence that pharmacological administration of nerve growth factor can

Figure 1 **A** Section through subnucleus interpolaris stained for cytochrome oxidase, osmicated and embedded in plastic, shows normal vibrissae pattern (Rows A-E, left) and an altered pattern (Row C removal, right). **B** Tissue from A (right side) after mounting on a plastic block for EM sectioning. **C** Tissue processed similarly to A and B, showing cytochrome oxidase-reactive mitochondria (M) and synaptic terminals with accumulations of synaptic vesicles (asterisks) on day 3. **D** Axon terminal of an HRP-labelled primary afferent in subnucleus intepolaris on day 2.

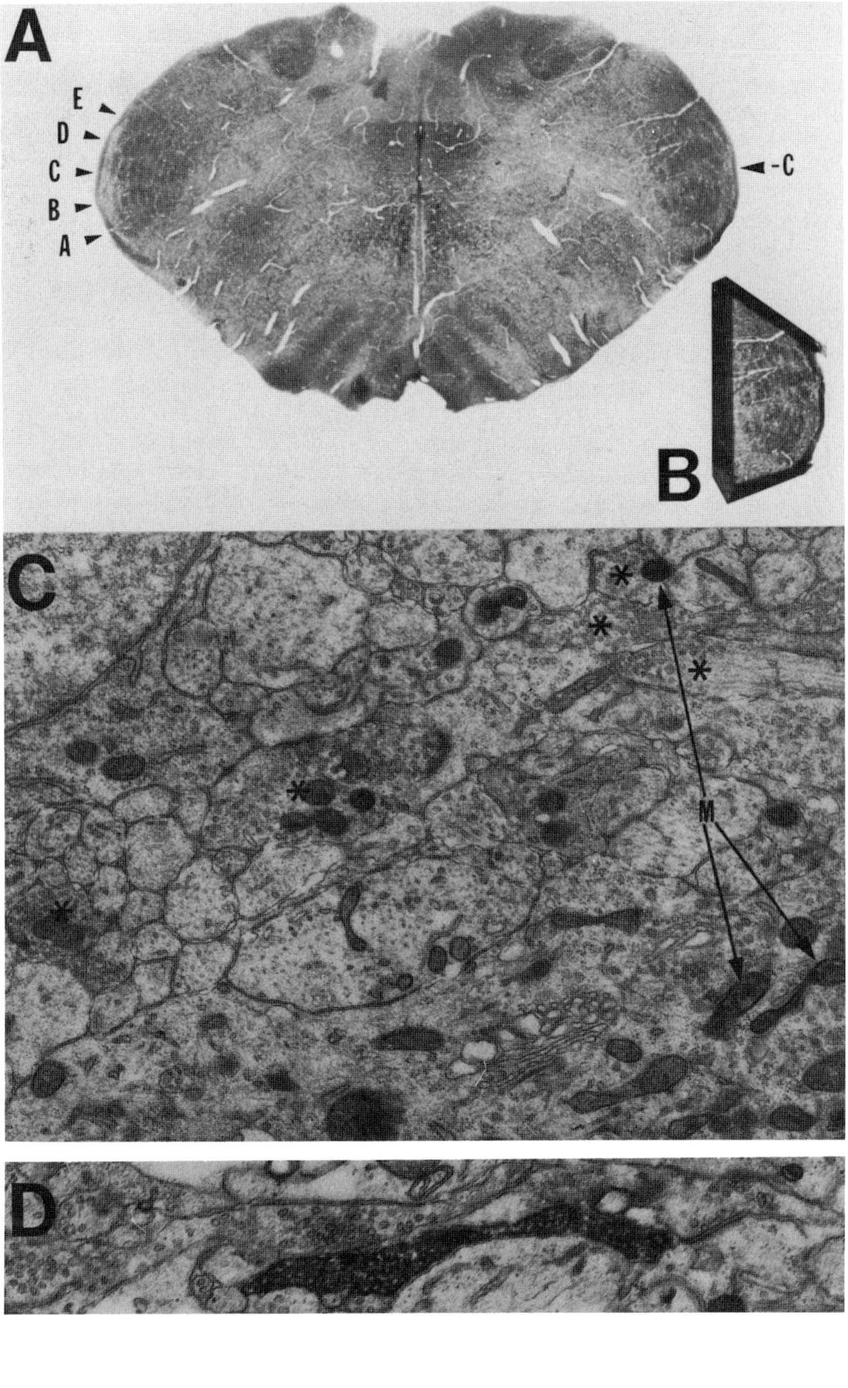
A
E
D
C
B
A
-C
B
C
M
D

prevent neuronal death in the dorsal root ganglion of the neonatal rat following nerve injury. Thus, cautery of a row of vibrissae may lead to a loss of trigeminal primary afferents because it separates these afferents from their peripheral source of nerve growth factor. Further, one can speculate that the application of nerve growth factor to neonatal vibrissae-damaged rats may counteract the effects of neonatal vibrissae damage on central pattern formation.

EARLY DEVELOPMENTAL PHASE

The effects of early fetal peripheral damage on the organization of the somatosensory system of mammals has not been well documented. We have recently extended our study of the organization and mutability of the cortical paw representations into the prenatal period. Previously, we had determined that if the paws or their innervation are damaged on the day of birth the cortical patterns usually associated with the paw representation are disrupted but occupy the same cortical area as normal (Dawson and Killackey, 1986a). All other portions of the pattern are normal and also occupy the same cortical area as in the normal animal. If the forepaw is removed on embryonic day 16, the resultant cortical pattern is highly disorganized and again occupies a normal area. However, the adjacent hindpaw pattern which is normal in terms of configuration expands to occupy up to twice its normal area (Dawson and Killackey, 1986b). This expansion appears to be specific to the hindpaw representation in that there are no changes in the lower lip representation which is also adjacent to the forepaw representation. The expansion seems to be at the expense of cortical areas which border on primary somatosensory cortex.

Our tentative interpretation of this phenomenon is that like the effects of later damage it can be best understood in terms of events occurring at the level of the brainstem. Forepaw damage on embryonic day 16 removes primary afferents before they have ever reached their target neurons in the cuneate nucleus. We hypothesize that under this condition primary afferents usually associated with the adjacent gracile nucleus are able to recruit some neurons of the naive cuneate nucleus into the hindpaw representation, and that this recruitment is maintained at more central stations.

MATURE PHASE

The concept of a "sensitive" or "critical" period referred to above implies that after a certain age peripheral damage will not have the same effect on central organization that it does during the developmental period. However, it does not follow that peripheral damage has no effect on central organization in the mature animal. There has been a number of recent reports of functional changes in the adult central nervous system following peripheral damage. Most pertinent to the present essay is an experiment by Wall and Cusick (1984). These authors report that sciatic nerve section in the adult rat results in a functional expansion of the adjacent saphenous nerve representation into the cortical region in which the sciatic nerve is normally represented. Our own results would indicate that these functional changes are not accompanied by morphological pattern changes (Dawson and Killackey, 1986a). The rapidity of this functional expansion in the adult (one or two days) suggests that this phenomenon may be largely due to the unmasking of previously existing but physiologically undetectable neuronal circuitry. Further, there is no reason to suppose that such expansion is either restricted to cortex or particularly dependent on the brainstem, as are developmental changes. Indeed, it is likely that peripheral damage in the adult may produce functional changes in local neuronal circuitry at all levels of the neural axis.

CONCLUSIONS

During its life span, an organism undergoes a series of commitments which then limits the range of the nervous system's response to a peripheral challenge. This short essay illustrates the differences in response to similar peripheral manipulations at different times and underscores the importance of defining the state of the organism at the time of a peripheral insult.

ACKNOWLEDGEMENTS

Work from my laboratory discussed here was funded by the National Science Foundation.

REFERENCES

Bates, C.A. and Killackey, H.P. (1985). The organization of the neonatal rat's brainstem trigeminal complex and its role in the formation of central trigeminal patterns. J Comp Neurol 240:265-287.

Belford, G.R. and Killackey, H.P. (1980). The sensitive period in the development of the trigeminal system of the neonatal rat. J Comp Neurol 193:335-350.

Dawson, D.R. and Killackey, H.P. (1985). Distinguishing topography and somatotopy in the thalamocortical projections of the developing rat. Dev Brain Res 17:309-313.

Dawson, D.R. and Killackey, H.P. (1986a). The organization and mutability of the forepaw and hindpaw representations in the somatosensory cortex of the neonatal rat. J Comp Neurol., in press.

Dawson, D.R. and Killackey, H.P. (1986b). Morphological changes in rat somatosensory cortex following prenatal limb removal. Soc Neurosci Abs, in press.

Erzurumlu, R.S. and Killackey, H.P. (1983). Development of order in the rat trigeminal system. J Comp Neurol 213:365-380.

Ide, L.S. and Killackey, H.P. (1985). Fine structural survey of the rat's brainstem sensory trigeminal complex. J Comp Neurol 235:145-168.

Jensen, K.F. and Killackey, H.P. (1986). Terminal arbors of axons projecting to the somatosensory cortex of the adult rat. II. The altered morphology of thalamocortical afferents following neonatal infraorbital nerve cut., manuscript submitted.

Johnson, E.M., Rich, K.M. and Yip, H.K. (1986). The role of NGF in sensory neurons in vivo. TINS 9:33-36.

Killackey, H.P. and Belford, G.R. (1979). The formation of afferent patterns in the somatosensory cortex of the neonatal rat. J Comp Neurol 183:285-304.

Killackey, H.P. and Fleming, K. (1985). The role of the principal sensory nucleus in central trigeminal pattern formation. Dev Brain Res 22:141-145.

Van der Loos, H. and Woolsey, T.A. (1973). Somatosensory cortex: structural alterations following early injury to sense organs. Sci 179:395-398.

Wall, J.T. and Cusick, C.G. (1984). Cutaneous responsiveness in primary somatosensory (S-I) hindpaw cortex before and after partial hindpaw deafferentation in adult rats. J Neurosci 4:1499-1515.

Effects of Injury on Trigeminal and Spinal Somatosensory Systems, page 371

DEAFFERENTATION-PRODUCED METABOLIC ALTERATIONS WITHIN RAT SI.

P.J. Hand and S.-C. Scheu

University of Pennsylvania, Philadelphia, PA, USA (PJH) and National Yang-Ming Medical College, Taipei, Taiwan, ROC (SCS)

Developmental effects associated with different ages and postoperative survival times on a vibrissae deafferentation-produced metabolic (functional) reorganization in rat SI cortex (n=35) were examined by stroking spared (SC3) and control (CC3) C3 vibrissae and followed by (^{14}C)-deoxyglucose (2DG) labelling of metabolic activity. In the age effect series, all follicles, excepting SC3, were unilaterally ablated on postnatal days (PND) 0-12, 21. In the postoperative survival time series, deafferentations were performed on PND2. Postoperative survival times varied from 1-12 weeks. The vibrissa stroking-2DG experiments were performed 90 days postdeafferentation. Age effect series results were as follows: 1) in PND 0-3 deafferented rats, the SC3 metabolic representation was enlarged and diffuse; 2) in PND 4-11 lesioned rats, multiple SC3 representations were present in SI; and 3) in PND 12, 21 (also adults) lesioned rats, the SC3 representation in SI was enlarged, but remained focal. Postoperative survival time series results were as follows: 1) the size of the SC3 SI representation (as compared to CC3) increased from 25%-133% whereas the SC3 anatomical "barrel" only increased in size from 24-36% over the 12 week period and 2) the SC3 SI representation exhibited no increase in size between weeks 3-4 and 5-7. In conclusion, the vibrissa deafferentation-produced metabolic reorganization in rat SI is a very labile process heavily dependent upon dynamic developmental factors.

Effects of Injury on Trigeminal and Spinal Somatosensory Systems, pages 373–379

SUMMARY AND CRITIQUE OF SESSIONS ON THALAMUS AND CEREBRAL CORTEX

W.D. Willis

Marine Biomedical Institute

University of Texas Medical Branch, Galveston, TX

ISSUES CONCERNING THE THALAMUS

1. Location of Nociceptive Neurons In and Around the Ventrobasal Complex

In the experiments reported by Yokota and his group, nociceptive neurons with restricted receptive fields in the vicinity of the ventrobasal complex of both the cat and the monkey were found to be exclusively in the shell region. Ralston pointed out that this was consistent with the distribution of the projections of the spinothalamic and trigeminothalamic tracts in the cat but not with those in the monkey, since the spinothalamic tract ends on rods of neurons within the monkey VPL nucleus. Furthermore, the results in the monkey appeared to differ from findings previously reported by the Willis group. Yokota responded by noting that previous work emphasized spinal projections, whereas his group has examined chiefly the trigeminal ones. He also cautioned that some of the spinothalamic projections may relate to tactile rather than to nociceptive neurons.

Vahle-Hinz observed that in studies done in her laboratory on the trigeminal system of the cat, most of the nociceptive cells were distributed broadly in an area below VPM and the external medullary lamina, not just in the shell region. The cells did not have the somatotopic arrangement described by Yokota, nor were nociceptive specific and wide dynamic range cells segregated as he found. Yokota replied that he had similar results initially but that with years of experience he has finally been able to obtain the results he reported on ventrobasal thalamic neurons with restricted receptive fields. Nociceptive neurons with nonrestricted, sometimes bilateral, receptive fields have been found in many locations by many people, for example in centralis lateralis, parafascicularis, subparafascicularis, the fields of Forel, and the thalamic reticular nucleus.

Willis commented that in studies done in his laboratory, nociceptive units recorded in the primate ventrobasal complex had hindlimb receptive fields, whereas Yokota's units had receptive fields chiefly on the face, trunk and upper extremity. This might lead to differences between the two studies. However, both wide dynamic range and nociceptive-specific neurons were found within VPL proper, and these could be activated antidromically from the SI cortex. Yokota pointed out that some of his neurons were rostral in VPL, perhaps in VPLo, which forms part of the shell region. Willis responded that both histological evidence and the fact that the cells could be backfired from the SI cortex showed that the nociceptive cells in the study from his laboratory were in VPLc.

2. The Role of the Dorsolateral Spinothalamic Tract

Hodge and his associates have found that part of the spinothalamic projection in the cat ascends in the dorsal part of the lateral funiculus. This component of the spinothalamic tract originates from neurons of lamina I. Besson stressed that most of the emphasis of Hodge's group has been on the cat. The organization of nociceptive pathways is often different in the cat as compared with the rat and monkey. For example, there are many nociceptive neurons within the VPL nucleus in the rat and monkey but not in the cat. Furthermore, the organization of lamina I projections is complex in that these distribute not only to the thalamus but also to the nucleus cuneiformis, the periaqueductal gray and the parabrachial region, and there are many collaterals of the spinothalamic tract that enter the reticular formation. A second point was that in the rat the nociceptive responses of VPL neurons are largely blocked by a lesion of the ventrolateral quadrant of the spinal cord, whereas a lesion of the dorsal lateral funiculus has only a slight effect. Hodge responded that the recordings made by his group could not distinguish between thalamic responses to direct input from lamina I and those due to input relayed in other brainstem structures. A dorsolateral projection of lamina I cells has now been found not only in the cat but also in the squirrel monkey and in the rat. It appears that the possibility of conduction of nociception information in the dorsolateral quadrant needs reexamination. Peschanski enlarged upon the results of experiments in which spinal cord lesions were made in rats while recording from nociceptive neurons in the ventrobasal complex. These responses were decreased only after a lesion of the ventrolateral quadrant. However, in arthritic rats, such a lesion was insufficient to reduce the nociceptive responses. Thus, nociceptive information ascends in more than one pathway under these pathological conditions.

Willis cited evidence from Kennard and also from Morrow and Casey that is consistent with transmission of nociceptive information in both the dorsolateral and ventrolateral quadrants of the cat spinal cord. Vierck indicated that in his experience on changes in pain responsiveness in monkeys following spinal cord lesions it appears that the ventral pathways are the most important. It would be desirable to know if the squirrel monkey projections resemble those of other monkeys and of the human. Vierck also observed that animals with complete lesions of the dorsolateral and ventrolateral white matter on one side showed recovery of pain sensitivity, indicating alternative nociceptive pathways.

The question of plastic changes following cordotomy was broadened to the case of humans by Berkley. Hodge indicated that there are two different postcordotomy pain problems. There may be the rapid onset of "denervation dysaesthesia" and there may be a gradual return of pain. Berkley asked what pathway is responsible for the return of pain. Hodge replied that every ascending somatosensory pathway is a candidate. However, the propriospinal system is perhaps a leading candidate. Evidence for this is the effectiveness of a midline myelotomy at C1 in relieving pain.

Perl addressed further the question of recovery of function after a spinal cord lesion. He pointed out that there are ipsilateral ascending projections in the ventrolateral part of the cord. This can be shown in monkeys by retrograde labeling with horseradish peroxidase, as well as by recovery of pain following a unilateral lesion.

Willis raised the question of whether studies of the effects of lesions that sever descending inhibitory pathways in the dorsolateral funiculus are confounded by the simultaneous interruption of an ascending nociceptive transmission system. Sessle pointed out that this could also be a problem in the trigeminal system where nucleus caudalis projections to more rostral trigeminal nuclei would be interrupted by trigeminal tractotomies.

3. Spinothalamic Synaptic Terminals in the Primate Thalamus

Berkley noted that in the anatomical experiments of Ralston and Ralston, degenerating spinothalamic tract endings in the central lateral nucleus included both large and small profiles containing round vesicles. Ralston indicated that there may be more than one type of neuron projecting to this nucleus. Willis suggested that these may correspond to spinothalamic neurons that bifurcate to supply both VPL and CL and those that project only to CL.

Csillik inquired of Ralston what might be the function of the triadic arrangements seen in the VPL nucleus that closely resemble those found in the substantial gelatinosa. Ralston agreed that these might play a role in limiting excitatory drive by converting the initial excitation to a long-lasting inhibition, since the local synaptic connections are likely to be from GABAergic inhibitory neurons.

4. Growth Cones in the Rat Ventrobasal Complex Following Kainic Acid Lesions

Peschanski and Besson reported observations of profiles resembling growth cones in the rat ventrobasal complex following kainic acid lesions. Munger stressed that it is necessary to demonstrate the absence of ribosomes to be confident that the profiles really are growth cones. This will be particularly difficult for structures containing granuled vesicles, as was the case in many of the examples illustrated. Peschanski felt confident that the profiles really were growth cones, based in part on the apparent absence of ribosomes after a careful search. Furthermore, the profiles are axonal, since they can be labeled anterogradely and myelin sheaths can be demonstrated in some cases on processes leading to the putative growth cones.

Berkley wondered about retrograde changes in neurons projecting into the area lesioned by the kaianic acid injections. Peschanski indicated that they had expected cell loss in the dorsal column nuclei but found instead only a shrinkage of the neurons. This shrinkage is difficult to relate to the presence of growth cones in the thalamus.

ISSUES CONCERNING THE CEREBRAL CORTEX

1. The Analysis of Brainstem Processing by Recordings of Somatosensory Evoked Potentials

Dong and his colleagues reported on the use of far-field components of somatosensory evoked potentials to examine brainstem processing of sensory information. Sessle raised the question of whether or not evoked potential recordings could demonstrate activation of both a rostral trigeminal trigeminothalamic path and a caudal one following tooth pulp stimulation. Dong indicated that the resolution of the technique did not permit this, although it was possible to show signals derived from spinal levels over both the lemniscal and extralemniscal systems.

2. Alternations in Somatosensory Receptive Fields in cerebral Cortex Following Peripheral Nerve Lesions

Wall described alterations in the somatosensory representation of the monkey hand following peripheral nerve lesions. Zimmermann noted that there appeared to be considerable inter-animal variation in the maps of the receptive fields of cortical neurons responsive to stimulation of the monkey hand. He asked what criteria were used to determine if peripheral nerve lesions really caused changes and if recovery then ensued. Wall replied that it was difficult to study large numbers of animals, and so statistical tests were hard to do. However, it was possible to describe consistent features of the normal representation and to demonstrate changes in these following lesions. Zimmermann suggested that it might be helpful to use a naive observer in the mapping experiments. Wall responded that two individuals participated in the mapping and that he did not know where the electrode was placed when he mapped a receptive field. Juliano added that the animals served as their own controls, since the same individual animal is remapped over a long period of time. However, she wondered if normal animals had been mapped repeatedly to determine if changes occurred over time. Wall pointed out that maps of the representation of areas that were not denervated served the same purpose.

Ochoa asked about the perceptual implications of the work. Cortical neurons were responding to stimulation of innervated skin rather than to stimulation of the denervated skin that had previously formed the receptive field. Does this mean that in humans sensation in the denervated area should be evoked by stimulation of an adjacent innervated region? Wall suggested that the receptive field change did not really represent a substitution but rather an enhancement of a capability that was normally present. Thus, a false localization does not result from stimulation of the skin adjacent to a denervated region because the brain does not interpret that there is a gross change. You can get false localization after nerve repair because the brain has no way to cross-check for this kind of change.

Devor asked if Wall had determined changes in thresholds of the neurons whose receptive fields were mapped. Wall responded that thresholds were not quantitated. However, they were certainly low enough to be sure that the neurons were activated by low threshold mechanoreceptors. Another question raised by Devor was whether the changes in cortical maps following peripheral nerve injury were taking place because of changes in the spinal cord, brainstem or cortex. Wall agreed that there seemed to be changes occurring in the spinal cord and the dorsal column nuclei, but there was too little evidence to be sure about changes within the cortex. Hand felt that his 2-DG material provided support for the idea that there are cortical changes, although the data have been insufficiently analyzed.

3. Absence of Cell Death of Corticospinal Neurons Following Lesions of the Pyramids

Munger questioned Kalil's assertion that the number of corticospinal neurons was not reduced following interruption of the pyramid in immature hamsters. Kalil responded that the cell counts and also the fact that the sectioned axons regrow argue that the cells are not lost. Although the neurons lose their spinal cord targets, there are still collateral projections in the brainstem and cortex, and many of the axons regrow to establish new connections in the spinal cord.

4. 2-Deoxyglucose Study of Somatosensory Cortex

Munger wondered if the neuromata formed by removal of mystacial vibrissae in the neonatal rat affect the development of the pathway. Hand indicated concern about the possibility that activity originating from the wound produced by removal of a single vibrissa might affect the 2-DG results. However, complete removal of the vibrissae did not change the amount of metabolism determined by the 2-DG technique.

Willis asked whether the label in the 2-DG experiments is in synaptic terminals or in postsynaptic structures. Hand responded that this was not known but probably both. Electron microscopy would be needed to resolve this question, but this may not be feasible because of the signal-to-noise ratio.

IV
PATHOPHYSIOLOGY AND BEHAVIOR

Effects of Injury on Trigeminal and Spinal Somatosensory Systems, pages 383–388

HYPERALGESIA FOLLOWING PERIPHERAL NERVE INJURY

Richard A. Meyer, James N. Campbell and Srinivasa N. Raja

Departments of Neurosurgery (RAM, JNC) and of Anesthesiology (SNR) and Applied Physics Lab (RAM), Johns Hopkins University, Baltimore, Maryland 21205

INTRODUCTION

One of the complications of nerve injury is the development of chronic pain. In addition to varying degrees and time periods of ambient pain (pain without apparent exogenous stimulation), cutaneous hyperalgesia may develop. The hyperalgesia is characterized by a decrease in the threshold for pain from mechanical stimuli, and an increase in the pain to suprathreshold stimuli. This mechanical hyperalgesia is readily demonstrated in that light stroking of the skin elicits pain. For some patients, movement of a single hair follicle is painful.

The goal of this study was to characterize the hyperalgesia that follows a nerve injury. In one series of experiments, we sought to determine whether the hyper-algesia to mechanical stimuli is signalled by activity in large or small diameter primary afferents. In another series of experiments, we sought to determine whether sensory testing could be helpful in the diagnosis of these patients.

AFFERENTS WHICH SIGNAL HYPERALGESIA

Under normal circumstances, pain is thought to be signalled by activity in C-fiber and small-diameter

A-fiber nociceptive afferents (for review see Meyer, et al, 1985). Do these fibers also signal the hyperalgesia that occurs following a nerve injury? To determine if large or small diameter afferents signal the hyperalgesia, we performed an ischemic block of the nerves in the affected extremity. Such a block induces an orderly loss of sensation corresponding to the loss of large fiber function prior to loss of small fiber function. Thus touch sensation is lost first, followed by loss of the sense of coolness and warmth, corresponding to a loss of A-beta, A-delta and C-fiber function respectively.

Patients were selected for study who had chronic pain following peripheral nerve injury in the distal part of an extremity and who had hyperalgesia to mechanical stimuli. In each patient, light stroking of the affected skin elicited pain. To obtain an ischemic block, a sphygmomanometer cuff was placed on the proximal part of the affected extremity and inflated to a pressure which was 50-100 torr above systolic pressure. By performing sensory testing in an area of normal skin adjacent to the hyperalgesic area, we were able to monitor which fibers were affected by the block at a given time. Touch sensation was assessed by observing whether subjects could detect light stroking of the skin with a cotton swab or a camel's hair brush. Temperature sensation was assessed by determining whether subjects could distinguish between a warm and a cool probe placed on the skin. The presence and severity of hyperalgesia was monitored by asking subjects to describe sensations elicited by stroking the usually hyperalgesic skin and to compare these sensations to those they felt prior to implementation of the block.

Fourteen patients participated in this study. All, but one, experienced complete relief of their mechanical hyperalgesia during the block. The pain relief began 4 to 20 minutes after inflation of the cuff with complete elimination of pain occurring 15 to 30 minutes after inflation of the cuff. The affected area could be handled vigorously without pain. At the time that the hyperalgesia was eliminated, only touch sensation was affected in the normal skin adjacent to the hyperalgesic zone. Cold and warm stimuli still felt normal and could be readily distinguished. The hyperalgesia returned beginning several minutes after release of the cuff.

These data indicate that hyperalgesia was gone when A-beta fibers which signal touch sensation were blocked but when A-delta (cold sensation) and C-fibers (warmth sensation) were still conducting. These preliminary results are similar to those described by Wallin et al (1976) and Ochoa (1982) and suggest that hyperalgesia following nerve injury is signalled by activity in large-diameter myelinated afferents. Thus, the C-fiber and small-diameter A-fiber nociceptive afferents which signal pain under normal circumstances are not involved in signalling the hyperalgesia that follows a nerve injury.

SYMPATHETICALLY MAINTAINED PAIN

In some patients, the mechanical hyperalgesia is accompanied by signs of sympathetic hyperactivity in the affected limb (e.g., lowered skin temperature, skin discoloration, hyperhidrosis and trophic changes). The abnormal sympathetic activity is associated with the pain state since an anesthetic block of the appropriate sympathetic ganglia can result in temporary pain relief particularly when performed at an early stage in the disease. Following the suggestion of Roberts (1986), we use the term sympathetically maintained pain (SMP) to refer to this population of patients in order to avoid the imprecise definitions associated with causalgia, reflex sympathetic dystrophy, and Sudeck's atrophy. There are some patients who have mechanical hyperalgesia but do not have SMP. Because a sympathectomy can be curative for SMP patients but has no beneficial effect for other patients, it would be helpful to develop techniques to diagnose differentially SMP.

We sought to determine if sensory testing could be used to distinguish between sympathetically maintained pain (SMP) and non-sympathetically maintained pain (Non-SMP). Sixteen patients who suffered from chronic pain and mechanical hyperalgesia participated in this study. Six patients had signs of sympathetic overactivity and relief of pain following a sympathetic block and were therefore classified as having SMP. The remaining 10 patients did not have SMP.

Mechanical and thermal stimuli were applied to the hyperalgesic skin and to normal skin on the contralateral limb. Detection and pain thresholds for mechanical stimuli in the normal and affected extremities were tested using von Frey hairs. Thresholds for heat pain were tested using a non-contact laser thermal stimulator (Meyer, et al, 1976). The presence or absence of pain for cold was tested by placing a drop of ice water, alcohol and/or acetone on the skin. Since the pressure of the fluid drop might elicit mechanical hyperalgesia, a 38°C water drop was also applied as a control stimulus.

Pronounced hyperalgesia to mechanical stimuli was observed in all patients. The mean (±S.E.M.) touch and pain thresholds on the affected limb are compared to those of the contralateral limb in Table I. The pain thresholds on the affected limb were similar for the 2 patient groups, and were significantly lower than the pain thresholds on the contralateral limb (t-test: $p<0.01$ for SMP group; $p<0.001$ for Non-SMP group). For 2/3 of the patients in each group, the von Frey threshold for pain and detection of the stimuli were equivalent on the affected side.

Table I

		SMP (n=6)	NON-SMP (n=10)
Touch Threshold (bars)	Normal	2.1 ± 0.4	1.8 ± 0.2
	Affected	1.8 ± 0.5	1.6 ± 0.3
Pain Threshold (bars)	Normal	8.1 ± 1.7	9.4 ± 1.7
	Affected	2.5 ± 0.5	2.1 ± 0.4

All 6 SMP patients showed some form of thermal hyperalgesia. For 3 (of 4 tested), the heat threshold for pain was lower on the affected limb relative to the contralateral limb. For 3 (of 4 tested), a drop of ice water or acetone on the affected limb was painful, whereas it was not painful on the contralateral limb. In contrast, only 1 of 10 patients without SMP showed thermal hyperalgesia. None (of 9 tested) had a lower heat pain threshold on the affected limb compared to the contralateral limb. One (of 6 tested) reported that cold stimuli were painful.

Our preliminary results indicate that thermal testing may aid in the differential diagnosis of sympathetically maintained pain. These results are consistent with those of Lindblom and Verillo (1979) who reported that chronic neuralgia patients could be divided into two groups by whether they were hypo- or hypersensitive to thermal stimuli.

ACKNOWLEDGEMENTS

Some of the A-fiber block data was kindly provided to us by Dr. Susan E. Mackinnon. We also greatly appreciate the technical support of Sheila A. Frost, Adil A. Khan, and Timothy V. Hartke. This research was funded by NIH grant NS-14447.

REFERENCES

Lindblom U, Verillo RT (1979). Sensory functions in chronic neuralgia. J. Neurology, Neurosurgery, and Psychiatry 42: 422-435.

Meyer RA, Campbell JN, Raja SN (1985). Peripheral neural mechanisms of cutaneous hyperalgesia. In Fields HL, Dubner R, Cervero F (eds.): "Advances in Pain Research and Therapy, Vol. 9", New York, Raven Press, p. 53-71.

Meyer RA, Walker RE, Mountcastle VB (1976). A laser stimulator for the study of cutaneous thermal and pain sensations. I.E.E.E. Trans. Biomedical Engineering, BME-23: 54-60.

Ochoa J (1982). Pain in local nerve lesions. In Culp WJ, Ochoa J (eds.): "Abnormal Nerves and Muscles as Impulse Generators", New York: Oxford University Press, p. 568-587.

Roberts WJ (1986). A hypothesis on the physiological basis for causalgia and related pains. Pain 24: 297-311.

Wallin G, Torebjork E, Hallin R (1976). Preliminary observations on the pathophysiology of hyperalgesia in the causalgic pain syndrome. In Y. Zotterman (ed.): "Sensory Functions of the Skin", Oxford: Pergamon Press, p. 489-502.

Effects of Injury on Trigeminal and Spinal Somatosensory Systems, pages 389–397

PAIN AND PARESTHESIAS PROVOKED MECHANICALLY IN HUMAN CERVICAL ROOT ENTRAPMENT (SIGN OF SPURLING). SINGLE SENSORY UNIT ANTIDROMIC RECORDING OF ECTOPIC, BURSTING, PROPAGATED NERVE IMPULSE ACTIVITY.

J. Ochoa, M. Cline, R. Dotson, & P. Marchettini
Departments of Neurology, Good Samaritan Hospital and Medical Center, Portland, Oregon 97210 (J.O., M.C.), and Oregon Health Sciences University, (R.D.), Portland, Oregon 97201, and University of Milano, Italy (P.M.).

INTRODUCTION

A relatively underrated priority in research on injury to somatosensory systems is distorted sensation. This deficiency stems from two facts. First, it remains close to impossible to adequately explore subjective sensation in the experimental animal. Second, until recently it was impossible to document the pathophysiological basis for sensory aberrations of positive character, originating in the primary sensory unit in man. Microneurography (Hagbarth and Vallbo, 1967; Vallbo and Hagbarth, 1968; Vallbo et al., 1979), fulfilled the long sought aim "to correlate both stimulus and sensation with the messages which pass up the sensory fibres" (Adrian, 1931), making those subjective positive sensory phenomena accessible to scientific study. Indeed, in the past decade, ortho- or antidromic microneurographic recordings from human primary sensory units have established ectopically generated impulses as the basis for (a) postischemic paresthesias in normal volunteers (Torebjörk, Ochoa and McCann, 1979; Ochoa and Torebjörk, 1980); (b) ongoing spontaneous paresthesias symptomatic of nerve injury (Ochoa et al., 1982; Ochoa, 1985); (c) recurrent mechanosensitive pain in traumatic neuroma (sign of Tinel) (Ochoa et al., 1982); recurrent mechanosensitive paresthesias in entrapment of peripheral nerve, brachial plexus and nerve roots (Nordin et al., 1984); and even for (d) the mechanosensitive sign of Lhermitte, in focal demyelination of the central branch of primary sensory neurons in the spinal cord (Nordin et al., 1984).

The present communication adds another definitive example to the series. As in previous reports, injury to the primary sensory neuron gave rise to somatosensory dysfunction of positive character, and concomitant, abnormal nerve impulse activity was recorded from nerve fascicles supplying symptomatic skin. Again, there was an unambiguous temporal correlation between sensory symptoms and the abnormal paroxysmal nerve impulse activity. Such activity, triggered by a provocative clinical maneuver involving mechanical irritation of nerve, was unique in that its single unit components were fortuitously recorded.

METHODS

The subject for these investigations was Mr. Emmett W., Ph.D., a school principal with excellent capacity to observe, describe and endure hardship. He had a characteristic neurological syndrome involving weakness of muscles supplied mostly by spinal cord segment C8, loss of triceps reflex and "numbness" of the ulnar side of the hand, medial forearm and upper arm on the left. By "numbness" he meant to describe a combination of (a) spontaneous, intermittent tingling and pins and needles, (b) vaguely distorted sensory quality and reduced subjective magnitude in response to natural cutaneous stimuli, and (c) episodic spells of intense paresthesias and pain consistently provoked by certain movements of the neck. Clinical diagnosis of cervical radiculopathy, most likely due to entrapment of nerve root by intervertebral pathology, was confirmed by routine electrodiagnosis and cervical myelography, and was eventually cured by anterior discectomy.

The clinical confirmation of a strikingly reproducible foraminal sign (Spurling maneuver), and the patient's willingness to consent to microneurography, prompted us to implement a protocol to achieve the following: (i) a unitary recording of identified afferent units in a fascicle supplying symptomatic skin (ulnar nerve at wrist level), and (ii) a demonstration of changes in baseline neural activity in response to impinging upon the vulnerable cervical nerve root by positioning the neck through Spurling maneuver.

Conventional intraneural tungsten microelectrode sampling (microneurography) was carried out using custom made equipment for microneurography (Department of Clinical Neurophysiology, Academic Hospital, Uppsala, Sweden) plus a standard oscilloscope, FM tape recorder and electrostatic chart recorder. The sessions were videotaped yielding unique, real time, simultaneous documentation of (i) the provocative clinical maneuver, (ii) the articulate description of abnormal subjective somatosensory experience by the patient, and (iii) bursting impulse activity propagated antidromically to the intraneural recording electrode.

RESULTS AND DISCUSSION

On two occasions a stable intraneural recording was successfully achieved from two different ulnar nerve fascicles projecting to symptomatic skin and, at the same time, recordable ectopic discharge was elicited by Spurling maneuver. On the first occasion no particular single unit stood out from multi-unit background activity evoked normally by natural stimulation of the skin. As such, the abnormal nerve impulse activity subsequently triggered by the mechanical Spurling maneuver, although obvious in its occurrence, was not as sharp and impressive as with the single unit recording attained on the second occasion. The latter is shown in Figure 1. It may be seen that a quarter of a minute after displacing the cervical spine there is abrupt onset of high frequency (90 Hz) unitary discharge. It is steady for approximately half a minute, and then it breaks into recurrent bursts. Seconds after initiation of Spurling maneuver and before the onset of discharge, the patient started describing a sequence of abnormal sensations which was stereotyped in subjective quality and, like a focal epileptic marche, in its spatial spread. Qualitatively it featured "tingling", "pins and needles" and pain. Spatially the projected sensations spread proximo-distally from shoulder to hand, along the medial aspect of arm and forearm. It was only when the abnormal sensations "reached" the hand that the abnormal discharge, recorded from fascicles projecting to skin of fingers, was initiated. The bursting discharge persisted for several seconds following discontinuation of the provocative mechanical maneuver. The paresthesias began to fade before discontinuation of the Spurling

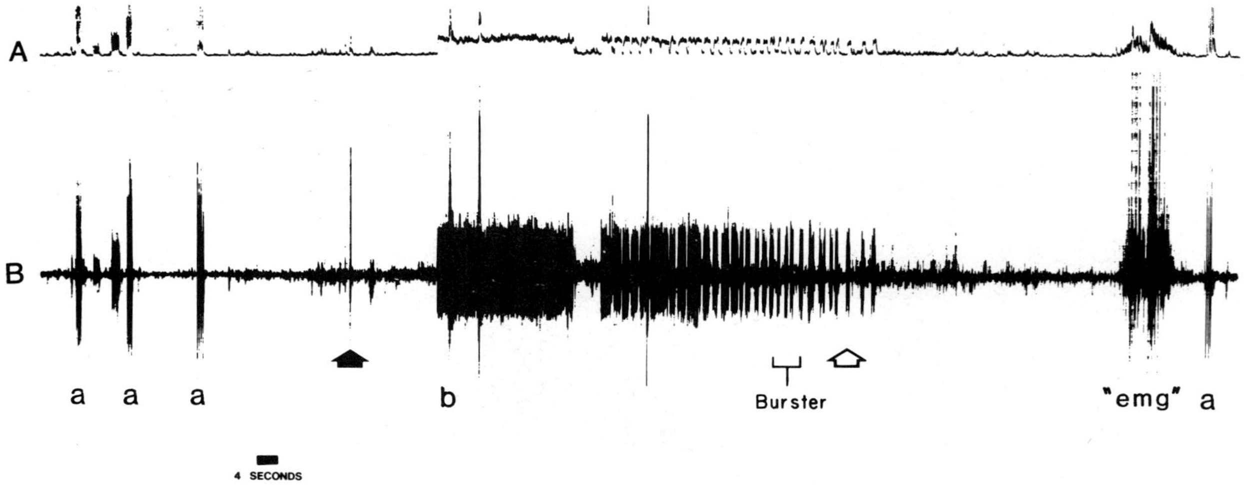

FIGURE 1: Recording from left ulnar nerve at wrist level. A = integrated neurogram; B = simultaneous discriminated neurogram. Symbols: a = stimulation of receptive field in little finger; solid arrow = head flexed to left and extended; b = onset of abnormal unitary bursting, temporally correlating to verbalized report of paresthesias reaching the hand; open arrow = head returned to neutral position; "emg" = voluntary muscle artifact; a = original receptive field reconfirmed.

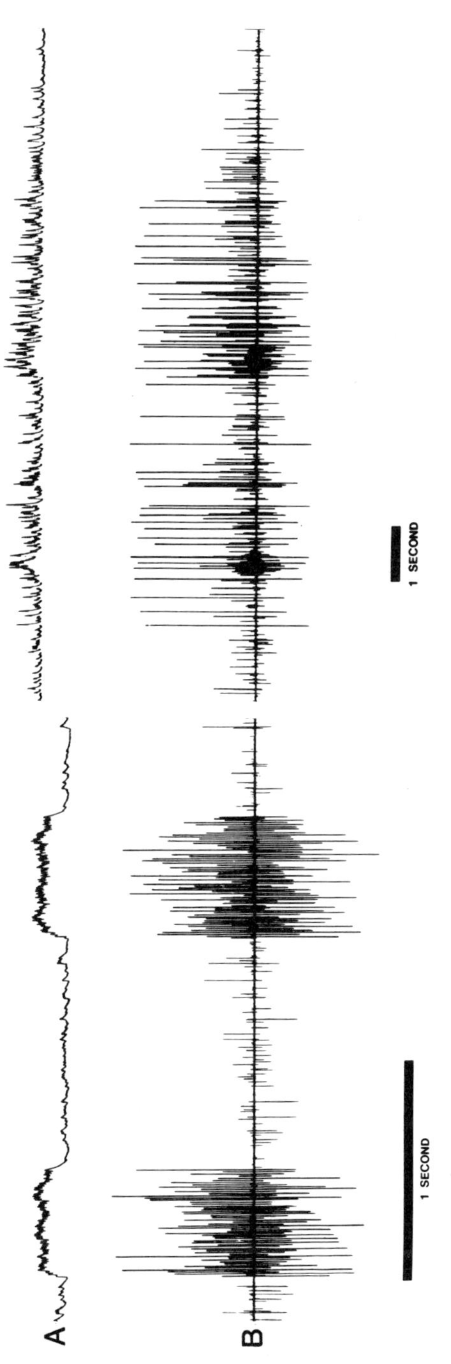

FIGURE 2: Same recording as Figure 1. A = integrated neurogram; B = simultaneous discriminated neurogram. Details of spontaneous bursts (Left) and electromyogram (Right), extracted from Figure 1. Note how the two records differ in burst morphology (see text). Gain for neural signals equals three times emg gain.

maneuver, but nevertheless, outlasted the bursting discharge in the particular unit illustrated.

It may also be seen in Figure 1 that a preidentified low threshold mechanoreceptor unit (a) is in excellent position for intraneural electrode recording. It responds with repetitive impulses to light stroking of its receptive field on three occasions. It again responds in a consistent manner at the end of the record (on the right), after termination of the mechanical maneuver. This indicates that despite neck movement and minor unavoidable displacements of the explored limb, the intraneural microelectrode retained its spatial relation to one particular nerve fiber. It is therefore unlikely that the bursting was an injury discharge due to accidental electrode movement.

Towards the end of the tracing, at "emg", there is a double burst of impulse activity. This is the electromyogram, voluntarily initiated by mild contraction of intrinsic hand muscles, in response to the examiner's command. It was elicited in order to contrast the characteristics of those signals with the bursting neural activity. It can be seen that multiunit EMG signals do not start abruptly and they recruit and de-recruit in a manner typical for EMG and different from the relatively steady single nerve unit response. This is best shown in the integrated neurogram above and in Figure 2. This indicates that the abnormal bursting displayed in the Figures is not a misinterpreted electromyogram.

The fact that the projecting territory of paresthesias extended so broadly, covering several textbook dermatomes from axilla to hand, could be taken to indicate that several roots participate in the generation of the sensory dysfunction. However, it must be remembered that conventionally accepted dermatomes (Foerster, 1933) map restricted single root territories, where no overlap exists. The clinical translation of those territories is expressed through sensory deficit. But for positive sensory phenomena, sensations would be projected anywhere within the broader territory of actual maximal innervation, similar to those mapped in Keegan's dermatomes (Keegan and Garrett, 1948) which were actually delineated in man for the area of abnormal sensation arising from root irritation.

The site of origin of the abnormal bursting discharge cannot be exactly determined. It must lay within the primary sensory unit, but whether at the comparatively easier to excite dorsal root ganglion cells (Kirk, 1974; Howe et al., 1977; Calvin, 1982), or in nerve fibers at either side of it, remains uncertain. The consistent sensory marche is intriguing and suggests a somatotopic arrangement of the neural structures excited at the locus of irritation. This is perhaps anatomically consistent with intraspinal distribution of sensory fibers or cells, but is rather surprising for the more peripheral sensory components which are not known to be orderly arranged in human roots or spinal nerves. However, in the spider monkey there is some evidence of rostrocaudal subdermatomal organization of rootlets (Pubols and Pubols, 1969).

As to the nerve fiber types engaged in discharge, judging from the subjective quality of the paresthetic sensations, (Torebjörk and Ochoa 1980; Ochoa and Torebjörk, 1983; Ochoa et al., 1984), it can be accepted that the fibers responsible for initiating the afferent activity are of various specific types. The bursting neural activity displayed in the Figures clearly reflects myelinated fiber origin, in view of its high frequency and relative sustainment (Culp et al., 1982). No convincing C-fiber discharge was observed. However, unmyelinated fibers are bound to be able to engage in ectopic discharge of their own, too, as recorded in animals (Blumberg and Jänig, 1984).

SUMMARY

A unique, real time, simultaneous documentation of the provocative clinical maneuver of Spurling, the abnormal subjective sensory experience, and ectopic impulse generation recorded antidromically from peripheral sensory nerve fibers is presented. Every feature was consistently reproduced on separate occasions and the single unit character of the discharge was clearly recorded. Identification of site of origin and fiber types involved is attempted.

ACKNOWLEDGMENT

Supported by NINCDS grant No. RO1 NS24740-01 and NIH-NRSA grant No. 5 T32 NS07026-09.

REFERENCES

Adrian ED (1931). The messages in sensory nerve fibers and their interpretation. Proceedings of the Royal Society B 109:1.

Blumberg H, Jänig W (1984). Discharge patterns of afferent fibers from a neuroma. Pain 20(4):335-353.

Calvin WH (1982). To spike or not to spike? Controlling the neuron's rhythm, preventing the ectopic beat. In Culp WJ, Ochoa JL (eds): "Abnormal nerves and muscles as impulse generators," New York, NY: Oxford University Press, pp 295-321.

Culp WJ, Ochoa J, Torebjörk E (1982). Ectopic impulse generation in myelinated sensory nerve fibers in man. In Culp WJ, Ochoa JL (eds): "Abnormal nerves and muscles as impulse generators," New York, NY: Oxford University Press, pp 490-512.

Foerster O (1933). The Dermatomes in Man. Brain, 56:1-39.

Hagbarth K-E, Vallbo AB (1967). Mechanoreceptor activity recorded percutaneously with semi-microelectrodes in human peripheral nerves. Acta Physiol Scand, 69:121-122.

Howe JF, Loeser JD, Calvin WH (1977). Mechanosensitivity of dorsal root ganglia and chronically injured axons: a physiological basis for the radicular pain of nerve root compression. Pain, 3:25-41.

Keegan JJ, Garrett FD (1948). The segmental distribution of the cutaneous nerves in the limbs of man. Anatomical Record, Philadelphia, 102:409-437.

Kirk EJ (1974). Impulses in dorsal spinal nerve rootlets in cats and rabbits arising from dorsal root ganglia isolated from the periphery. J Comp Neurol, 2:165-176.

Nordin M, Nyström B, Wallin U, Hagbarth K-E (1984). Ectopic sensory discharges and paresthesiae in patients with disorders of peripheral nerves, dorsal roots and dorsal columns. Pain, 20:231-245.

Ochoa JL, Torebjörk HE (1980). Paraesthesiae from ectopic impulse generation in human sensory nerves. Brain, 103:835-853.

Ochoa JL, Torebjörk HE, Culp WJ, Schady W (1982). Abnormal spontaneous activity in single sensory nerve fibers in humans. Muscle and Nerve, 5:S74-S77.

Ochoa JL, Torebjörk HE (1983). Sensations evoked by intraneural microstimulation of single mechanoreceptor units innervating the human hand. J Physiol, 342:633-654.

Ochoa JL, Torebjörk E, Culp W (1984). Determinants of subjective attributes of normal cutaneous sensation and of paresthesiae from ectopic nerve impulse generation. In Franzén O, Ottoson D, von Euler C, Lindblom U (eds): "Somatosensory Mechanisms," Wenner-Gren Center International Symposium 40, New York and London: Plenum Press, pp 379-387.

Ochoa JL (1985). Pain and paresthesiae from neuropathy: intraneural microrecording and microstimulation studies and a proposed strategy for pathophysiological assessment. In Delwaide PJ, Gorio A (eds): "Clinical Neurophysiology in Peripheral Neuropathies," New York: Elsevier Science Publishers, pp 57-65.

Pubols BH, Pubols LM (1969). Forelimb, hindlimb, and tail dermatomes in the spider monkey (Ateles). Brain Behaviour and Evolution, 2(2):139-159.

Torebjörk HE, Ochoa JL (1980). Specific sensations evoked by activity in single identified sensory units in man. Acta Physiol Scand, 110:445-447.

Torebjörk HE, Ochoa JL, McCann, FV (1979). Paraesthesiae: Abnormal impulse generation in sensory nerve fibers in man. Acta Physiol Scand, 105:518-520.

Vallbo AB, Hagbarth K-E (1968). Activity from skin mechanoreceptors recorded percutaneously in awake human subjects. Exp neurol, 21:270-289.

Vallbo AB, Hagbarth K-E, Torebjörk HE, Wallin BG (1979). Somatosensory, proprioceptive and sympathetic activity in human peripheral nerves. Physiol Rev, 59:919-957.

Effects of Injury on Trigeminal and Spinal Somatosensory Systems,
pages 399–410

SPARED ROOT DEAFFERENTATION OF CAT SPINAL CORD: BEHAVIORAL RECOVERY

Michael E. Goldberger
Department of Anatomy, Medical College of Pennsylvania, Philadelphia, Pennsylvania

Sprouting in the adult brain and spinal cord consists of a local increase in the density of spared projections that overlap most intimately with those that have degenerated (see Cotman et al., 1981; Goldberger and Murray, 1978, 1986; Murray et al., this volume for reviews). Unlike the aberrant pathways sometimes seen when the developing nervous system is damaged (Bregman and Goldberger, 1982; Bernstein and Stelzner, 1984; see Goldberger and Murray, 1985 and Goldberger, 1986 for reviews), plasticity in the adult appears to result in the formation of connections that are quite similar to those formed during normal development; i.e. specificity is maintained to a considerable extent. The functional correlates of this type of plasticity require elucidation but one prediction might be an increase in the normal function of the spared pathways rather than the development of some new function mediated by the spared pathways. The physiological correlate of the anatomical plasticity would probably be the strengthening of a pre-existing synaptic input (Goldberger 1981, 1983; Mendell, 1984; Devor et al., 1986). The importance of the anatomical changes for behavior and recovery of function is that an understanding of the anatomical sequellae of CNS damage might have predictive value for the kind of behavior that may be expected to recover after a specific lesion. We (Murray and Goldberger, 1986; Murray et al., 1986; Murray et al., this volume) have found that plasticity after complete lumbosacral deafferentation in lamina II of cat spinal cord results in the maintenance of normal numbers of terminals. The number of terminals after partial deafferentation, we presume, is not further reduced and is therefore also normal. The resulting synaptic organization is not normal however after spared root or complete deafferentation and the synaptic organization after complete deafferentation differs from that observed after a spared root deafferentation. The behavioral sequellae of these two kinds of deafferentation were therefore studied to determine if any functional consequences of the two patterns of reorganization could be detected.

Lumbosacral Deafferentation in Cats

Extradural unilateral section of all the lumbar and first two sacral dorsal roots and removal of their ganglia eliminates most or all of the afferent input from the hindlimb. The initial (1-2 days) postoperative effect of deafferentation on hindlimb motor function is devastating. For example, when the animals attempt locomotion, the affected hindlimb does not participate but drags passively behind. The initial loss of all motor function in the deafferented hindlimb is a most dramatic expression of reflex depression (spinal shock), since spinal neurons on the lesioned side receive bilateral descending input and contralateral polysynaptic reflex input, from the undamaged side, but still cannot be activated to produce movement at this stage. Movements of the limb during locomotion are first seen on the second or third postoperative day. We have studied locomotion by conditioning the animals, for food reward, to cross runways - either simple 35 cm-wide runways that require only locomotion or more difficult, e.g. 5 cm wide, runways that add the requirement of accurate limb placement during locomotion (Goldberger, '77). During the first week, after quadripedal locomotion has returned and become rapid, the deafferented hindlimb is still not placed under the center of gravity at the end of the stance phase of locomotion. Predictably then, the animals cannot perform on those runways requiring accurate limb placement at this time. During this period, although reflexes commonly elicited by ipsilateral peripheral stimulation are abolished if the deafferentation is complete, crossed segmental and ipsilateral descending reflexes (vestibular, scratch reflex) have returned.

Accurate placement of the deafferented limb during

locomotion returns on the 8th (7th-9th) post-operative day. It is initially slow with many errors or misplacements. The recovery of accurate placement under the center of gravity permits adequate performance on a narrow (5 cm-wide) runway and the limb now provides weight support. After this time, speed increases and the number of errors in placement per trial decreases. Thus, the animals are now able to use non-topographic feedback to guide limb movements after the elimination of somatosensory, topographic feedback. These other cues are inadequate during the first week since accurate movement only returns during the second week. The failure of accurate movement to return during the first week cannot be attributed to spinal shock since a number of reflexes, as well as locomotion have been present since the second or third day post-operative. The recovery does not appear to be related to ventral root afferents since most or all of these have been eliminatedd by ganglionectomy and no difference in recovery is seen when rhizotomy and ganglionectomy are compared (Goldberger, 1977). Rather, the input of those systems which are identified only as ipsilateral descending systems (see Goldberger, 1977, 1983) that mediate the substituted cues must be strengthened by some mechanism such as sprouting or supersensitivity during the first week. Our evidence that sprouting contributes to this process is circumstantial. We have evidence for example that small simple terminals proliferate to maintain synapse number, that the descending systems on the deafferented side of the cord increase the density of their projection (Goldberger and Murray, 1978, 1982; Goldberger and Paige, 1986) and that these ipsilateral descending systems are essential for recovery after deafferentation (Goldberger, 1977). We do not know the time-course of the sprouting but it occurs quite early, (Murray and Goldberger, 1986); certainly within the first post-operative week i.e. the period during which accurate locomotion recovers. When the deafferentation is incomplete and one root is spared, the recovery is altered in many respects. The anatomical sequellae are also different. For example, our light-microscopic evidence suggests that the descending pathways do not increase their projection if one root is spared and our EM evidence suggests that the small simple terminals do not proliferate when one root is spared. These observations would lead us to predict that a dorsal root when spared, may be most important for recovery, taking precedence over the descending systems.

Spared Root Preparation

When all lumbosacral dorsal roots but one are sectioned (in most of our preparations the L_6 root is the spared one) both sparing and recovery of function can be demonstrated. The initial motor deficit, although severe, is not so profound as that seen after complete lumbosacral rhizotomy. Locomotion, although severely impaired, can be elicited within twenty-four hours post-operatively. Repetitive flexion-extension sequences are seen as the animal appears to search for the missing somatosensory input. On the second day, they can cross the wide runway, slowly. Unlike the animals with a completely deafferented hindlimb, they can cross some of the more difficult runways during the first week but accurate limb placement has not yet returned. If the number of misplacements per crossing is counted, it is quite apparent that successful placements are at a chance level. Bizarre limb positions are also often seen during locomotion in this period. Thus, the spared root's input is not adequate to guide limb movements to appropriate positions at this time. Observations on postural reflexes support the idea that the spared root does not yet contribute fully to the elaboration of movement at this early post-operative stage. Low threshold placing, tested within the spared root's dermatome is dramatically reduced or abolished. The threshold for placing is tested with a force transducer that serves as the stimulus for placing as well as measuring the force required to elicit placing. The threshold is clearly raised and almost all placing at this time is proprioceptive. Other postural reflexes e.g. monopedal hopping and vestibular placing, are also deficient at this time as is the force of support (positive supporting response). Thus, as in the deafferented preparation, the spared pathways are not yet capable of mediating the recovery of somatosensory postural reflexes and accurate limb placement.

Consistent accurate limb placement recovers on the seventh day in most animals, but occasionally on the sixth or eighth day. The number of misplacements on narrow or other challenging runways decreases during the second post-operative week, often rather abruptly, and speed increases. The recovery of low-threshold (hair-contact) placing almost always precedes the recovery of accurate limb placement by a day or a part of a day. The force of support also recovers, at this time, to almost normal levels. The residual somatosensory input conveyed by the spared root is therefore sufficient to mediate the recovery of contact placing and positive supporting responses but not until the end of the first week. Thus, it seems reasonable to suggest that the spared root's input has become strengthened during that recovery period. Whether the recovery of accurate limb placement during locomotion is mediated by this spared and strengthened somatosensory input is uncertain. However, the recovery of somatosensory reflexes and the recovery of accurate limb placement are very closely related temporally. Furthermore, the recovery of accurate placement is only temporarily reversed by lesions destroying the descending pathways on the side of the spared root deafferentation. This implies that, unlike the deafferented hindlimb, recovery in the spared-root hindlimb is independent of the descending pathways. Finally, we have presented evidence (Goldberger and Murray, 1982; Wu et al., 1986; Murray et al., this volume) that reactive reinnervation is mediated by terminals arising from the spared root's scalloped terminals rather than by the small terminals that increase after complete deafferentation. Our hypothesis is therefore that anatomical plasticity of the spared root mediates an increase in reflex input to the spinal cord which is used in the recovery of accurate limb placement during locomotion.

<u>Comparison of deafferented and spared root preparations</u>:

There are some similarities between the two preparations. Both display an initial period of profound reflex depression either of spared segmental reflexes or brainstem-spinal reflexes or both. Both recover locomotion very quickly - around the second post-operative day but the locomotion lacks accuracy. Both recover accurate limb placement at about seven or eight days post-operative. There are many differences in the motor behavior of the two groups however. The obvious difference is the presence of somatosensory reflex behavior in the spared root preparation. The input of the spared root becomes enhanced during the first post-operative week; after deafferentation, in contrast, descending reflexes become enhanced. Recovery after deafferentation, with or without ganglionectomy depends on ipsilateral descending pathways; in the spared root preparation recovery is not dependent on those pathways. These observations suggest that although in both preparations, recovery of accurate movement occurs, the pathways by which this recovery is achieved might differ, and therefore the movements themselves might differ in the two preparations.

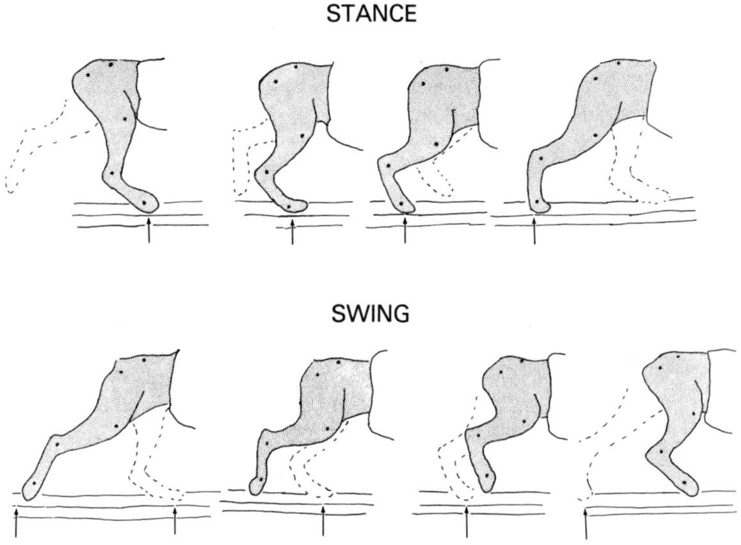

Fig 1. The phases of the cat step cycle. Swing is divided into flexion (F) and extension (E1). Stance is that part of the cycle during which the foot is in contact with the surface (E1-E2). For kinematic studies the excursion for each joint is measured as the limb passes from the end of Ec to the end of F; from the end of F to touchdown; from touchdown to the end of E3. Bony prominences are marked with dots which are filmed, projected and digitized in order to measure excursions.

An animal's movements can be characterized by measuring the excursion made at each joint during the phases of the locomotor cycle (e.g. Goslow et al., 1973). A kinematic pattern is thus obtained which provides some information about the contribution of each limb segment to the overall movement. A normal cat will exhibit a consistent kinematic pattern during the performance of overground locomotion although considerable differences occur from animal to animal. Furthermore, an animal will use comparable kinematic patterns regardless of whether locomotion does or does not require accurate limb placement (Olivier and Goldberger, 1986).

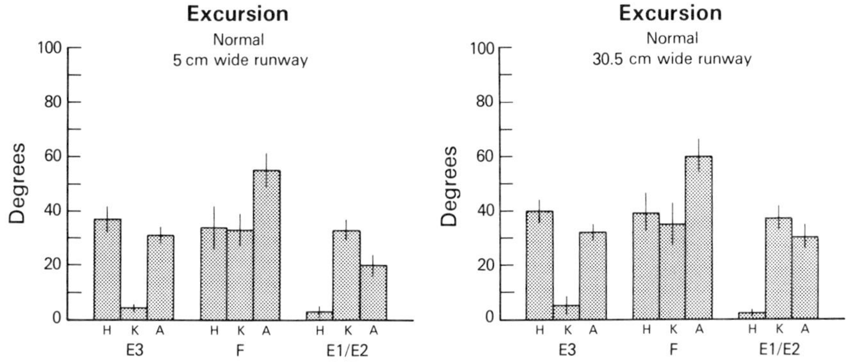

Fig. 2. Kinematic pattern for one normal cat. Each bar represents the mean excursion (± SD) for the joint designated for five complete locomotor cycles of the right hindlimb. These excursions were measured from films made while the animal crossed a three-meter long runway. For the upper group of cycles a wide runway was used to assess uncomplicated locomotion. The lower group shows the pattern used for a narrow runway which required accurate placement of the limb. The kinematic pattern is very similar for the two tasks.

In this respect the spared root animals resemble normal cats, since after recovery they display very similar kinematic patterns on wide and narrow runways. The deafferented hindlimb, in contrast, uses two different patterns, one for simple locomotion on a wide runway, and another forlocomotion with the additional requirement that the limb be placed accurately on a narrow runway to prevent falling. These two different patterns are used throughout the chronic period by the deafferented limb. These differences support the idea that the pathways mediating recovery in the two preparations differ somewhat.

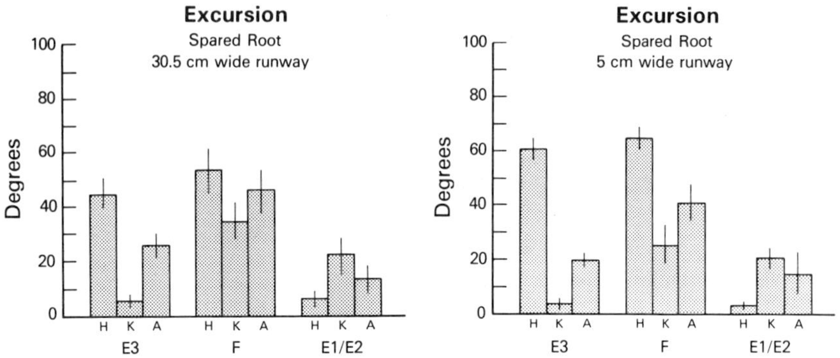

Fig. 3. Kinematic patterns for one chronic L6 spared-root cat. The right hindlimb was the partially deafferented one and the measurements shown here were from the right hindlimb's movements. Note that the kinematic patterns used for the wide and narrow runway are similar, as they are in normal animals. They are also similar to this animal's preoperative patterns (not shown). The pattern was altered during the first post-operative week but returned to normal during the second.

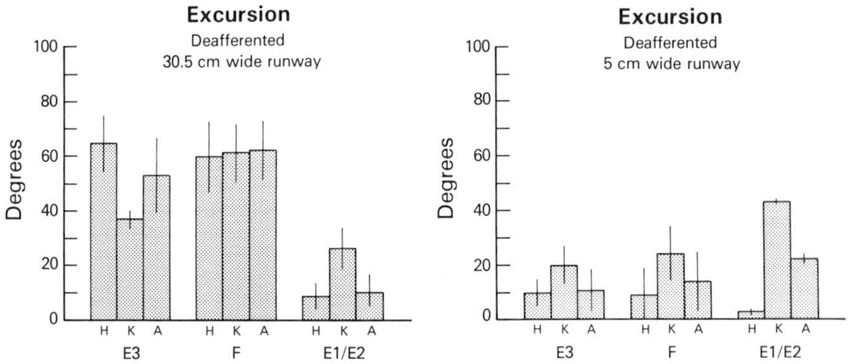

Fig. 4. Kinematic pattern after chronic deafferentation. From the beginning of the second post-operative week when accurate locomotion recovered, onwards different kinematic patterns were used for locomotion and locomotion requiring accuracy respectively.

Locomotion, in its simplest form, is mediated by the Spinal Pattern Generator for Locomotion (SPGL) (Grillner, 1986; Smith et al., 1986; Rossignol et al., 1986; Robinson and Goldberger, 1986) and requires neither afferent input nor descending control. Nevertheless, in the normal cat, (and in the spared root preparation), there is a constant inflow of somatosensory information during locomotion (Loeb, 1981). Thus, normal cats and spared-root cats, in which topographic somatosensory input is available, do not require a change in motor pattern in situations in which this feedback takes on greater importance, i.e. on a difficult terrain. The feedback is present during both types of locomotion. After deafferentation, however, the SPGL, without topographic somatosensory input, is sufficient for simple locomotion (Grillner and Zangger, 1984), but not for locomotion requiring accurate limb placement (Goldberger, 1977). Rather, in the deafferented group accurate locomotion requires input from descending pathways after peripheral input is eliminated. Thus, the kinematic motor pattern used for accurate movement is different from that used in simple locomotion because it is mediated by a system that is different from that subserving ordinary locomotion. Here, locomotion is altered by the additional input from descending tracts.

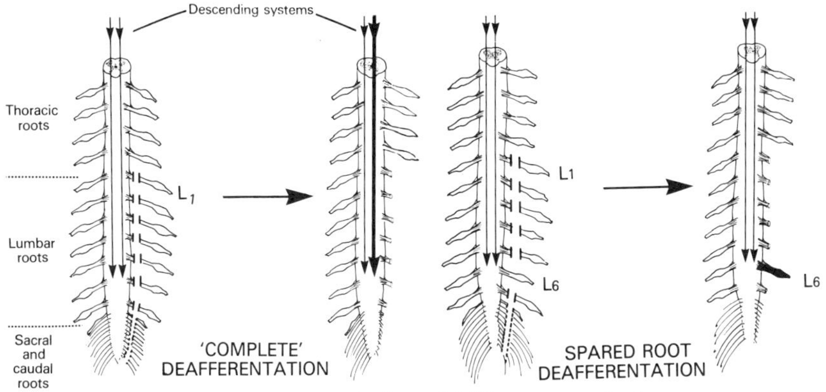

Fig. 5. Diagrams summarizing differences between deafferentation with and without spared root, After complete deafferentation descending (and intraspinal) axons sprout and recovery depends on ipsilateral descending pathways. When one root is spared recovery is independent of ipsilateral descending pathways and these do not sprout. Reinnervation comes from the spared root which also mediates recovery.

Thus the two preparations recover in somewhat different ways. When a single root is present, it is able, in time, to guide not only the parts of the limb it represents but all parts of the limb resulting in movement that is similar to normal movement. The dermatome represented must increase its sphere of influence over spinal neurons by the end of the first post-operative week (cf Pubols and Goldberger, 1980). This suggests a substitution of one set of somatosensory cues for movement when the normal complement of input is eliminated. The deafferented hindlimb in contrast recovers by substituting some new motor patterns for the lost normal ones to meet the demands of a more altered spinal cord organization. Our anatomical results suggest that normal synapse numbers can be maintained by reactive reinnervation but the type of anatomical plasticity may differ depending on some characteristics of the responding system. Our behavioral results suggest that the recovery of accurate limb movements may be achieved by the use of somewhat novel motor patterns which may reflect an altered synaptic organization.

REFERENCES

Bernstein DR, Stelzner DJ (1984). Plasticity of the corticospinal tract following mid-thoracic spinal cord injury in the neonatal rat. J Comp Neur 221:382-401.

Bregman BS, Goldberger ME (1982). Anatomical plasticity and sparing of function after spinal cord damage in neonatal cats. Science 217:553-555.

Cotman CW, Nieto-Sampedro M, Harris EW (1981). Synapse replacement in the nervous system of adult vertebrates. Physiol Rev 61:684-782.

Devor M, Basbaum AI, Seltzer Z (1986) Spinal somatotopic plasticity: Possible anatomical basis for somatotopically inappropriate connections. In Goldberger ME, Gorio A, Murray M (eds): "Development and Plasticity of the Mammalian Spinal Cord," Liviana Press, Springer-Verlag, pp 211-225.

Goldberger ME (1977). Locomotor recovery after unilateral hindlimb deafferentation in cats. Brain Res 123:59-74.

Goldberger ME (1981). The role sprouting might play during recovery of function. In Flohr H, Precht W (eds): "Lesion-Induced Neuronal Plasticity in Sensorimotor Systems," New York: Springer-Verlag, pp 130-140.

Goldberger ME (1986). Segmental and suprasegmental contributions to development and recovery of motor function in cats. In Grillner S (ed): "The Neurobiology of Vertebrate Locomotion," MacMillan, London. In Press.

Goldberger ME (1983). Recovery of accurate limb movements after deafferentation in cats. In Kao CC, Bunge R, Reier P (eds): "Spinal Cord Reconstruction," New York, Raven Press.

Goldberger ME, Murray M (1978). Axonal sprouting and recovery of function may obey some of the same laws. In Cotman C (ed): " Neuronal Plasticity," Raven Press, pp 73-96.

Goldberger ME, Murray M (1982). Lack of sprouting and its presence after lesions of the cat spinal cord. Brain Research 241:227-239.

Goldberger ME, Murray M (1985). Recovery of function and anatomical plasticity after damage to the adult and neonatal spinal cord. In Cotman C (ed): "Synaptic Plasticity," Guilford Press, pp 77-110.

Goldberger ME, Murray M (1986). Patterns of sprouting and implications for recovery of function. In Waxman S (ed): "Physiological Basis for Functional Recovery in Neurological Disease," In press.

Goldberger ME, Paige E (1986). Anatomical plasticity of serotonin (5HT) projections after deafferentation of cat spinal cord. Neurosci Abstr 12:512.

Goslow GE, Jr., Reinking RM, Stuart DG (1973). The cat step cycle: Hindlimb joint angles and muscle lengths during unrestrained locomotion. J Morphol 141:1-41.

Grillner S (1986). Locomotion in spinal vertebrates. Physiology and Pharmacology. In Goldberger ME, Gorio A, Murray M (eds): "Development and Plasticity of the Mammalian Spinal Cord," Liviana Press, Springer-Verlag, pp 311-321.

Grillner S, Zangger P (1984). The effect of dorsal root transection on the efferent motor pattern in the cat's hindlimb during locomotion. Acta Physiol Scand 120:393-405.

Loeb GE (1981). Somatosensory unit input to the spinal cord during normal walking. Can J Physiol Pharmacol 59:627-635.

Mendell LM (1984). Modifiability of spinal synapses. Physiol Rev 64:260-324.

Mendell LM, Sedivic MJ, Traub RJ (1986). Response of an identified population of spinal cord neurons to partial deafferentation. In Goldberger ME, Gorio A, Murray M (eds): "Development and Plasticity of the Mammalian Spinal Cord," Italy, Liviana Press, pp 111-112.

Murray M, et al (this volume).

Murray M, Goldberger ME (1986). Replacement of synaptic terminals in lamina II and Clarke's nucleus after unilateral dorsal rhizotomy in adult cats. J Neurosci. In press.

Olivier J, Goldberger ME (1986). Spared root deafferentation of spinal cord: Behavioral recovery. Neurosci Abstr 12:114.

Pubols LM, Goldberger ME (1980). Recovery of function in dorsal horn following partial deafferentation. J Neurophysiol 43:102-117.

Robinson GA, Goldberger ME (1986). The development and recovery of motor function in spinal cats. I. The Infant Lesion Effect. Exp Brain Res 62:373-386.

Rossignol S, Barbeau H, Julien C (1986). Locomotion of the adult chronic spinal cat and its modification by monaminergic agonists and antagonists. In Goldberger ME, Gorio A, Murray M (eds): "Development and Plasticity of the Mammalian Cord," Liviana Press, Springer-Verlag, pp 323-345.

Smith JL, Bradley NS, Carter MC, Giuliani CA, Hoy MG, Koshland GF, Zernicke RF (1986). Rhythmical movements of the Hindlimbs in spinal cat: Considerations for a controlling nework. In Goldberger ME, Gorio A, Murray M (eds): "Development and Plasticity of the Mammalian Spinal Cord," Liviana Press, Springer-Verlag, pp 347-361.

Effects of Injury on Trigeminal and Spinal Somatosensory Systems, pages 411-418

EFFECTS OF EXPERIMENTAL CONCUSSION ON SPINAL CORD INTEGRATION OF SENSORY INPUT: RELATIONSHIP TO ACUTE TRAUMATIC UNCONSCIOUSNESS

Ronald L. Hayes, Yoichi Katayama, and Henry H. Stonnington

Departments of Surgery (R.L.H.) and Rehabilitation Medicine (H.H.S.), Medical College of Virginia, Richmond, Virginia 23298-0001; Nihon Univeristy, Tokyo, Japan (Y.K.)

INTRODUCTION

Coma is usually associated with abolition or suppression of all responses to external stimulation. This suppression of responses can occur without gross structural changes and can include even spinally mediated reflex activity. Thus, this form of coma has been described as paralytic coma (Denny-Brown, 1945; Denny-Brown and Russell, 1941; Ommaya and Gennarelli, 1974; Walker et al, 1944). It is certainly possible that the abolition of brain stem reflexes by concussive injury may be attributable to suppression of neural responses produced by direct mechanical stress (Groat et al, 1944; Groat et al, 1945). However, concussion may not produce sufficient mechanical stresses within the spinal cord to interfere with neural function (Denny-Brown, 1945; Walker et al, 1944). Alternatively, it is possible that the concussion-produced suppression of flexion reflexes is related to decreased excitability of spinal cord motor neurons following a period of intense excitation (Walker et al, 1944). However, at least in the period immediately following injury, an enhancement of spinal monosynaptic reflexes has been reported (Rhines et al, 1945; Katayama et al, 1985). Thus, it is possible that suppression of flexion reflexes immediately following head injury may be due to depressed transmission of sensory input within the spinal cord.

The data presented here (Katayama et al, 1985a; Katayama et al, 1985b) indicate that concussion can depress sensory transmission within the dorsal horn of the spinal cord. Suppressed segmental sensory transmission may also contribute to suppression of ascending sensory transmission. This suppression of sensory transmission within the spinal cord may be attributable to changes in neural function within the bulbar brain stem.

METHODS

Twenty adult cats weighing 2-3 kg were used. Experimental concussion was produced by a fluid-percussion head injury model (Sullivan et al, 1976). Previous research has established that this model is able to produce biomechanically well-controlled, momentary mechanical stress transmitted to the brain stem and resultant concussive responses indistinguishable from those obtained by acceleration head injury (Sullivan, 1976) (see also Denny-Brown, 1945; Denny-Brown and Russell, 1941; Walker et al, 1944). In addition, fluid-percussion head injury reproduces a number of features of human head injury observed clinically (see refs. Hayes et al, 1983a; Hayes et al, 1983b). While detailed electrophysiological studies are generally impractical in studies of experimental head injury, fluid-percussion models minimize artifactual movement at the moment of injury and thus allow stable recordings of spinal root potentials. Detailed procedures have been described elsewhere (Hayes et al, 1983a; Sullivan et al, 1976). Briefly, animals were paralyzed with pancuronium bromide (0.08 mg/kg, i.v.), mechanically ventilated and anesthetized with a gas mixture of 75% N_2O and 25% O_2 supplemented with methohexital sodium (Brevital, 30 mg/kg, i.v.). Depth of anesthesia was confirmed by absence of sympathetic cardiovascular responses to intense somatosensory stimulation. All wound margins and pressure points were repeatedly infused with lidocaine. Concussive head injury was administered by a pressure-fluid pulse (peak intensity, 2.2-2.4 atm; duration, 21-24 ms) transmitted to the epidural space via a hollow metal injury screw placed through a circular craniectomy (11 mm in diameter), the center of which was located along the midline at A 5.5. This level of injury consistently produces a concussive syndrome characterized by initial, generalized reflex suppression (i.e., unconsciousness) followed by a more prolonged comatose or stuporous state.

These responses are not associated with prolonged apnea, profound circulatory collapse, or overt intraparenchymal hemorrhage (Sullivan, 1976). Body temperature, end-tidal CO_2, arterial gas tension and pH were monitored and maintained within the physiologically normal ranges. Blood pressure, heart rate and intracranial pressure were also monitored.

The dorsal roots L6, L7 and rostral S1 were sectioned. The dorsal root L6 was mounted on a bipolar Ag/AgCl wire electrode for recording of dorsal root potentials. In order to evoke L6 dorsal root potentials, dorsal root L7 or rostral S1 was placed on a bipolar Ag/AgCl wire electrode for single pulse stimulation (frequency, 0.2-0.5 Hz; pulse duration 0.01 ms; supramaximal stimulation). One pole of the recording electrode was placed close to but not touching the cord and the other on the cut peripheral end. In 10 experiments, a glass-insulated, tungsten stimulating microelectrode was also inserted in the terminal field of primary afferent fibers in the internuncial cell group of L6 in order to evoke an antidromic L6 dorsal root potential (frequency 0.5 Hz, pulse duration 0.01 ms, submaximal intensity). Another bipolar Ag/AgCl wire electrode was placed for tetanic stimulation of dorsal root L6 (frequency 200 Hz; duration 0.01 ms, pulse for 10 seconds; submaximal stimulation). In all cases, the amplitude of PAD (recorded as the dorsal root potential) and each weave of the early near-field cortical potentials were measured as the averaged amplitude (peak to baseline) of each recorded potential taken either from photographs of storage oscilloscope tracings (four sweeps superimposed) or potentials averaged by a signal processor (four to eight sweeps averaged for dorsal root potentials and 36 to 90 sweeps for cortical potentials), and displayed by an ink-writing recorder. In 8 animals, midpontine transections were performed approximately 3 hours before injury by radio frequency lesions delivered through a 4-pronged lesion rake (Greenberg et al, 1981). Additional details have been reported elsewhere (Greenberg et al, 1981). Transection was made at a 45° angle from the coronal plane at the caudal aspects of the trigeminal motor nucleus. Transection of the spinal cord at the level of T4 was also performed in 2 animals 2 days before the experiment through a small incision in the dura which was subsequently closed.

RESULTS

Afferent-induced primary afferent depolarization (PAD), recorded as dorsal root potentials evoked by adjacent dorsal root stimulation, was consistently depressed immediately following injury (latency to maximal suppression 1-3 seconds), and depression continued for a few minutes in both intact (n=4) and midpontine-transected (n=4) animals (2-5 minutes). Depression of afferent-induced PAD following concussive head injury was also detected as attenuation of adjacent dorsal root-evoked augmentation (Wall, 1958) of antidromic dorsal root potentials in both intact (n=3) and midpontine-transected (n=3) animals. In contrast, spontaneous potentials of dorsal roots showed no discernible change following injury. In fact, concussive head injury appeared to stabilize the spontaneous dorsal root potential which commonly showed fluctuations before injury. Likewise, concussive head injury did not significantly change the resting amplitude of antidromic dorsal root potentials. In addition, reduction of the antidromic dorsal root potential for 30 seconds following tetanic stimulation of the same root (Eccles and Krnjevic, 1959) was not altered 1 minute following injury, indicating that post-tetanic hyperpolarization of primary afferent terminals was unchanged by concussion. These lines of evidence suggest that concussive head injury can suppress PAD without altering functions of primary afferent fibers. Thus, depression of afferent-induced PAD in the initial few minutes following injury may result primarily from depression of interneuronal transmission.

The depression of afferent-induced PAD was not observed in spinalized preparations (n=2) despite the occurrence of concussive responses in systemic arterial pressure, heart rate and intracranial pressure which were identical to those observed in intact animals. Thus, PAD depression appears to be a neurally produced phenomenon rather than reflecting changes in cardiovascular parameters or humoral factors. Furthermore, data from spinalized cats indicate that PAD depression is attributable to concussion-produced changes originating at supraspinal sites rather than to changes occurring within the spinal cord. Previous research has established that the neural arc mediating PAD produced by stimulation of flexion reflex afferent is tonically inhibited by a descending pathway arising in the brain stem. Thus, spinalization immediately produces potentiation of afferent-induced PAD (Carpenter et al, 1963; Lundberg, 1964). The PAD depression observed in the present study, therefore, is not well explained by a massive depression of functions in the brain stem following injury, since this depression would be expected to potentiate PAD. Thus, it is possible that descending impulses from the brain stem to the spinal cord may be responsible for depression of afferent-induced PAD following concussive head injury. Since PAD depression produced by concussion can be seen in midpontine transected animals, such descending impulses appear to originate in the bulbar brain stem. Since recording of somatosensory near-field cortical potentials (SSEP's) requires the averaging of a large number of potentials, multiple recordings were not possible within the period in which profound changes in PAD were observed. However, we were able to determine that all components of SSEP's were transiently abolished during the period in which PAD was also profoundly depressed. The amplitude of the initial positive early near-field potential (P_1) of SSEP's recorded in three animals within 3 minutes after injury was significantly depressed ($p<0.01$). The magnitude of depression of the P_1 wave generally corresponded with the average value of the PAD depression recorded simultaneously following injury ($r=0.75$, $p<0.01$). The depression of late near-field potentials (N_2) showed a similar time course. Although the limited number of averaged potentials precludes definitive statements regarding far-field SSEP's, four positive waves, which are presumably equivalent to waves IIa, IIb, III, and IV reported by others (Dong et al, 1982) were distinguished prior to P_1. All of these waves were depressed in recordings taken within the initial 3 minutes following injury.

CONCLUSIONS

The data presented here (Katayama et al, 1985a; Katayama et al, 1985b) have demonstrated that concussion can depress sensory transmission even at the level of the spinal cord. In contrast, earlier studies have emphasized changes in sensory transmission within supraspinal structures (Foltz and Schmidt, 1956; Hayes et al, 1983b; Letcher et al, 1973; Ommaya and Gennarelli, 1974; Tsubokawa et al, 1981). Importantly, concussion also depressed sensory transmission in ascending pathways since somatosensory near-field cortical potentials were also reduced. As we have pointed out elsewhere (Katayama et al, 1985b), neural changes within the bulbar brain stem producing this suppression may reflect nonspecific activation of interneuronal systems. This nonspecific activation of bulbar systems may have a predominantly inhibitory effect, via descending pathways, on sensory input to the spinal cord.

However, nonspecific activation of neural systems may not mediate other behavioral and electrophysiological disturbances associated with concussion. Concussive injury may result in the activation of pontine cholinergic sites resulting in the profound behavioral suppression characterizing a transient comatose state (Hayes et al, 1983b; Hayes et al, 1984). Activation of this cholinergic system could also contribute to suppression of spinal cord motor output (Katayama et al, 1985b) or disruption of higher order processes related to disturbances in orienting or attention (Katayama et al, 1985c; DeSalles et al, in press). Thus, perturbations in neural function related to suppression of sensory input following concussion may be importantly different than functional changes mediating other characteristics of comatose-like states including motor suppression and stuporous inattention (Hayes et al, in press).

REFERENCES

Carpenter D, Engberg I, Fundenstein H, Lundberg A (1963). Decerebrate control of reflexes to primary afferents. Acta Physiol Scand 59:424-437.

Denny-Brown, D (1945). Cerebral concussion. Physiol Rev 25:296-325.

Denny-Brown D, Russell WR (1941). Experimental cerebral concussion. Brain 64:7-164.

DeSalles AAF, Kayayama Y, Newlon PG, Dixon CE, Becker DP, Hayes RL (in press). Transient suppression of event-related evoked potentials in the cat produced by mild head injury. J Neurosurg.

Eccles JC, Krnjevic K (1959). Presynaptic changes associated with post-tetanic potentiation in the spinal cord. J Physiol (Long) 149:274-287.

Foltz EL, Schmidt RP (1956). The role of the reticular formation in the coma of head injury. J Neurosurg 13:145-154.

Greenberg RP, Stablein DM, Becker DP (1981). Non-invasive localization of brain stem lesions in the cat with multimodality evoked potentials: correlation with human head injury data. J Neurosurg 54:740-750.

Groat RA, Magoun HW, Dey FL, Windle WF (1944). Functional alterations in motor and supranuclear mechanisms in experimental concussion. Am J Physiol 141:117-127.

Groat RA, Windle WF, Magoun HW (1945). Functional and structural changes in the monkey's brain during and after concussion. J Neurosurg 2:26-35.

Hayes RL, Galinat BJ, Kulkarne P, Becker DP (1983a). Effects of naloxone on systemic and cerebral responses to experimental concussive brain injury in cats. J Neurosurg 58:720-728.

Hayes RL, Lewelt W, Yeatts ML, Jenkins LW, Katayama Y, Newlon PG, Pechura CM, Povlishock JT, Becker DP, Miller JD (1983b). Metabolic, behavioral and electrophysiological correlates of experimental brain injury in the cat. J Cerebral Blood Flow Metabol 3:539-540.

Hayes RL, Stonnington HH, Lyeth BG, Dixon CE, Yamamoto T (in press). Metabolic and neurophysiological sequelae of brain injury: A cholinergic hypothesis. J Central Nervous System Trauma.

Hayes RL, Pechura CM, Katayama Y, Povlishock JT, Giebel ML, Becker DP (1984). Activation of pontine cholinergic sites implicated in unconsciousness following cerebral concussion in the cat. Science 223:301-303.

Katayama Y, Becker DP, Hayes RL (1985a). Depression of afferent-induced primary afferent depolarization at the lumbar spinal cord following concussive head injury. Brain Res 335(2):392-395.

Katayama Y, Glisson JD, Becker DP, Hayes RL (1985b). Concussive head injury producing suppression of sensory transmission within the spinal cord. J Neurosurg 63:97-105.

Katayama Y, Reuther S, Dixon CE, Becker DP, Hayes RL (1985c). Dissociation of endogenous components of auditory evoked potentials following carbachol microinjection into the cholinoceptive pontine inhibitory area. Brain Res 334(2):366-371.

Letcher FS, Corrao PG, Ommaya AK (1973). Head injury in the chimpanzee. Part 2. Spontaneous and evoked epidural potentials as indices of injury severity. J Neurosurg 39:167-177.

Lundberg A (1964). Supraspinal control of transmission in reflex paths to motor neurons and primary afferents. In Eccles JC, Schade JP (eds): "Progress in Brain Research," Amsterdam: Elsevier, pp 198-221.

Ommaya AK, Gennarelli TA (1974). Cerebral concussion and traumatic unconsciousness. Correlation of experimental and clinical observations on blunt head injuries. Brain 98:633-654.

Rhines R, Magoun HW, Windle WF (1946). The bulbar inhibitory mechanism in concussion. Am J Physiol 146:344-347.

Sullivan HG, Martinez J, Becker DP, Miller JD, Griffith R, Wist AO (1976). Fluid-percussion model of mechanical brain injury in the cat. J Neurosurg 45:520-534.

Tsubokawa T, Yamamoto T, Miyazaki S, Kondo T, Katayama Y, Tomizawa N, Sugawara T, Moriyasu N (1981). Pathogenetic mechanism of cerebral concussion due to rotational angular acceleration impact. Neurol Med Chir 21:657-668.

Walker AE, Kolloros JJ, Case TJ (1944). The physiological basis of concussion. J Neurosurg 1:103-116.

Wall PD (1958). Excitability changes in afferent fiber terminations and their relation to slow potentials. J Physiol (Lond) 142:1-21.

Supported by NIH grant NS21458

Effects of Injury on Trigeminal and Spinal Somatosensory Systems, pages 419–427

MOTOR CAPACITIES AND DEFICIENCIES AFTER INTERRUPTION OF THE DORSAL SPINAL COLUMNS IN PRIMATES

Charles J. Vierck, Jr., Brian Y. Cooper and Christiana M. Leonard

Department of Neuroscience and Center for Neurobiological Sciences University of Florida College of Medicine, Gainesville, FL 32610, U.S.A.

INTRODUCTION

Somatosensory input to the motor cortex originates from the dorsal column-lemniscal system (Brinkman and Porter, 1978; Waters et al., 1985), and the corticospinal system is crucial for facile control of the hands (Beck and Chambers, 1970; Tower, 1940). Therefore, it is expected that somatomotor deficits of the hands (and feet) would result from interruption of the dorsal columns. However, the motor performance of monkeys with dorsal column (DC) lesions has been described as normal on apparently demanding tasks (Asanuma and Arissian, 1984; Brinkman and Porter, 1978). Visual control of the movements was permitted in these behavioral tests, and deficits that resulted from interruption of proprioceptive and tactile feedback may have been compensated for by the presence of visual cues. Thus, to fully describe the consequences of DC interruption, it is necessary to observe animals in situations that restrict visual inputs and/or permit analyses of different aspects of movement control. This report summarizes data from a series of previous investigations and ongoing experiments that are defining the conditions required to reveal an absence of DC-lemniscal modulation of motor control. More comprehensive accounts of the anatomical and physiological properties and the sensory functions of the dorsal columns have appeared previously (Vierck, 1978a, 1978b, 1982b, 1984).

MATERIALS AND METHODS

Macaca arctoides monkeys have been trained on tasks requiring directed movements of the arms, hands and fingers to targets that varied in location, size and resistance to movement. In addition, stump-tailed monkeys have been observed from close range and videotaped as they groomed themselves and conspecifics that lived in outside enclosures. After performance on the motor task(s) was stabile, the dorsal column was interrupted surgically on one side. The lesions were at upper cervical levels, involving tactile and proprioceptive afferents supplying the forelimbs and tactile input from the hindlimbs; or they were at mid- to upper-thoracic levels, interrupting cutaneous afferents in the long projection system of fasciculus gracilis (Whitsel et al., 1969). Under deep halothane anesthesia, dorsal laminectomies exposed two segments of the spinal cord for transection of one dorsal column with precision forceps. The animals were rested at least one week before resumption of behavioral testing. After completion of the behavioral experiments, the animals received an overdose of Nembutal and were perfused for histological analysis of the spinal lesions. Only data from animals with complete transection of the ipsilateral dorsal column are included in this report.

RESULTS AND DISCUSSION

Within the first few days after surgical interruption of one dorsal column, tone is reduced in the ipsilateral forelimb (Schneider et al., 1977), and then the arm and hand are held in flexed postures. Use of this limb in manipulation of the environment is reduced. For example, grooming activities can cease entirely. However, in the early postoperative period it is particularly difficult to separate a reluctance of the animals to use the limb from an inability or deficit in performing motor acts. In order to elicit and observe motor capacities, it is helpful to train the animals to use the partially deafferented limb to perform specific movement sequences, but the animals are rested for at least a week before instituting formal postoperative testing. Therefore, accurate descriptions of recovery within the first postoperative week are not available. But observations of spontaneous behaviors and neurological examinations clearly indicate that there is gross ataxia. The ipsilateral limbs can be misdirected in reaching or stepping, and the hand or foot can be placed and maintained in abnormal positions (Ferraro and Barrera, 1934; Gilman and Denny-Brown, 1966; Liu and Chambers, 1975; Schneider et al., 1977).

Within the first few weeks postoperatively, considerable recovery of gross motor ataxia occurs, and spontaneous behavior of the DC-lesioned animal approaches normal form. It is likely that there is a discrete recovery process, involving visuomotor coordination, that occurs primarily within the first few postoperative days and eventually restores adaptive ambulation, climbing and posturing. The reduction of proprioceptive and tactile feedback temporarily disrupts motor contol by intact visuomotor circuits, but recovery is rapid, as indicated by formal testing within the second postoperative week. When monkeys are trained to project a limb on cue to different locations in space when vision is unrestricted, impairments of latency, speed or accuracy of the goal directed reaching are minimal and transient. Under visual control, complex movements involving sequential actions of different muscle groups can be programmed and run off by DC-lesioned animals, including grasp of an object at the endpoint (Vierck, 1975, 1978c). The recovery of forelimb projection is understandable, since these movements have been characterized as "open loop", indicating that they are preprogrammed and do not require moment-to-moment monitoring of proprioceptive information (Evarts, 1985). The visual information is sufficient to identify the origin and the goal of a ballistic movement that also can be directed accurately following interruption of the corticospinal tract (Beck and Chambers, 1970; Illert et al., 1978; Lawrence and Kuypers, 1968; Laursen and Wiesendanger, 1967). However, when the position and movement of the responding limb must be derived from somatosensory cues, a different result is obtained.

When vision of the responding limb is prevented, trial times for reaching to different targets from different positions are elevated by DC section. Macaca arctoides monkeys were trained to project a forelimb to different locations that were specified by placing a metal peg in one of 64 holes in a 3 ft by 3 ft surface in front of the animals. The target location was observed by the monkeys in bright lighting and then, 1 to 5 sec after the lights were extinguished, one arm was released (from variable start positions). The time from release of the arm to contact of the hand with the peg was increased more than four-fold by section of the ipsilateral fasciculus cuneatus (Vierck, 1978c, 1982a), demonstrating an important role for the DC-lemniscal system in programming directed movements when visual cues are not available to determine the relative positions of the hand and the goal. The limb projection was quickly initiated after release of the limb, but it was inaccurate, necessitating searching (groping). This deficit in dynamic motor adjustment is consistent with a critical role for the DC-lemniscal system in temporal and spatiotemporal coding (Vierck et al., 1985).

Within the first several months of postoperative practice, the deficit in directing arm and hand movements attenuated substantially (Vierck, 1978c), and normal response latencies were obtained eventually. The proprioceptive deficit recovered in two stages: as a short term event at 2-4 weeks, and over subsequent months of practice on the task. This return of fast and accurate limb projection occurred for the hindlimbs and the forelimbs. The short term recovery of reaching accuracy correlates with the timing of a loss and recovery of HRP transport by DC-lemniscal projection neurons in the brainstem (Berkley and Vierck, 1977). After recovery from a transneuronal effect of partial deafferentation, intact pathways emanating from the dorsal horn of the spinal cord can support dynamic motor programming. Based upon demonstrations of highly convergent systems of control over reaching movements of the limbs (Illert et al., 1978), recovery from partial deafferentation of movements primarily involving proximal musculature is understandable.

On the reaching task, the required movement involved accurate projection of a limb to a target that was simply to be contacted. The task did not demand a precision grip or a precise orientation of the hand or a rapid sequence of adjustive movements of the hand or fingers. Based on a presumed role of the corticospinal system in fractionation of movements by the digits (Lawrence and Kuypers, 1968), it is expected that DC lesions would impair finely regulated movements of the distal extremities. Considering first the purely temporal aspect of generating rapid sequences of hand movements, monkeys were trained to press a lever on several fixed ratio schedules (FR 5 and FR 50) that promoted rapid rates of alternating flexion and extension at the wrist. Interruption of the dorsal columns produced little or no deficit on this task (Vierck, 1978c), demonstrating that rapid sequences can be performed when a high degree of sensory feedback is not required for regulating the force or precision of each flexion and extension component of the motor pattern. The bar was fixed in place for all trials and was pushed to a mechanical stop; and therefore, precise control of hand positions was not required.

As tests of the extent to which the dorsal columns contribute to facile orientation of the hands during movements not under visual control, monkeys were trained to project a hand or foot from a fixed start position to one of several vertical compartments. The compartments were situated behind an opaque vertical panel with lights that indicated the position of the correct compartment (behind the panel). To obtain food reinforcement, the monkeys: projected a hand (below an opaque horizontal panel) to the opening of the specified compartment (32 mm by 80 mm), oriented the fingers vertically (in a frontal plane) and reached inside the compartment to touch a metal rod. After interruption of the dorsal columns, they projected the ipsilateral hand rapidly and accurately to the opening of the compartment. The animals could visualize the start position of the limb and the position of the goal, and a correctly aimed response could be programmed. However, at the end of the ballistic arm movements, the animals were not successful in orienting the hand to fit through the opening (Vierck, 1978c). In order for them to obtain reinforcement, it was necessary to enlarge the compartments so that their hands would fit through without orienting their fingers in a frontal plane. Normal trial durations on trials with the large compartments were obtained within a few weeks after DC section. The deficit in hand or foot orientation to the small compartments recovered substantially with careful retraining, but normal latency values were not obtained after as many as 560 days of practice.

In another series of tests of naturalistic movements that could be evaluated in terms of accuracy and speed, monkeys performed reaching movements that terminated in a grasp response. The hindlimbs were tested, to evaluate the effects of lesions that involved only cutaneous, DC-lemniscal afferents (interruption of fasciculus gracilis at upper thoracic levels). For these tasks, direct visualization of the foot and the object was permitted, but at the terminal phase of the limb projection, the foot obscured the goal object (a food pellet), so that evaluation of the success of the grasp came from cutaneous cues. When a pellet was placed on a slick surface and then a limb was released, the foot of a DC-lesioned animal was directed quickly and accurately to come down over the pellet, but the success rate for securing the pellet with the first grasp was reduced considerably. Often the pellet would be knocked out of reach when contacted by the foot. Similarly, if the pellet was placed on a trap door, requiring that the animals grasp the morsel securely before exerting downward pressure, lesioned animals frequently triggered the door before grasping with the toes.

Deficits on these tasks that require a well-timed grasp at the termination of a ballistic movement could result: (a) from poor braking of the ballistic response, (b) from poor form or timing of the grasp or (c) from insufficient feedback concerning the moment or force of contact with the object. Sensory deficits of cutaneous force discrimination are produced by DC interruption (Vierck, 1977), suggesting the latter as a factor contributing to the decreased effectiveness of grasp responses by the feet. The load compensation that must occur with contact of the skin and object is expected to depend upon cutaneous receptors (Evarts, 1985) - a component common to the gracile and cuneate fasciculi (Whitsel et al., 1969). Interruption of fasciculus cuneatus involves proprioceptive afferents in addition, and therefore more severe deficits in somatomotor coordination are expected to result for the hands than for the feet (Ferraro and Barrera, 1934; Gilman and Denny-Brown, 1966).

In order to evaluate the capacities of monkeys to use the hands for manipulative actions, they have been tested on a variant of the classical dexterity board (Cole, 1952). The monkeys were presented raisins in each of 10 wells that were 12 mm in diameter and 6 mm deep. Normal performance on the task involved precise apposition of the thumb and forefinger. Because the raisins were eaten one at a time, the task produced a sequence of ballistic movements of the hand from the mouth to the board, followed by a facile grasp and immediate return to the mouth. Following ipsilateral interruption of fasciculus cuneatus, the monkeys could project the hand precisely to loaded wells, but prehension was clumsy. Trial times were elevated more than three-fold during the early postoperative period (Vierck, 1975). Eventually, performance became more efficient, but the animals generally adopted a strategy of scraping the raisin out with the thumb, followed by grasp of the morsel on the surface of the board. This is consistent with results suggesting that lesions of the corticospinal system produce an inability of monkeys to fractionate movements of individual fingers (Lawrence and Kuypers, 1968; Tower, 1940).

The precision grip could be dependent upon proprioceptive feedback if the recruitment order for specific intrinsic muscles of the hand depends critically upon feedback concerning the relative positions of each phalanx of the fingers involved (Muir, 1986). That is, formation of certain configurations of the fingers may not be possible without proprioceptive feedback provided by the dorsal columns. Alternatively, the timing and location of cutaneous stimuli may be insufficiently specified for evaluation of the consequences of the grasp. The act of grooming involves stereotyped sequences of prehension that provide another opportunity to observe capacities for executing precision grasps.

Close range videotaping of grooming bouts by monkeys has revealed several distinct motor patterns that interact to comprise the overall pattern. Sweeps of one hand are used in an exploratory phase that exposes the skin by rubbing movements that are directed against the grain of the hair. The palm and fingers are swept gently over hairy skin with the fingers relaxed and splayed out. Then one hand "pinches" up a fold of skin that is explored by a series of prehensions by the other hand. For the monkey described here, the precision grasps typically consisted of a pick-pluck sequence involving: (a) apposition of the thumb and forefinger at the skin surface, followed by a quick flexion at the wrist and then (b) another precision grasp, followed by supination and flexion at the wrist. The head is held at close range, and sometimes the hand is brought to the mouth.

Detailed analysis of video tapes of a monkey who received an upper cervical lesion of the left DC have documented the following sequence of deficits and recovery: (a) The frequency of grooming dropped to or near zero for 10 weeks, and other social interactions were reduced. (b) When grooming resumed, there were subtle alterations in the form and patterning of the individual motor acts, but examples of apparently normal sweeps, picks and plucks were observed for the left hand. Clearly this animal could precisely appose the thumb and forefinger in a precision grasp. (c) Despite the return of grooming movements of apparently normal form, the frequency of grooming has remained low for 20 postoperative months, and grooming bouts are initiated less frequently by the female conspecifics of the lesioned male. Judging from their reactions, grooming by the DC-lesioned monkey can be aversive, suggesting that force regulation is impaired.

Observations of grooming indicated that the form of prehensile grasp with the thumb and forefinger can be normal after DC section, in contrast to the results of form-board testing, where prehension was disrupted. The form of grooming movements may be less susceptible to disruption because it is a relatively stereotyped motor act for which detection of successful grasp of an object is less important than the social functions served by gentle and repetitive tactile stimulation. Also, it is easier to direct the apposed thumb and forefinger to contact a fold of skin that is clearly observable than it is to sense effective closure on a soft object that is imbedded in a small compartment and is not observable during the motor act. Finally, prehension may not require a high degree of proprioceptive feedback from distal phalanges. Successful apposition of the thumb and forefinger can be accomplished by a simple movement at the proximal joints of the thumb and/or the forefinger. In contrast, by training animals to depress a recessed key with only the forefinger, a movement is required that involves flexion at the metacarpophalangeal joint and extension of the interphalangeal joints, without concomitant movements of other fingers.

The same animal that was observed during grooming was trained to place either hand on a horizontal tray such that the tips of 3 fingers rested above 3 holes (7mm in diam). Within each hole a disc (5mm diam) was supported by a lever arm. At the fulcrum of each lever was a transducer that monitored degrees of rotary movement. The surface of each disc was formed by a force transducer. Schmidt triggers in circuits supplying the force transducers were set to define key contacts and measure applied force. Criterion key depressions of 10.5mm (for the forefinger) or 7mm (the middle finger) were defined by microswitches. In order to receive food reinforcement, it was required that key 1, in contact with the forefinger, be depressed to the criterion point, without an associated criterion depression of key 2, in contact with the adjacent finger. With difficulty, the monkey learned preoperatively to depress only key 1 to the criterion level, and ipsilateral interruption of the dorsal column eliminated this well-learned response. Throughout 20 months of postoperative testing, this animal flexed all the phalanges of fingers 1-4 in concert. In spite of the ability to appose the thumb and forefinger in the context of grooming, differentiation of flexion vs. extension at different joints of the forefinger did not occur, and the animal was not capable of isolating a flexion to only the index finger, even when visual control was available. Thus, a specialized role in the control of digital fractionation that has been accorded to the corticospinal system is highly dependent upon feedback from the DC-lemniscal system that uniquely supplies the motor cortex.

CONCLUSIONS

Observations of naturalistic behaviors and trained motor actions have revealed a sequence of recovery following spinal injury that is characterized as follows: (a) An early period of partial functional restoration occurs primarily within the first few postoperative days. (b) A precipitous improvement of some skills occurs over several days within the third or fourth postoperative weeks, regardless of intervening practice on the motor task. (c) A gradual process of recovery depends absolutely on task-specific practice.

The model system presented here involved selective interruption of the dorsal spinal column. Recovery proceeded as follows: (a) Gross ataxia of the limbs under visual control was clearly observable in the first few postoperative days, but ambulation, climbing and visuomotor coordination recovered rapidly in the first few days and could appear normal within several weeks. (b) Somatomotor coordination of whole limb actions, however, was severely impaired for 2-4 weeks after DC interruption. Without the aid of visual cues, projection of a limb to different targets from variable start positions was impaired substantially, and then a rapid change in proficiency brought performance near to normal levels. The animals could project the limb toward the target and then locate it with corrective orientations of the distal extremity. (c) Fine adjustive movements of the distal extremities were impaired "permanently" after interruption of the dorsal columns, but considerable improvement in the facility of hand orientation and precision grasp occured with task-dependent practice.

Fractionation of fine movements of the fingers and load compensation with prehension did not recover substantially with practice. Correct sequencing of proximal flexion and distal extension by the index finger did not recover on a task requiring a key press with one finger. Also, a DC-lesioned animal could not restrict proximal flexion to the index finger. When DC-lesioned animals grasped objects, control of and adjustment to contact with the object were impaired, and force regulation of active palpation also appeared to be deficient.

REFERENCES

Asanuma H, Arissian K (1984). Experiments on functional role of peripheral input to motor cortex during voluntary movements in the monkey. J Neurophysiol 53:212-227.

Beck CH, Chambers WW (1970). Speed accuracy and strength of forelimb movement after unilateral pyramidotomy in rhesus monkeys. J Comp Physiol Psychol 70:1-22.

Berkley KJ, Vierck CJ Jr (1987). Transient reduction in retrograde labeling of diencephalic-projecting neurons in monkey dorsal column nuclei following removal of their dorsal column input. This volume.

Brinkman J, Bush BM, Porter RJ (1978). Deficient influences of peripheral stimuli on precentral neurones in monkeyus with dorsal column lesions. Physiol 276:27-48.

Brinkman J, Porter R (1978). Movement performance and afferent projections to the sensorimotor cortex in monkeys with dorsal column lesions. In Gordon G. (ed.) "Active Touch." Pergamon, Oxford, pp. 119-138.

Cole J (1952). Three tests for the study of motor and sensory abilities in monkeys. J Comp Physiol Psychol 45:226-230.

Evarts EV (1985). Transcortical reflexes: their properties and functional significance. In "Hand Function and the Neocortex." Goodwin AW, Darian-Smith I (eds.) Exper Brain Res (Suppl 10) Springer-Verlag, Berlin, pp. 130-154.

Ferraro A, Barrera SE (1934). Effects of experimental lesions of the posterior colum;ns in Macaca rhesus monkeys. Brain 57: 307-332.

Gilman S, Denny-Brown D (1966). Disorders of movement and behavior following dorsal column leions. Brain 89:397-418.

Illert M, Lundberg A, Padel Y, Tanaka R (1978). Integration in descending motor pathways controlling the forelimb in the cat. 5. Properties of and monosynaptic excitatory convergence on C3-C4 propriospinal neurons. Exp Brain Res 33: 101-130.

Lawrence DG, Kuypers HGJM (1968). The functional organization of the motor system in the monkey. 1. The effects of bilateral pyramidal lesions. Brain 91:1-14.

Laursen AM, Wiesendanger M (1967). The effect of pyramidal lesions on reponse latency in cats. Brain Res 5:207-220.

Liu CN, Yu J, Chambers WW, Ha H (1975). The role fo the medial lemniscal and spinocervicothalamic pathways on tactile reactions in cats. Acta Neurobiol Exp 35:149-157.

Muir RB (1986). Small ha;nd muscles in precision grip: a corticospinal prerogative? In Goodwin AW, Darian-Smith I (eds) "Hand Function and the Neocortex." Springer-Verlag, Berlin, pp. 155-174.

Schneider RJ, Kulics AT, Ducker TB (1977). Proprioceptive pathways of the spinal cord. J Neurol Neurosurg Psychiat 40:417-433.

Tower SS (1940). Pyramidal lesions in the monkey. Brain 63:36-90.

Vierck CJ Jr (1975). Proprioceptive deficits after dorsal column lesions in monkeys. In Kornhuber H (ed) "The Somatosensory System." Thieme, Stuttgart, pp. 310-317.

Vierck CJ Jr (1977). Absolute and differential sensitivities to touch stimuli after spinal cord lesions in monkeys. Brain Res 134:529-539.

Vierck CJ Jr (1978a). The somatosensory system. In Masterton RB (ed) "Sensory Integration; Handbook of Behavioral Neurobiology." Plenum, N.Y., pp. 249-309.

Vierck CJ Jr (1978b). Interpretations of the sensory and motor consequences of dorsal column lesions. In Gordon GG (ed.) "Active Touch." Pergamon, Oxford, pp. 139-159.

Vierck CJ Jr (1978c). Comparison of forelimb and hindlimb motoric deficits following dorsal column section in monkeys. Brain Res 146:279-294

Vierck CJ Jr (1982a). Comparison of the effects of dorsal rhizotomy and dodrsal column section on motor performance of monkeys. Exper Neurol 75:566-575.

Vierck CJ Jr (1982b). Plasticity of somatic sensations and motor capabilities following lesions of the dorsal spinal columns in monkeys. In Morrison AR and Strick PL (eds) "Changing Concepts of the Nervous System." Academic, N.Y., pp. 151-169.

Vierck CJ Jr (1984). The spinal lemniscal pathways. In Davidoff R (ed) "Handbook of the Spinal Cord." Vols. 2 and 3, Dekker, N.Y., pp. 673-750.

Vierck CJ Jr, Cohen RH, Cooper BY (1985). Effects of spinal lesions on temporal resolution of cutaneous sensations. Somatosensory Res 3:45-56.

Waters RS, Tamai Y, Asanuma H (1985). Caudal cuneate nucleus projection to the direct thalamic relay to the motor cortex: an electrophysiological study. Brain Res 360: 361-365.

Whitsel BW, Petrucelli LM, Sapiro G (1969). Modality representation in the lumbar and cervical fasciculus gracilis of squirrel monkey. Brain Res 15:67-78.

Effects of Injury on Trigeminal and Spinal Somatosensory Systems, pages 429–436

TRANSIENT REDUCTION IN RETROGRADE LABELING OF DIENCEPHALIC-PROJECTING NEURONS IN MONKEY DORSAL COLUMN NUCLEI FOLLOWING REMOVAL OF THEIR DORSAL COLUMN INPUT

Karen J. Berkley and Charles J. Vierck, Jr.

Dept. of Psychology, Florida State Univ., Tallahassee, FL 32306-1051 (K.J.B.) and Dept. of Neuroscince, Univ. of Florida College of Medicine, Gainesville, FL 32610 (C.J.V.) USA

A constellation of behavioral deficits are often an immediate consequence of injury to a portion of the central nervous system. Although many or all of these deficits frequently recover, the time course of recovery is variable. In general, there appear to be three recovery rates (Mendell, 1982). Some deficits, thought to be due to "shock" of the injury (e.g. "spinal shock"; Sherrington, 1906 or "diaschesis"; von Monakow, 1914) recover rapidly over a period of 1-7 days. Others recover within a longer, but still relatively short time period (2-6 weeks), while still others recover much more slowly over a period of many months.

As shown below in Fig. 1, lesions of the dorsal columns in the upper thoracic segments of the monkey spinal cord produce different behavioral deficits with approximately three recovery rates. Thus, recovery from dorsal column lesions provides a model for studies of neural mechanisms underlying recovery of function.

The present experiment was part of a series examining potential anatomical correlates of the behavioral recovery patterns in this model system. The studies are focused on diencephalic-projecting neurons in the dorsal column nuclei (DCN) since they are the major central target of dorsal column fibers. Specifically, the present experiment examined whether changes in the retrograde transport characteristics of diencephalic-projecting DCN neurons occurred as a consequence of dorsal column lesions and, if so, whether they varied over time to correlate with some aspect of the behavioral recovery pattern.

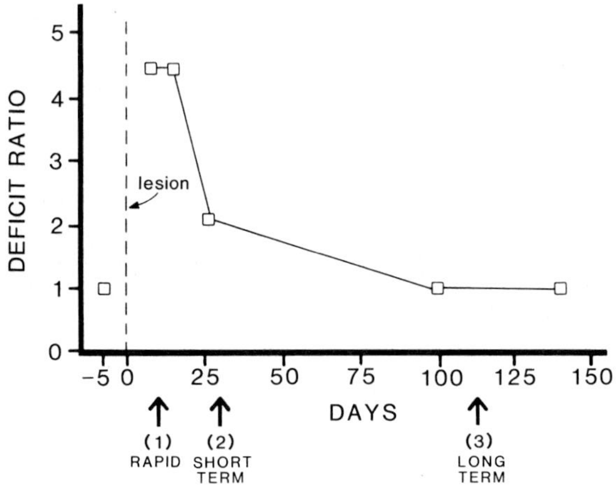

Figure 1. Effects of dorsal column lesions on motor performance in the monkey. Dorsal column lesions in the upper thoracic cord produce (A) gross ataxia of the ipsilateral hindlimb as well as deficits (B) in visuomotor coordination, (C) in coordination of proximal ballistic movements (without vision) and (D) in coordination of precise distal movements (grasping and finger fractionation). Deficits A and B usually recover within 1-7 days following the lesion (arrow: RAPID <1>). (The graph shows how deficit C recovers in two stages. "Deficit Ratio" = postoperative latencies/ preoperative latencies. Each point represents the mean from 6 subjects with 11 lesions.) In the first stage, there is a precipitous general improvement within 2-5 weeks (arrow: SHORT TERM <2>), followed, in the second stage, by a slower improvement with task-specific practise (arrow: LONG TERM <3>). Deficit D does not recover. (See Vierck et al., this volume for more details.)

METHODS

The studies were done on 8 adult monkeys (6 M. mulatta; 2 M. nemestrina). In each barbiturate-anethetized monkey, 4.4 ul of horseradish peroxidase (50% HRP: 5 cases) or HRP conjugated with wheatgerm agglutinin (10% WGA:HRP; 3 cases) was injected bilaterally into the diencephalon at various intervals (7, 7, 13, 17, 21, 210, 255, 315 days) following a unilateral lesion of the dorsal columns at levels varying from T3 - T8. Thirty six to 48 hrs later, the monkey was sacrificed and perfused transcardially with 1.0 % paraformaldehyde, 2.0 % glutaraldehyde and 4 % sucrose. The brainstem was removed, frozen, and 50um-thick sections were cut through DCN and processed using tetramethylbenzidine (Mesulam, 1982). The sections were examined at 250-500 X magnification under bright field conditions, sometimes with cross polarizers. Retrogradely labeled neurons were plotted using an X-Y pantograph apparatus. Tissue processing and plotting were performed without knowledge of when or on which side the dorsal column sections had been made.

RESULTS

As shown in Fig. 2, few neurons in the deafferented part of DCN (i.e. the ipsilateral gracile n.) were labeled in the first two weeks following the dorsal column lesion. This lack of labeling stood in striking contrast to the dense labeling observed in the ipsilateral cuneate and contralateral gracile and cuneate nuclei. By 17 to 21 days post-lesion, many more neurons in the deafferented region became labeled (Fig. 3 A). It was still the case, however, that there was less labeling in the deafferented region. Not only were there fewer labeled neurons, but the intensity of labeling within each labeled neuron was lower in the deafferented regions (Fig. 3 C,D). By 7 months post-lesion (Figs. 3 B), even though the deafferented region was shrunken, labeling in it was comparable to labeling in the other regions.

DISCUSSION

These results demonstrate that short term behavioral deficits resulting from lesions of the dorsal columns in the primate (Fig. 1, <2>) are accompanied by a similar short term change in retrograde transport of HRP by the deafferented diencephalic-projecting neurons in DCN.

The mechanisms that might underly this reduction and recovery of retrograde labeling are unclear. Reductions in the retrograde HRP labeling of deafferented neurons have been observed in two other similar studies. In 1977, Singer et al. observed that retrograde labeling of lateral geniculate nucleus neurons was reduced in adult cats that had been

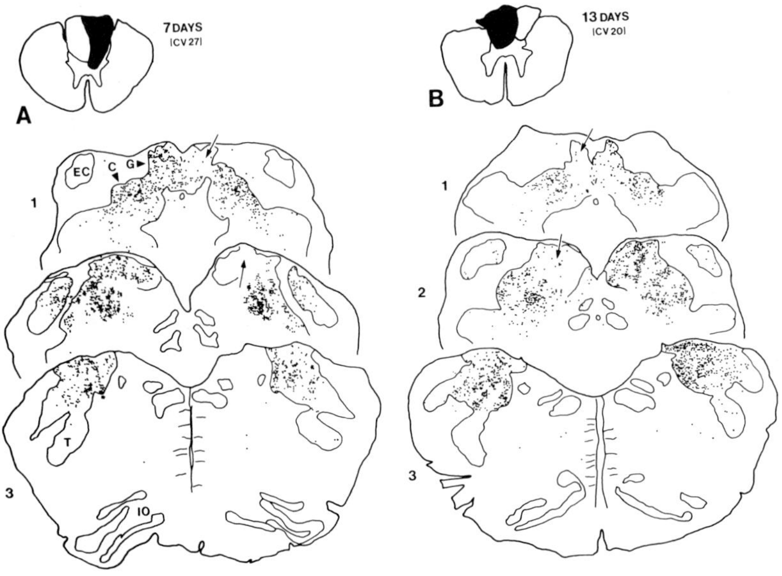

Figure 2. Retrograde transport of HRP in diencephalic-projecting DCN neurons 7 days (A) and 13 days (B) following unilateral lesions of the thoracic dorsal columns (shown at top of figure). In both cases, the bilaterally comparable HRP injections had filled the ventroposterior nucleus and surrounding regions on both sides. The charts are sections through caudal (1), middle (2) and rostral (3) levels of DCN. Each dot represents one labeled neuron. Within DCN, note the paucity of labeled neurons only in the deafferented gracile nucleus (arrows). Abbreviations: C, cuneate n.; EC, external cuneate n.; G, gracile n.; T, trigeminal nucleus; IO, inferior olive.

unilaterally enucleated immediately following injection of HRP into striate cortex. The authors hypothesized that this reduction in labeling was related to the then presumed, but now documented (Eysel, 1979) "low activity" of the deafferented neurons. No attempt was made to determine if the labeling returned at any time after the enucleation. Presumably, however, such recovery might occur, since the deafferented neurons recover some spontaneous activity within 10 weeks (Eysel, 1979). On the other hand, if recovery of labeling reflects recovery of behavioral functions, rather than the simple presence of neuronal activity, then labeling might not recover (since cats can never regain vision in an enucleated eye).

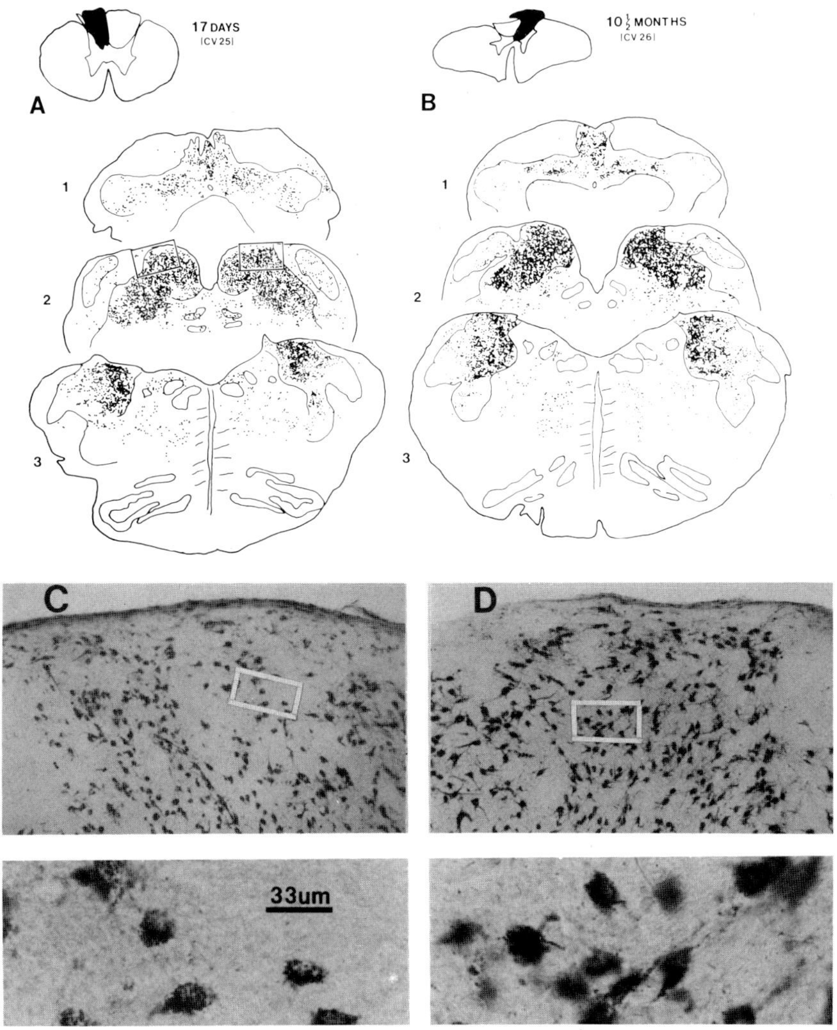

Figure 3. Retrograde transport of HRP in diencephalic-projecting neurons 17 days (A) and 10.5 months (B) following unilateral lesions of the thoracic dorsal columns. Injections and charts in these cases are like those in Fig. 2. The photomicrographs were taken from the areas outlined on the left (C) and right (D) sides of section A2.

In 1983, Peyronnard and Charron reported that although bilateral sectioning of the L3-L5 dorsal roots in rat had no effect on the number or characteristics of motor axons, there was a significant decrease in the number of motoneurons retrogradely labeled by HRP through the L4 spinal nerve. Unlike the deafferented lateral geniculate nucleus neurons, however, this longlasting reduction in labeling did not appear until 4 months after the rhizotomies, despite the immediate (and permanent) motor impairments they produced.

Like Singer et al, Peyronnard and Charron hypothesized that the reduction in motoneuronal labeling might be related to reduced "activity" of the motoneurons. No conclusive evidence exists, however, to support this hypothesis, particularly since primary afferents constitute only a small proportion of the total synaptic input to motoneurons (e.g. Ralston and Ralston, 1979), and the reduction in labeling took several months to develop. In addition, as discussed by the authors, inputs converging on motoneurons are complex and heterogeneous (e.g. see Henneman and Mendell, 1981), making any general conclusions regarding the effectiveness of removing one of them (e.g. the primary afferents) on their overall "activity" oversimplifications.

Thus, in these very different studies, deafferentation clearly resulted in a reduced retrograde labeling of the deafferented neurons. It remains unclear, however, how well this reduction correlates with behavioral deficits and their recovery or with some aspect of the overall "activity" of the deafferented neurons.

With regard to the present results, electrophysiological studies in cat have shown that deafferentation of DCN by sectioning dorsal roots (Millar et al., 1976; Dostrovsky et al., 1976) or by cold block of dorsal columns (Dostrovsky et al., 1976) results in an immediate alteration of the response properties of many neurons in the deafferented region. Although such neurons acquire "new" receptive fields and an unusual bursting spontaneous activity, there are "no consistent differences" in their overall spontaneous activity rate from normal neurons. The authors did not report whether overall spontaneous activity continued unchanged at longer intervals after deafferentation, but, presumably, no changes occurred, because 8 months after dorsal root section, the only major change reported was an increase in the percent of neurons with "new" receptive fields.

If these results in the cat can be applied to those of the present study in the monkey, the most logical conclusion would be that the reduction and recovery of retrograde labeling was not related to the overall activity level of DCN neurons. However, this conclusion must remain tentative, because of incomplete electrophysiological evidence for the dorsal column nuclei and because studies in other regions levels have indicated that there are clear decreases followed by increases in the activity of neurons following their deafferentation (Kjerulf and Loeser, 1973).

CONCLUSION

One intriguing aspect of the present study was the apparent correlation in time between the reduction and recovery of retrograde labeling with the loss and recovery of certain sensorimotor abilities. It will thus be of interest to examine in more detail the precision of this correlation (e.g. how soon after deafferentation it occurs and precisely when it recovers in relation to the sequence of behavioral changes), whether such changes (both in labeling and behavior) occur with more extensive deafferentation of DCN (e.g. rhizotomies, dorsal column lesions that extend into the dorsolateral funiculus sensorimotor cortical lesions), and how these labeling changes are related to the synaptic rearrangements (e.g. Kjerulf et al., 1973; Ganchrow et al., 1981) and sprouting (Goldberger and Murray, 1978) that appear to occur during the period of recovery.

ACKNOWLEDGEMENTS

This work was supported by NIH grants R01 NS 11892 and R01 NS 07261. We thank S. Core, L. Rinaman, E. Wood and H. R. Harris for help with histology and plotting, and R. J. Budell, D. Yeomans, M. S. Bull and Dr. R. Cohen for suggestions and assistance during the conduct of the experiments.

REFERENCES

Dostrovsky JO, Millar J, Wall PD (1976). The immediate shift of afferent drive of dorsal column nucleus cells following deafferentation: A comparison of acute and chronic deafferentation in gracile nucleus and spinal cord. Exp Neurol 52:480-495.

Eysel UT (1979). Maintained activity, excitation and inhibition of lateral geniculate neurons after monocular deaf-

ferentation in the adult cat. Brain Res 166:259-271.
Ganchrow D, Margolin J, Perez L, Bernstein JJ (1981). Patterns of reafferentation in rat nucleus gracilis after thoracic dorsal column lesions. Exp Neurol 71:437-451.
Goldberger ME, Murray M (1978). Recovery of movement and axonal sprouting may obey some of the same laws. In Cotman CW (ed): "Neuronal Plasticity," New York: Raven Press, pp 73-96.
Henneman E, Mendell LM (1981). Functional organization of motoneuron pool and its inputs. In Brookhart JM, Mountcastle VB, (eds): "Handbook of Physiology: Sec 1. The Nervous System: Vol II. Motor Control, Part 1," Bethesda: American Physiological Society, pp 423-507.
Kjerulf TD, Loeser JD (1973). Neuronal hyperactivity following deafferentation of the lateral cuneate nucleus. Exp Neurol 39:70-85.
Kjerulf TD, O'Neal JT, Calvin WH, Loeser JD, Westrum LE (1973). Deafferentation effects in lateral cuneate nucleus of the cat: correlation of structural alterations with firing pattern changes. Exp Neurol 39:86-102.
Mendell L (1982). Temporal changes after spinal cord injury. In Nicholls JG (ed): "Repair and Regeneration of the Nervous System," Berlin: Springer-Verlag, pp 255-268.
Mesulam M-M (1982). "Tracing Neural Connections with Horseradish Peroxidase." New York: John Wiley and Sons.
Millar J, Basbaum AI, Wall PD (1976). Restructuring of the somatotopic map and appearance of abnormal neuronal activity in the gracile nucleus after partial deafferentation. Exp Neurol 50:658-672.
Monakow, C von (1914). "Die Lokalisation in Grosshirnrinde und der Abbau der Funktion durch Korticale Herde." Wiesbaden: J. F. Bergmann.
Peyronnard J-M, Charron L (1983). Decreased horseradish peroxidase labeling in deafferented spinal motoneurons of the rat. Brain Res 275:203-214.
Ralston HJ, Ralston DD (1979). Identification of dorsal root synaptic terminals on monkey ventral horn cells by electron microscopic autoradiography. J Neurocytol 8:151-166.
Sherrington, CS (1906). "The Integrative Action of the Nervous System." New York: Charles Scribner's Sons.
Singer W, Hollander H, Vanegas H (1977). Decreased peroxidase labeling of lateral geniculate neurons following deafferentation. Brain Res 120:133-137.
Vierck CJ Jr, Cooper BY, Leonard CM (1987). Motor capacities and deficiencies after interruption of the dorsal spinal columns in primates. This volume.

Effects of Injury on Trigeminal and Spinal Somatosensory Systems, pages 437–449

DEVELOPMENT OF TACTILE FUNCTION FOLLOWING DAMAGE TO SOMATIC SENSORY CORTEX IN INFANT *MACACA*

Harold Burton, Mary Carlson and Susan Warren

Departments of Neurobiology (H.B.), Psychiatry and McDonnell Center for Studies of Higher Brain Function,(M.C., S.W.), Washington University School of Medicine, Saint Louis, Missouri 63110

INTRODUCTION

Studies of tactile capacities after either partial (Semmes and Porter, 1972; Randolph and Semmes, 1974; Carlson, 1981) or total (Semmes, Porter and Randolph, 1974) removals of the hand area in the primary somatic sensory cortical projection area, SI, of adult macaques have shown severe tactile discrimination deficits. Removal of the more posterior SI areas, 1 and 2, produces selective but persistent deficits on texture and size-shape discriminations, respectively, and damage to area 3b interferes with all forms of tactile discriminations. The secondary somatic sensory area, SII, is another parietal cortical area that receives cutaneous and non-cutaneous inputs into a somatotopically organized map (Robinson and Burton, 1980). Lesions of SII in adult macaques also produce deficits across the same range of texture and size-shape tasks affected by SI lesions (Murray and Mishkin, 1984). In contrast, infants receiving either partial or total ablations of SI fully recover the ability to perform size and texture discriminations (Carlson, 1984b,c). In a search for the source of this recovery of tactile function, we have compared the discrimination capacities of normal and SI-lesioned infants to that of infants with SII or combined SI-SII lesions.

MATERIALS AND METHODS

An automated tactile discrimination apparatus was developed to present paired objects to infants as young as 6 weeks of age (Carlson, 1984a). Infants were removed from their natural mother soon after birth, and raised on infant formula with surrogate mothers in heated incubators for the first months of life. On weekdays all formula was obtained by performing on the apparatus. Animals were initially given small amounts of formula for repeatedly contacting the objects (vertically oriented handles) and eventually only in response to correctly discriminating the smallest size or smoothest surface of paired handles on a forced-choice trial. Infants were first trained on an easy size (7-18 mm diameter) or texture discrimination (320-40 grains/linear inch abrasive papers) until they reached a criterion of 80% correct in a single session of 50-200 trials. After criterion was reached on the initial comparison, a more difficult comparison was presented (7-12mm or 320-80 gr/in) until criterion was reached. The most difficult comparisons (7-9mm and 320-120 gr/in) were chosen to approximate the size and texture thresholds of normal adult animals determined in previous studies (Randolph and Semmes, 1974). Finally all other combinations of these four size and texture handles were presented until all levels were learned to criterion; ACQUISITION curves of percent correct across days illustrate the course of learning and the total number of errors to criterion was used as a measure of efficiency of ACQUISITION. Subsequently, a measure of performance was introduced, the ALLS test. In this test all six pairs were presented together in the same session to measure the performance on easy, moderate and difficult comparisons. In this more complex task, where levels of difficulty changed on every trial and where the "correct" choice also changed, the average percent correct over five sessions was used as a measure of performance.

Following completion of all behavioral testing the animals were given an overdose of sodium pentobarbital and immediately perfused transcardially with saline and neutral formalin. The brains were subsequently photographed and sectioned frozen at 50 μm; the mounted sections were stained with thionin. Lesion sites were reconstructed from the sections and the cytoarchitectonic areas surviving in the vicinity of the lesions were noted. The thalamic nuclei showing retrograde cell degeneration were also identified.

RESULTS

Normal infants were able to learn the most difficult size and texture discriminations as early as 9-10 weeks of age; this demonstrated mature tactile acuity at the earliest age that the infants had the motor capacity to respond (Carlson, 1984a). Errors to criterion on the most difficult size tasks decreased as a function of age (between 7 and 25 weeks, $r=-0.57$, n.s.) whereas total errors for the six tasks actually increased significantly as a function of age ($r=+0.80$, $p<.005$). The average errors to criterion for the six size tasks was 115 and for texture tasks was 249. ACQUISITION curves for one normal infant and averages on ALLS performance are illustrated in Fig. 1A and 1E. Note that ACQUISITION occurred within 5-6 sessions and that performance on even the most difficult comparisions during the ALLS test was between 60-70% correct.

Four SI-lesioned infants were prepared with partial SI lesions (either 3b or areas 1 and 2) to determine the role of these areas in tactile acquisition and performance with the expectation of more recovery of tactile function than seen after similar lesions in adult macaques. Infants with either type of partial lesion were delayed in ACQUISITION by 2-3 months compared to normal infants but all eventually mastered even the threshold level tasks. Their performance levels were equal to or slightly below normal infants (Carlson, 1984b). In order to determine how the remaining areas in the damaged SI may mediate the recovered function, infants with total SI lesions were prepared. Contrary to all expectations these SI-lesioned infants learned size and texture comparisons over the same time and with the same efficiency as normal infants. Furthermore, when tested on the ALLS task their performance was at the level of normal infants (Carlson, 1984c). The ACQUISITION scores and ALLS performance of a typical unilateral SI-lesioned infant are presented in Fig. 1B and 1F.

SII-lesioned infants received either unilateral or bilateral lesions between 5.6 and 8.8 weeks of age. Results from one infant with a unilateral and four infants with bilateral lesions were consistent in showing that infants with SII lesions have no deficits on size ACQUISITION (Fig. 1C). In fact, average errors to criterion on size ACQUISITION were consistently lower for SII-lesioned (Fig. 1C) than normal infants (28.6 vs. 115.1 errors). It is important to

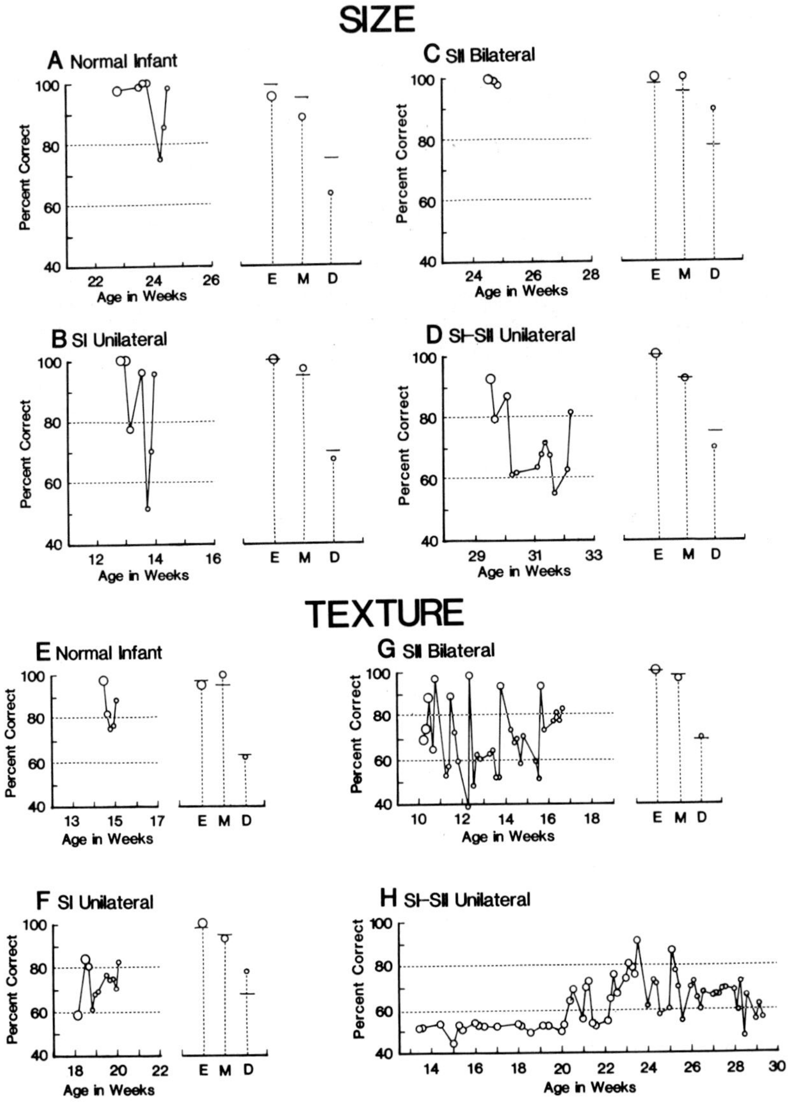

Figure 1. ACQUISITION and ALLS curves for size and texture comparisons in normal and lesioned infants. Difficulty of comparisons indicated by circle sizes (largest= easiest,E; smallest=most difficult,D). Average performance for normal infants shown as horizontal bars through ALLS curves (on right of each panel).

emphasize that age is a factor in efficiency of size ACQUISITION. SII-lesioned infants were tested between 20-40 weeks of age as compared to an average testing age of 8-30 weeks of age for normal infants. Performance on the size ALL tasks by SII-lesioned infants was equal to or better than the average for normal infants.

ACQUISITION of texture discrimination in SII-lesioned infants was protracted; error scores for one of these lesioned infants (Fig. 1G) were 1737, four times that of normal infants. Although SII-lesioned infants were tested on texture prior to size, in contrast to normal infants, the inflated errors could not be accounted for by procedural differences alone. Performance on texture ALLS was normal.

Combined lesions of SI and SII were of three types: SI and SII removed simultaneously in infants and older juveniles, SII-SI sequentially in older infants and SI-SII sequentially in older juveniles. Regardless of the lesion sequence or whether animals were infants or juveniles, the consequences of combined SI-SII lesions were devastating for texture but not size discrimination capacity. The one SI-SII lesioned infant to show some retardation of size ACQUISITION is illustrated in Fig. 1D; the performance on size ALLS tasks for this and all other SI-SII lesioned animals was normal. In contrast, a two-year old juvenile macaque given a SI-SII lesion was so impaired that it never relearned even the easiest size comparison during ACQUISITION. Two 6-month old infants with sequential SII-SI lesions made, on average, 376 errors to criterion on size ACQUISITION, but size ALLS performance was normal.

The consequences of the combined SI-SII lesion were much greater when measured on the texture tasks. The SI-SII infant illustrated in Fig. 1H made thousands of errors on the easiest texture test and never mastered the moderate levels. The remaining three infants with simultaneous SI-SII lesions showed inflated errors on the ACQUISITION of easy and moderate level comparisons and failed to learn the difficult level tasks. Overall performance on the texture ALLS task was inferior compared to normal infants, particularly on the difficult texture comparisons. Infants with combined SI-SII lesions never recovered the ability to appreciate small differences in texture.

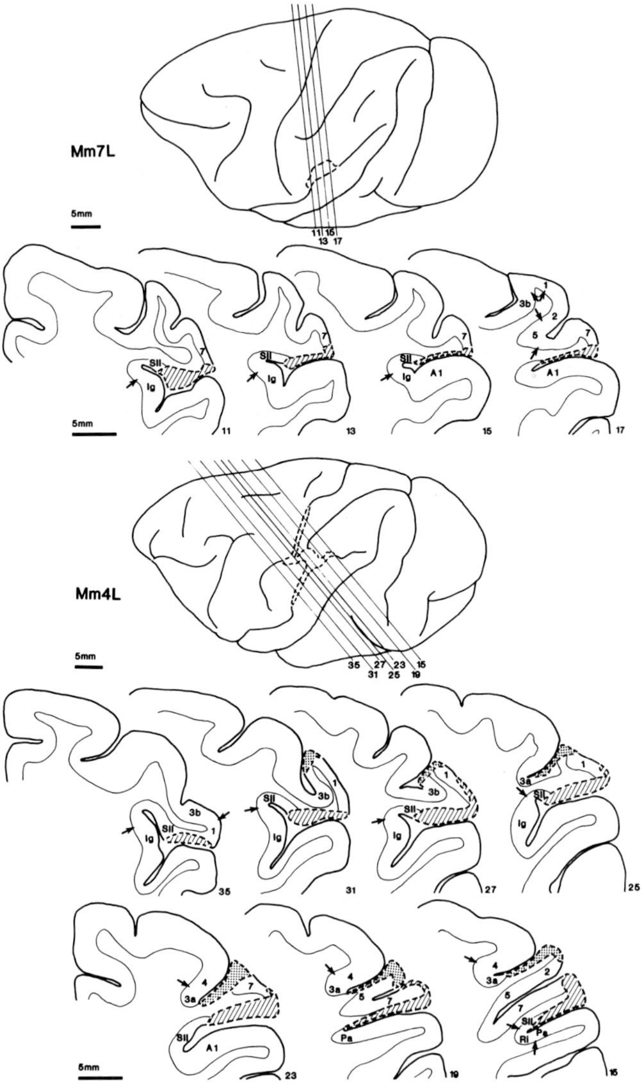

Figure 2. SII lesioned infant (Mm7L) and combined SI-SII lesioned infant (Mm4L). Lesions shown with dashed line on surface views, on sections with dots in SI and with cross-hatching in SII. Corresponding numbers on lines and sections. A1, primary auditory area; Ig, granular insula; Pa, postauditory area; Ri, retroinsular area; SII, second somatic sensory area; 3a, 3b, 1, and 2, areas of SI; 5 and 7, parietal association areas; 4, primary motor cortex.

Anatomy

An example of a total SI lesion is shown in Fig. 2, (Mm4) where SI and SII had been removed simultaneously at 7.6 weeks in the left hemisphere. The lesion across the postcentral gyrus extended from the fundus of the central sulcus (CS) to the fundus of the intraparietal sulcus (IPS). The lesion also extended laterally past the IPS but without reaching the fundus of CS. Medially the lesion narrowed to the exposed surface of the gyrus. The lesion partially invaded area 3a, and totally destroyed all of areas 3b, 1 and 2 in the vicinity of the SI hand area.

The SII lesions varied in extent across the different cases; in all but one case, however, all or most of the hand area located near and immediately posterior to the insula was damaged. As shown in Fig. 2 (Mm4), the lesion in the lateral sulcus (LS) blanketed all of the outer face of the sulcus along the posterior third of the insula, extended posteriorly from the insula along the full extent of the upper bank of the LS and spread over the adjoining inferior parietal lobule to the lateral edge of the IPS. This lesion totally destroyed SII except for a small wedge of tissue

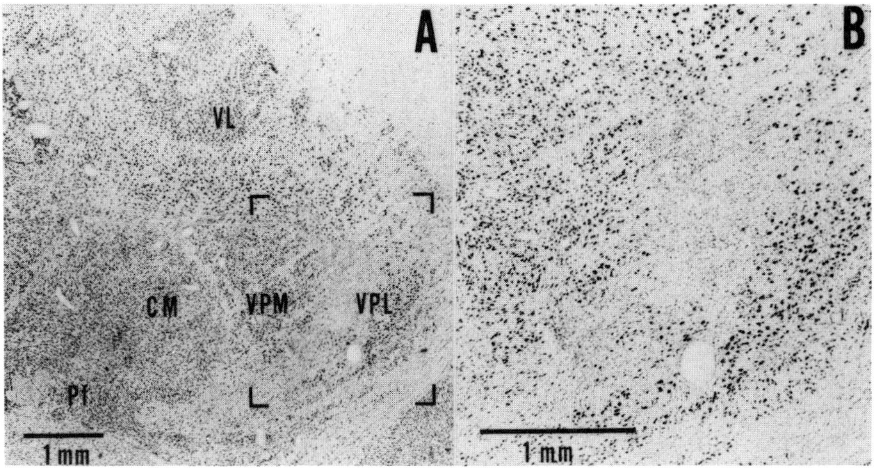

Figure 3. Photomicrographs of horizontal section through thalamus of Mm4L. Region bracketed in A shown in B. Note absence of any cells in central portion of gliotic zone in B. CM, centrum medium n.; Pf, parafascicular n.; VL, ventrolateral n.; VPL, ventroposterior lateral n.; VPM, ventroposterior medial n.

anteriorly near the superior limiting sulcus (SLS). In this and all other cases (Fig. 2, Mm7), the insula, temporal operculum, and most of the posterior tip of the LS were spared. Lesions into the LS also ablated portions of area 7b but frequently spared lateral SII (mostly lower limb and trunk regions) near the SLS and the rostral SII face region.

Retrograde cell degeneration was present throughout the medial half of the ventroposterior lateral nucleus (VPL) to all boundaries of the nucleus in cases involving lesions of SI and SII. In the case illustrated (Fig. 3, Mm4), no surviving cells were found in the center of the zone of maximum degeneration. Small islands of surviving cells were noted, however, near the borders of non-gliotic portions of the ventroposterior nuclei. The VP medial nucleus also contained gliosis along its lateral border. This was more evident through the dorsal half of VPM. At the dorsal, posterior boundary of VPL, a small patch of gliosis was additionally traced into the anterior pulvinar. Along the ventral and posterior boundary of VPL a greater number of surviving, small cells were seen. No degeneration was detected in the region of the posterior nucleus. In contrast, there was no clear zone of gliosis noted in cases with lesions restricted to SII.

DISCUSSION

Studies of tactile function in normal macaques indicated that the ability to detect small differences in the size or texture of objects was at adult levels by two months of age (Carlson, 1984a). Although these results imply that the somatic sensory cortex matures early, the behavioral consequences of lesions at this age suggest that the functional organization of SI and SII differs in infant and adult macaques (Carlson, 1984b,c). Infants receiving either partial or total ablations of SI or SII may show some delay in the acquisition of fine discriminations but recover normal performance even on difficult threshold tasks.

The results indicate that for texture tasks recovery only occurs when SI or SII is spared. Other cortical regions possibly involved with tactile behavior (commissural SI and SII, motor cortex, parietal association areas) do not mediate the behavior when both SI and SII are gone. The potential of any distribution of texture discrimination abilities is thus limited. In addition, a general substitution of intact portions of SI or SII also does not occur indicating that these cortical regions are not pleuripotential for the hand areas in the damaged regions. However, some revision of strategies is likely as the ACQUISITION curves for texture discrimination were prolonged when one of the cortical somatic sensory areas was damaged in infants.

Contrary to previous findings in adults, size discriminations were spared after SII lesions in infants and recovered after SI-SII lesions. Part of this difference may be due to the recovery capacities of infants. Additionally, however, the recovery of size discrimination abilities may reflect that the potential for making size comparisions is more widely distributed to cortical areas not ablated; candidate regions may be areas 3a, 5 or 4.

Recovery of function after early brain damage has been reported for other cortical systems (Kennard, 1942; Goldman, 1974) and a considerable literature has developed on the possible mechanisms underlying this phenomenon. Some interest has focused on the possibility of collateral sprouting in the central nervous system under certain conditions of deafferentation. Considerable data has also shown that regressive changes (i.e., cell death and synapse elimination) are important mechanisms in the development of the central nervous system (Purves and Lichtman, 1985). The age range during which recovery was obtained in the present experiments overlapped with the period when maximum synaptic exuberance has been found throughout the cerebral cortex of primates (Rakic et al., 1986). This coincidence of time may be far more significant as a potential explanation for recovered behavior in primates than the recurrence of collateral sprouting.

Synapse elimination is observed both in pre- and postnatal development and extends over the same period as the formation of ocular dominance columns and the recovery of behavioral function after cortical lesions. Previously, we suggested that the presence of exuberant connections in the immature primate cortex may play a role in the observed tactile recovery (or sparing) after total SI lesions (Carlson, 1984c). Recent findings on the elimination of exuberant synapes in the cortex of macaques over the first 3-4 months of life provide even greater support for the contention that early lesions may result in a modification of synapse elimination in related cortical areas such that the uninjured areas may continue to mediate normal functions. This hypothesis would suggest that in the infant macaque SI and SII are more similar in function than at a later age. Given the complete removal of one area, the remaining area may serve to mediate what might become the specialized functions of the two areas in a normal juvenile or adult. In the framework of altering synaptic densities, one might suggest that this recovery may rely on the persistence of connections that would have competed unsuccessfully with the normal cortical connections that were removed by the lesions. Three categories of connections may persist: commissural from the same somatic sensory areas in the opposite hemisphere, association and numerous subcortical, including thalamic (specific and intralaminar nuclei), striatal, locus coeruleus and basal nucleus of Meynert.

CONCLUSION (SEE FIG. 4)

These studies have shown that the capacity to discriminate fine differences in the size and texture of objects was at mature levels by two months of age; this was the earliest that infants could be trained to perform the tasks. When partial SI lesions were made at this age, the acquisition of size discrimination was slightly retarded compared to normal infants; the acquisition of texture discrimination was markedly retarded. Partial SI lesioned infants frequently required 2-3 months longer than normal infants and made thousands of errors in the process of acquisition. In contrast to juveniles with partial lesions, these infants mastered all difficult comparsions. Infants with total SI lesions also recovered normal capacities even more rapidly. This left SII as the most likely area to be mediating recovery after total SI lesions in infants. When either unilateral or bilateral SII lesions were made in infants no deficits were seen on size tasks, delayed acquisition was found on texture tasks, but no performance deficits were evident for texture on the ALLS test. The unilateral combination of a SII lesion with a SI lesion in infants had devastating consequences for texture discrimination. No consistent delays were seen in size ACQUISITION or size ALLS performance. It appears that the "sparing" or "recovery" of texture discrimination capacity after either SI or SII lesions is dependent upon the complementary somatic sensory area in the damaged hemisphere but size discrimination may recover through other

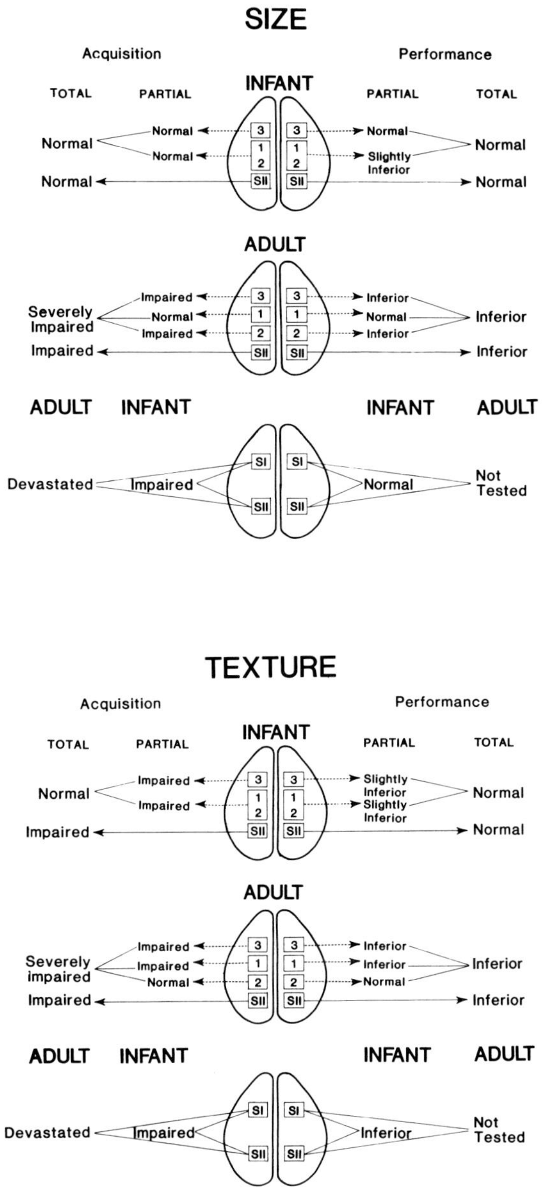

Figure 4. Summary of ACQUISITION and performance on size and texture discrimination ALL tasks in infant and adult macaques following lesions to indicated parts of SI (3,1,2) and SII.

cortical areas. The rapid time course of recovery to normal levels of function seen in these studies do not suggest the formation of novel pathways as a mechanism. Rather the recovery in most cases following SI or SII lesions may relate to the maintenance of certain exuberant connections in the somatosensory cortex of the infant macaque in response to perinatal injuries that remove competing connections.

REFERENCES

Carlson M (1981). Characteristics of sensory deficits following lesions of Brodman's areas 1 and 2 in the postcentral gyrus of Macaca mullata. Brain Res 204:424-430.

Carlson M (1984a). Development of tactile discrimination capacity in Macaca mulatta. I. Normal infants. Dev Brain Res 16:69-82.

Carlson M (1984b). Development of tactile discrimination capacity in Macaca mulatta. II. Effects of partial removal of primary somatic sensory cortex (SmI) in infants and juveniles. Dev Brain Res 16:83-101.

Carlson M (1984c). Development of tactile discrimination capacity in Macaca mulatta. III. Effects of total removal of primary somatic sensory cortex (SmI) in infants and juveniles. Dev Brain Res 16:103-117.

Goldman PS (1974). An alternative to developmental plasticity: Heterology of CNS structures in infants and adults. In Stein DG, Rosen JJ, Butters N (eds): "Plasticity and Recovery of Function in the Central Nervous System," New York: Academic Press, pp 149-174.

Kennard M (1942). Cortical reorganization of motor functions: studies on series of monkeys of various ages from infancy to maturity. Arch Neurol and Psychiat 47:227-240.

Murray EA, Mishkin M (1984). Relative contributions of SmII and area 5 to tactile discrimination of monkeys. Behav Brain Res 11:67-84.

Purves D, Lichtman JN (1985). "Principles of Neural Development." Sunderland, MA: Sinauer.

Rakic P, Bourgeois J-P, Eckenhoff F, Zecevic N, Goldman-Rakic PS (1986). Concurrent overproduction of synapses in diverse regions of the primate cerebral cortex. Sci 232:232-235.

Randolph M, Semmes J (1974). Behavioral consequences of selective subtotal ablations in the postcentral gyrus of Macaca mulatta. Brain Res 70:55-70.

Robinson CJ, Burton H (1980). Somatotopographic organization in the second somatosensory area of M. fascicularis. J Comp Neurol 192:43-67.

Semmes J, Porter LA (1972). A comparison of precentral and postcentral cortical lesions on somatosensory discrimination in the monkey. Cortex 8:249-264.

Semmes J, Porter LA, Randolph MC (1974). Further studies of anterior postcentral lesions in monkeys. Cortex 10:55-68.

ACKNOWLEDGMENTS

We thank E. Crader, J. Charlton, J. Hayes, J. Hoffmann, Z. Leventhal, P. Nystrom and G. Perry for their much appreciated technical assitance. Research supported by funds from NIH grants NS09809, NS12090, NS14261, NS15070, and MH14677

Effects of Injury on Trigeminal and Spinal Somatosensory Systems, pages 451–458

SUMMARY AND CRITIQUE

Barry J. Sessle

Faculty of Dentistry, University of Toronto, Toronto, Canada M5G 1G6.

Discussion first centered on specific aspects of each paper presented, and concluded with some more general questions related to mechanisms underlying central neural responses to injury. In the discussion of the papers on primary afferent processes involved in pathophysiological responses to injury in human subjects, questioning focussed initially on nerve blocks used by Meyer et al in their patients. Lynn asked what were the effects of nerve block on experimentally-induced mechanical hyperalgesia. Meyer cited recent studies by Lamotte and his colleagues which had indicated that the mechanical hyperalgesia induced by capsaicin injection into the skin was mediated by C fibres. However, these fibres and the A-delta fibres do not appear to be involved in the hyperalgesia associated with the peripheral nerve injury cases which were reported in the paper by Meyer et al; rather, their data indicate a role for A-beta fibres. In this connection, Perl emphasized the demonstrated existence of some A-beta nociceptive afferents which conceivably could be involved in this hyperalgesia.

Zimmermann questioned the selectivity of the method of ischaemia used by Meyer et al, or indeed of other methods such as local anaesthesia, in blocking different groups of afferent fibres. He cited his own earlier experiments showing that while arterial occlusion disrupts A-fibre low-threshold mechanoreceptors, A-fibre and C-fibre conduction may not be impaired. Torebjork doubted whether this method of arterial occlusion was indeed equivalent to the approach used by Meyer et al, i.e. ischaemia plus cuff compression, and Meyer and Campbell drew attention to their having other independent lines of evidence supporting their conclusions. They also pointed to the extensive data of long standing demonstrating the orderly manner in which sensations are differentially affected by ischaemic block.

Perl also questioned the use of cold sensation as an appropriate marker for A-delta fibre activity. Campbell stated that the cold afferents examined in their animal experiments regularly had a conduction velocity ranging between 5-15 m/sec, but Perl noted that A-delta afferents conducting at speeds greater than this range could have been affected by the ischaemic block and thereby contributed to the loss of mechanical hyperalgesia. Ochoa said that his own studies which used compression-ischaemia in patients with different types of peripheral neural injury, supported the conclusion of Meyer et al that large-diameter afferents are primarily responsible for the hyperalgesia. Nonetheless, he did note that some patients may have hyperalgesia associated with sensitized nociceptors which is C-fibre mediated, yet the post-ischaemic paraesthesia which occurs soon after the block is removed in these patients is large-fibre mediated, but is painless. Meyer noted that in their patients, the post-ischaemic paraesthesia may be painful. suggesting that large fibres are indeed involved.

Lindblom was asked by Wall if in his studies of sensory disturbances in humans after nerve injury, poor localization or referral phenomena were manifested in the fringe surrounding the denervated skin. Lindblom could not give a categorical no, but stated that he was impressed by the distinct border and good localization in skin areas immediately adjacent to the area supplied by the injured nerve.

In response to a question from L. Pubols, Ochoa replied that the unit associated with pain in the patient which he described was also myelinated, but he could not be certain if it was A-delta or A-beta, or indeed if it was not associated only with the 'pins and needles' type of paraesthesia and not with the pain. He pointed out in response to a question from Diamond that the ectopic or 'injury' discharges which he described seem to be much more prevalent in sensory fibres than motor fibres. Schmidt suggested that as far as the site of generation of these ectopic discharges, the discharge pattern seemed similar to that of the so-called dorsal root (or trigeminal tract) reflexes generated in primary afferent endings in the spinal cord (or trigeminal brainstem complex) and conducted antidromically back out along the peripheral nerve fibres. Ochoa cited a recent paper by Nordin et al (1984) which documented antidromically recorded discharges in patients with injuries at a variety of sites and which suggested several possible loci for generation of the ectopic discharges.

Since these antidromically recorded discharges have been linked to the same central mechanisms generating PAD and presynaptic inhibition in the CNS, Sessle turned the discussion briefly to the relatively unexplored area addressed by Hayes et al who had evidence suggesting that these presynaptic regulatory mechanisms in the spinal cord dorsal horn are affected by concussive head injury. Iggo asked how concussion was having its effects, and Hayes replied that the biomechanical features of this type of injury are poorly understood. While brainstem structures appear to be integrally involved, as his paper pointed out, it is uncertain whether these neural effects are due to relatively direct compression of the supraspinal structures, or to compression of neural tissue against skeletal structures or to some other biomechanical factor.

In the papers relating injury to somatosensory afferents and motor behaviour, first Goldberger was asked by Mendell about the level of performance of the movement pattern in the spared-root animal. Goldberger emphasized that the disruption in the pattern which he observed was only temporary and returned to normal levels. In response to a question by Dostrovsky of possible effects on motor performance of the surgery required to effect dorsal root sections, Goldberger indicated that no motor effects were seen in sham-operated controls. Dostrovsky also asked about possible contralateral changes, and Goldberger replied that his data indeed indicated contralateral as well as ipsilateral changes in the motor behaviours. The possibility of contralateral as well as ipsilateral consequences of a unilateral nerve injury or experimentally induced deafferentation was highlighted in other papers at the conference and underscored the caution needed in using the contralateral side as a control in anatomical, electrophysiological or behavioural studies of the effects of injury.

The next few questions were addressed to Vierck and Berkley. Vierck responded to a comment by Kalil about the involvement of the corticospinal system by suggesting that although many of the deficits could be attributed to loss of dorsal column afferent inputs to the motor cortex, dorsal column projections to other regions involved in motor behaviour could not be discounted. It should be noted that the importance of somatosensory inputs and also their loss through injury, has been demonstrated in other behaviours requiring sensorimotor integration, including complex patterned behaviours such as locomotion, mastication and feeding, and that this somatosensory information does not necessarily operate only at the cortical level to influence these behaviours (e.g. see Dubner et al, 1978; Zeigler et al, 1985).

Berkley was then asked by both Goldberger and Dostrovsky if there were any differences in the retrogradely labelled regions of the DCN that might reflect spatial differences between the different types of inputs to DCN. Berkley replied that although dorsal column and corticofugal inputs, for example, are spatially segregated in the cat's DCN, this pattern seems less obvious in the monkey, and in the present study there was no obvious difference in labelling in the rostrocaudal extent of the monkey's DCN after removal of one of these inputs (i.e. dorsal column). She also mentioned, in response to comments by Hand, that it would be interesting to see if the recovery revealed by the retrograde labelling could be prevented if the DCN were deafferented further (e.g. by removing corticofugal or dorsolateral funicular inputs) and that, given the limitations of the HRP methodology employed, she saw no obvious changes in DCN neuronal size as a result of the dorsal column lesion. Ralston questioned her on whether the changes she observed could be attributed to loss of the electrical activity to the DCN from the dorsal columns or to changes in axonal transport and recycling of synaptic vesicle membranes. Berkley could not make this distinction; however, since her observations were obtained with both HRP and wheatgerm HRP which are taken up by different endocytotic processes, she did point out that her data do not favour a change in a specific endocytotic mechanism and cannot rule out the possibility of a change in axonal transport mechanisms.

In commenting on the papers by Vierck et al and Burton et al, Munger reminded the audience of earlier dorsal column lesion studies that had introduced uncertainty about the somatosensory role of the dorsal column-lemniscal system. He highlighted the findings by Vierck and colleagues of sensorimotor deficits following dorsal column lesions which showed clearly the functional importance of this system, and he cited Burton's work as perhaps indicating that texture discrimination is dependent on finely tuned cutaneous afferent information carried in the dorsal columns whereas size discrimination is more dependent on deep inputs e.g. from joints and muscle spindles. Sessle noted that Burton et al had emphasized that cortical regions such as area 3a were spared in their lesion experiments, and so it is not too surprising that they found that sensory functions dependent on deep inputs may be relatively intact since area 3a may be the major receiving area of these inputs. He went on to cite studies of digital and oral sensory capacities for size discrimination which indicated that joint, muscle and perhaps even superficial receptors contribute to size discrimination in humans (e.g. for review, see Dubner et al, 1978; McCloskey, 1978), and Terzis referred to her clinical observations of patients with nerve injuries which indicated that several receptor systems may contribute. With respect to texture discrimination, Torebjork asked Burton which cutaneous receptors were involved in the primate responses to the stimuli used in their study. Burton referred to Johnson's recent work suggesting that SAI, RA (e.g. Meissner) and Pacinian receptors may subserve different spectra of the stimulus, depending on the area being contacted by the cutaneous stimulus (Johnson, 1983). As a consequence, he suggested that all three receptors might contribute to texture discrimination although, in their own primate study, the nature of the stimulus they used probably precluded the use of afferent information from the Pacinians.

Burton responded to a question by Hand on synaptic exuberance by referring to the study (Rakic et al, 1986) cited in their paper. This study had shown that synaptic density peaks around 2-4 months of age and has a similar time frame in all areas of the primate cortex. While this finding might explain the recovered behaviour Burton et al reported in the monkey, both Hand and Burton noted that there may be species differences, and Hand's own rodent data of initial focal metabolic reorganization following deafferentation of vibrissae are more easily explained by mechanisms other than one based on synaptic exuberance.

Prompted also by Juliano's question on the patterns and mechanisms underlying reorganization in the adult cortex, Burton further commented that the papers presented earlier in the meeting suggested to him that a peripheral injury places an onus on central reorganization above and beyond that imposed by a central lesion alone, so that the organizational patterns may not be re-established in the somatosensory cortex. On the basis of Merzenich's earlier studies and other presentations made at this meeting, he was led to suggest that injury to more central somatosensory relay sites (e.g. ventrobasal thalamus or cortex) may result in reorganization that can be explained in terms of existing thalamocortical and intracortical connectivity whereas peripheral lesions may result in abnormal somatosensory representations in the cortex, as studies such as those reported by Wall and Kaas exemplify. Meyers suggested that recovery manifesting somatotopically inappropriate patterns might relate to recent, unpublished studies by Snow who noted that VPL thalamic neurones with a receptive field restricted to one digit could be antidromically excited not only from the SI cortical area of representation of that digit but also from adjacent cortical areas representing other digits. Sessle observed that these data reminded him of studies carried out many years ago which showed that a considerable proportion of VPM or VPL neurons with localized mechanoreceptive fields could be antidromically activated from several cortical sites, not only in SI but also in SII or motor cortex (Rowe and Sessle, 1968; Manson, 1969); at the time this collateralization of thalamocortical axons was considered in the framework of the even earlier concept of "essential" and "sustaining" projections from thalamus to cortex (e.g. Rose and Woolsey 1958; Pubols, 1968), but which now might be re-considered in terms such as 'effective' and 'ineffective' synapses that are currently being bandied about. Killackey referred to some of his recent experiments with Rhoades which also point to a lesion-induced uncovery of existing, perhaps "ineffective" synapses carrying sensory information into the thalamus. Normally, most VPM neurones responding to whisker stimulation in the rat are activated by deflection of a single whisker; however, about 4 weeks after a kainic acid lesion of the V principal nucleus, considered to be the essential brainstem relay of the whisker mechanosensitive information to VPM, most VPM neurones respond to deflection of several whiskers. These VPM neurones thus appear to be showing properties comparable to those of more caudal V brainstem neurones (e.g. in subnucleus interpolaris) which also project to VPM.

Wall closed the discussion by first referring in greater detail to the work of Merzenich et al on effects of a lesion in a digit's representation in cortical area 3b of the adult monkey. He noted that their re-mapping of the lesioned area several months after the lesion revealed a re-emergence of the topographic representation of the digit, and inputs from adjacent digits moved in around the edge of the lesioned representation (Jenkins et al, 1982). Wall suggested that an analgous phenomenon reflecting such apparent exuberance of connections might be occurring in the types of experiments described by Burton et al, with recovery of sensory function after larger somatosensory lesions. Wall suggested mapping within and around the edges of the lesioned areas in these young animals to see if these regions developed abnormal inputs that may reflect over-exuberance of connections that subsequently, with maturation, drop off to 'sharpen-up' the hand representation.

With respect to Burton's comment on the differences between peripheral and central injuries, he agreed that a peripheral lesion could be more devastating as far as central reorganization is concerned since the CNS has no clear 'fix' on how correct the regeneration should be. However he pointed out that some of his own cited observations (e.g. Wall et al, J. Neurosci. 1986) suggest that both central and peripheral factors are involved in reorganization following peripheral nerve lesions. After a peripheral nerve cut and repair, the reestablished patterns in areas 3b and 1 may be different, despite the fact that the peripheral injury is common as far as both cortical areas are concerned.

In summary, the series of papers presented in this session and the ensuing discussion have given us important information on the features and mechanisms underlying the pathophysiological and behavioural consequences of injury to the somatosensory systems. Clearly the consequences of the injury and the processes involved in the recovery from injury may vary, depending on factors related to the site of the injury (i.e. peripheral or central), maturational age of the organism at the time of the injury, time for recovery, species, etc. Such a large number of factors may explain in part not only the differences in results that are sometimes generated from different laboratories, but also the variable and often unpredictable or even bizarre features of recovery which are seen clinically following somatosensory injury in humans. The provision of further insights into these mechanisms and factors represents a particular challenge for the neuroscientist interested in this area. In addition, since chronic pain may be a consequence of injury to the somatosensory systems, a greater emphasis in these future research endeavours should be given to the features and mechanisms of recovery in nociceptive pathways since most of the studies to date, at least in animals, have focussed on the effects of injury on non-nociceptive somatosensory functions. Furthermore, appropriately designed and experimentally controlled studies in humans must also be emphasized, given the valuable insights that are accumulating from clinical research approaches utilizing single unit recordings in humans and from the correlation of data obtained in psychophysical studies of humans with findings provided through related experiments in animals.

REFERENCES

Dubner R, Sessle BJ, Storey AT (1978). "The Neural Basis of of Oral and Facial Function." New York: Liss.

Jenkins WA, Merzenich MM, Zook JM, Fowler BC, Stryker MP (1982). The area 3b representation of the hand in oral monkeys reorganizes after induction of restricted cortical lesions. Neurosci Abstracts 8:141.

Johnson KO (1983). Neural mechanisms of tactile form and texture discrimination. Fed Proc 42:2542-2547.

Manson J (1969). The somatosensory cortical projection of single nerve cells in the thalamus of the cat. Brain Res 12:489-492.

McCloskey DI (1978). Kinesthetic sensibility. Physiol. Rev 58:763-820.

Pubols B (1968). Retrograde degeneration study of somatic sensory thalamocortical connections in brain of Virginia opossum. Brain Res 7:232-251.

Rose JE, Woolsey CN (1958). Cortical connections and functional organization of the thalamic auditory system of the cat. In Harlow HF, Woolsey CN (eds): "Biological and Biochemical Basis of Behavior," Madison: Univ Wisconsin.

Rowe MJ, Sessle BJ (1968). Somatic afferent input to posterior thalamic neurones and their axon projection to the cerebral cortex. J Physiol (London) 196:19-35.

Zeigler HP, Jacquin M. Miller MG (1985). The trigeminal system and ingestive behavior in the rat. Prog Psychobiol Psychol 11:63-196.

V
WORKSHOP SUMMARIES

Effects of Injury on Trigeminal and Spinal Somatosensory Systems, pages 461–465

WORKSHOP SUMMARY: MECHANISMS OF PLASTICITY

Paul B. Brown

Physiology Department
West Virginia University
Morgantown, WV 26506, U.S.A.

The workshop on mechanisms of plasticity consisted of four invited presentations and general discussion. The four presentations were:

M. Murray: collateral sprouting
M. Devor: unmasking of synapses
L. Mendell: postsynaptic consequences of plastic changes
J. Haring: transmitter changes

Dr. Murray divided responses to CNS damage into three categories: regeneration, pruning and collateral (or terminal) sprouting.

Regeneration, or the regrowth of severed axons, is rare in the adult mammalian CNS. Pruning refers to growth of spared collaterals of axons in which other collaterals have been cut. Regeneration and sprouting of the pruning type are both elicited by direct damage to the neuron and in both cases, growth may be demonstrable at some distance from the site of the lesion.

Collateral sprouting is the growth of intact axons, or terminals, in response to partial denervation of the postsynaptic target. The pioneering studies on dorsal root sprouting in cat spinal cord demonstrated an increased density but also a more extensive projection of the sprouting dorsal root. The latter was presumably related to the use of Nauta-Laidlaw degeneration staining which may have suppressed a small projection of the intact root (Liu and Chambers 1957). More recent studies (Goldberger and Murray, 1978, 1982) using less suppressive degeneration stains replicated the finding of increased density but not the more extensive projection of the sprouting dorsal root. Thus, sprouting in the adult CNS is local; additional connections are established within the normal projection zone of the sprouting axons. Therefore, no new projections are established. EM evidence has suggested that sprouting may act to conserve the normal density of innervation of the denervated target.

Both light and electron microscopic methods have been used to demonstrate sprouting. Light microscopic methods depend on demonstration of an increase in density of an existing projection while electron microscopic methods can be used to demonstrate directly a replacement of synaptic contacts by sprouting systems.

Although sprouting has been observed in many places in the CNS, in axons of different diameters, and in axons with different transmitters, it has been more readily demonstrated in small diameter axon systems with widespread terminal arborization. There are now several examples of a hierarchy of preferred candidates for sprouting in a specific target region. Surprisingly, there are now more examples of heterotypic than homotypic sprouting. the time course of reinnervation by collateral sprouts is highly variable, ranging from replacement contemporaneous with degeneration to replacement after delays of several weeks or months.

Dr. Murray concluded her presentation with the question of whether strengthening of latent or silent connections and sprouting are different phenomena or different manifestations of the same phenomenon.

Dr. Devor began his presentation by pointing out that the closure of gaps in central representations of the peripheral sensory sheet is ubiquitous. For me, this brought to mind the experience of stroke patients who may lose large parts of their visual fields with no awareness of gaps. In the dorsal horn, the invasion of the medial, or foot representation, region by fibers normally projecting to the lateral, or leg representation, region has been reported by several investigators and several other investigators have failed to replicate this result. He suggested that one reason for this discrepancy might lie in the fact that cells like the spinocervical tract neurons studied in some laboratories might be the least likely to show alterations of somatotopy due to their relative lack of subliminal fringes or changes of receptive field size when descending inhibition is removed.

As for the signal which elicits unmasking, there are several logical candidates, but each has arguments against it. Degeneration of severed axons is unlikely, because cutting a peripheral nerve may not cause degeneration even though reorganization takes place, and shifts of somatotopy have been reported at times before any degeneration can occur; and because after cutting a peripheral nerve, the old synapses can be demonstrated still to be effective. The loss of input activity appears not to be the signal which evokes unmasking, because tetrodotoxin cuffs applied to peripheral nerves do not cause reorganization. Colchicine experiments indicate that there may be some trophic effect mediated by axonal transport of substances from the periphery.

Dr. Devor, like Dr. Murray, made the distinction between local and long-distance sprouting. He argued that there is no evidence for sprouting of terminals outside their normal termination zones, or for long dendritic sprouts, but that many dorsal horn cells have a more widespread distribution of dendrites than would be expected from their receptive field geometries: Perhaps normally ineffective, somatotopically inappropriate synapses are present on the far-lateral dendrites of medial cells.

Thigh fibers often enter the dorsal horn via its medial aspect, sweeping laterally to arborize and terminate in the lateral dorsal horn. Dr. Devor examined the medial dorsal horn for HRP-labeled axons and terminals of thigh axons loaded from the posterior femoral cutaneous nerve, and displayed electron micrographs of several such HRP-labeled profiles.

In his conclusion, Dr. Devor suggested that it may be an error to consider only two candidate mechanisms for plasticity, sprouting and unmasking. He presented twelve examples of other possible mechanisms, suggesting that these are only a few of the many possibilities.

Dr. Mendell considered both known postsynaptic effects of partial deafferentation in spinocervical tract cells, as well as effects which have been observed in other systems and which might occur in the somatosensory system. His own computer reconstruction studies of a small number of cells have shown that SCT neurons' dendritic trees show little change in dendritic length, but their diameters increase, resulting in an increased surface area and volume.

Studies of the motoneuron-neuromuscular junction system were cited which indicate that changes in the size of the terminal distribution can result in a change in the quantal content of synapses. In cases of sprouting, the quantal content can be lower than normal not only at the sprouted synapses, but at the normally present ones as well. This might indicate a tendency to conserve total presynaptic quantal content. For studies of plasticity such studies indicate that elevated levels of transmission may not necessarily be a consequence of sprouting.

I find it interesting that there is evidence for preservation of both synaptic inputs to postsynaptic cells and synaptic output from presynaptic cells. In computer studies of simulated neuronal networks with modifiable synapses, modellers generally have to incorporate such conservation rules in order to obtain stable, adaptive behavior.

In the Ia-motoneuron system, the size of EPSP measured during low frequency stimulation is not a measure of synaptic efficacy under all conditions. When presynaptic trains are evoked to simulate normal bursts of activity, some connections show a gradual decrease in the peak amplitude of EPSPs, and others show a gradual increase. Generally, larger EPSPs appear to depress in amplitude, and smaller ones facilitate. Thus large-amplitude EPSPs may not provide more summation than smaller-amplitude ones, particularly if the larger EPSPs have shorter durations. Adjustments that alter EPSP shapes and amplitude following deafferentation might have surprisingly large effects on synaptic efficacy.

Introducing his presentation, Dr. Haring pointed out that for historical reasons, most studies of transmitter changes have been done in monoamine systems. Some of these do grow new collaterals of substantial length. After cutting the peripheral processes of dorsal root ganglion cells which produce a particular transmitter, there is normally a decrease of central concentration of that transmitter, which may or may not be followed by recovery to a normal level. One exception is vasoactive intestinal peptide (VIP), which increases in central levels as soon as the peripheral processes are cut. Dr. Haring pointed out that many studies are too short (a month or less) for us to be certain that the full time course of changes has been described; also, the use of colchicine may produce artifactual results. For a full appreciation of changes of central levels of polypeptides, it may be necessary to supplement immunohistochemical methods with other techniques, such as complementary DNA methods.

Transmitters may interact: several examples of serotonin-substance P interactions were presented. In most but not all cases, a change in level of one, regardless of its cause, resulted in a reciprocal change of the other.

The general discussion following the four presentations was lively, concentrating mostly on the issue of whether somatotopic reorganization in the dorsal horn occurs. Briefly, some discussants believed that the evidence for such reorganization was amenable to alternative interpretations, such as simple loss of input; recording from different populations of cells in control and experimental dorsal horns; or stimulating different receptor populations, such as deep receptors, in the experimental dorsal horns. Those who had had positive results suggested that others had studied inappropriate cell groups or had suppressed changes by use of inappropriate anesthesia or by not eliminating descending inhibition.

Dr. Iggo endorsed the collaboration of scientists with differing views in experiments directed at resolving such differences, and suggested that we concentrate on monosynaptic effects, which are better-defined and easier to study.

Dr. Pomeranz invited the participants to use his preparation to investigate reorganization in the dorsal horn: the use of a spared saphenous nerve preparation, in which he has observed reorganization over several segments in a repeatable fashion.

In conclusion, it was clear to me that the level of consensus generally required for acceptance of a phenomenon by the scientific community at large is not yet achieved with regard to reorganization of dorsal horn somatotopy. We are more likely to achieve such consensus one way or the other by further collaborative studies and by careful redesign of experimental methods to eliminate alternative interpretations, control for artifacts, and produce robust, reproducible results. Then, as we reach the point where mechanisms can be studied, the existence of the phenomenon of somatotopic reorganization will no longer be in doubt.

Effects of Injury on Trigeminal and Spinal Somatosensory Systems,
pages 467–473

Workshop: New Methodologies/Future Directions

Chaired and Summarized by Alan R. Light

Department of Physiology, University of North Carolina at Chapel Hill, Chapel Hill, North Carolina 27514

Introduction

The purpose of this workshop was to allow individuals to share new technologies which they had developed or had adapted, and to speculate on the use of these technologies in the future study of injury in somatosensory systems.

The workshop was informal in nature. Three scientists were asked to present new techniques and were limited to 20 minutes each. Participation by the audience was encouraged with presentations limited to 5 minutes each. As the summary indicates, most of the techniques in fact were not new but rather represented new and unique applications of older methodologies. In the following summary of the presentations no attempt is made to report all the suggestions which came from the audience. In those instances, however, where questions raised important issues or changed the interpretation of the presentor, they are indicated.

Proceedings

Dr. Ochoa and Dr. Cline described the use of microneurography (percutaneous recording of single primary afferent units in humans) to determine the mechanisms which cause hyperalgesia.

They presented a patient with reflex sympathetic dystrophy of the arm which developed following repeated sunburn and a rash. Hyperalgesia was present in the distribution of the radial nerve.

Microneurography demonstrated that the C-polymodal

primary afferents in this patient had highly unusual response properties. They responded not only to noxious heat and noxious mechanical stimuli, but also to normally innocuous stimuli such as stroking the skin with a cotton wisp. These units often demonstrated a prolonged discharge to light stroking of the skin.

Dr. Torebjork also assisted in testing units in this patient and observed units with these same properties. C-polymodal units with these unusual properties have not been observed in normal human subjects.

Drs. Ochoa and Cline demonstrated that the response characteristics of these abnormal C-polymodal units corresponded to the intensity and duration of pain which the patient experienced. They also provided additional evidence that this patient's hyperalgesia was mediated by C fibers in that: 1) heat-pain and mechanical-pain were both hyperalgesic; 2) blocking the superficial radial nerve abolished pain; 3) ischemic block of the arm resulted in persistence of hyperalgesic pain at a time when the A fibers had been totally blocked.

There was some discussion by Dr. Terzis as to whether the patient should have been diagnosed as sympathetic dystrophic. Dr. Ochoa agreed that this patient was probably not a typical case of reflex sympathetic dystrophy. Dr. Schmidt expressed reservations with the correlation between C-polymodal discharge and the patient's pain ratings, stating that the onset latency of the pain rating appeared to occur too rapidly to have been caused by C-fiber activity. General discussion by the audience and Dr. Ochoa led to the conclusion that the latencies were not in mismatch, but that it was difficult to discern from the presented slide whether a mismatch was present. However, other data indicated that the hyperalgesia was definitely mediated by C-fibers.

Dr. Ochoa's and Dr. Cline's presentation demonstrates that microneurography can be used in cases of clinical hyperalgesia and has several implications:

1) This technique can be used to distinguish peripheral from central hyperalgesias;

2) This technique may lead to a better understanding of receptor alterations in clinical hyperalgesia.

Dr. Perl presented two new methodologies which can be used to determine the chemical profiles of dorsal root ganglion cells whose somatosensory receptor has been physiologically characterized. The first technique involved using monoclonal antibodies which recognize cell surface antigens of particular groups of dorsal root ganglion cells. The monoclonal antibodies had been characterized by Jessell and Dodd and had been shown to mark certain groups of dorsal root ganglion cells in vitro. Dr. Perl demonstrated that these antibodies (SSEA-3 and SSEA-4), which are stage specific embryonic antibodies, could be used to label physiologically identified dorsal root ganglion cells. The cells were identified in vivo in the guinea pig by intracellular recording, marked with Lucifer Yellow, and then removed for immunocytochemistry. He showed that SSEA-3 marked D-hair and some Field dorsal root ganglion cells, but did not mark deep receptor dorsal root ganglion cells. He also showed that both SSEA-3 and SSEA-4 marked High Threshold Mechanoreceptor dorsal root ganglion cells.

This technique should prove useful when used in conjunction with other techniques which identify the putative neurotransmitters associated with SSEA-3 and SSEA-4.

The second technique presented by Dr. Perl was the use of C-DNA probes to label specific messenger RNA's in dorsal root ganglion cells. He used partial sequence oligomers of synthesized C-DNA's (derived by using published sequences of particular C-DNA's for peptides) to label mRNA's for somatostatin and CCK-8. To do this he used P^{32}-labeled C-DNA's and in situ hybridization in fixed tissue from rat dorsal root ganglia. He demonstrated selective labeling of dorsal root ganglion cells with the C-DNA probe for somatostatin, but considerable background when the probe for CCK-8 was used.

The implications of this technique are:

1) It should be possible to use situ hybridization concomitantly with intracellular labels so that mRNA's of physiologically identified dorsal root ganglion cells (or any neuron) should be determinable.

2) the technique is theoretically quantitative so that the amount of a specific mRNA in a particular cell (and therefore the amount of protein synthesized) may be determinable

3) this technique could be used in the future to look at changes in transcription of mRNA which could occur due to injury of neural tissue.

Dr. Pechanski described the technique of intracerebral grafting of embryonic neural tissue into adult CNS. He reminded us that this technique was not new (see Bjorkland et al for references). However, he was using it in a novel way: to determine whether somatosensory afferent fibers deprived of their target neurons would establish contacts with embryonic neural tissue implanted in the correct locations.

He used kainic acid to kill neurons of the ventrobasal thalamus in adult rats. He showed that point-to-point afferent fibers from the dorsal column nuclei and somatosensory cortex persisted in the region which had been VB following complete loss of their target cells in the VB thalamus. He then injected a suspension of $[H^3]$thymidine labeled embryonic neurons from the fetal VB region into the lesioned region of the adult VB with a Hamilton syringe under stereotaxic control. After allowing time for the neurons to mature, he demonstrated that diffuse monoaminergic afferents invaded the graft. He also showed that some point-to-point afferent fibers from the dorsal column nuclei and more fibers from the cerebral cortex invaded the grafted neurons. Synaptic contacts were established on graft neurons but he did not quantitate the number from point-to-point systems. He also demonstrated that axons from the graft grew into the cerebral cortex. However, the normal reciprocal organization was not re-established in that the afferent projections from the cortex did not grow to the VB neurons which projected their axons to the cortex.

The implications of this technique are:

1) Point-to-point neural afferent systems have the capability of re-establishing connections with neural grafts.
2) These grafts may also establish axonal connections with appropriate host regions.
3) This technique may enable the assessment of the potential plasticity of adult central nervous system tissue
4) Conceivably, with better understanding, embryonic neural grafts ultimately might be useful for the treatment of central nervous system damage in humans.

Dr. Csillik demonstrated the use of enzymatic markers for selective groups of dorsal root ganglion cells and their projections into the spinal cord. The first marker was TRPase which can be used to make a dark reaction product which marks only one population of small dorsal root ganglion cells in the rat. This marker is easily visible with the light microscope and is found in the Golgi apparatus and endoplasmic reticulum by electron microscopy. When viewed with the light microscope it also labels nerve terminals in the substantia gelatinosa in the spinal cord and labels afferent termination regions in the medulla. Dr. Csillik speculates that this marker may be specific for nociceptive neurons.

The second marker that he demonstrated was a lectin Ulex Europaeus-I which binds to fucose epitopes and also marks a population of small dorsal root ganglion cells. This marker also labels terminations in the substantia gelatinosa of the spinal cord not only in the rat, but also in human spinal cord tissue. The marker in the substantia gelatinosa disapears after dorsal root section, indicating its origin in the dorsal root gangia.

Dr. Csillik suggested that these two markers could be used to assess the injury or regeneration of nociceptive afferents in the spinal cord. However, since both of these markers labeled the inner substantia gelatinosa much better than the outer substantia gelatinosa it seems that the labeled terminations are primarily not nociceptive because nociceptive primary afferents end primarily in the marginal zone and outer substantia gelatinosa.

Dr. Apkarian presented the use of a cold block technique introduced by Salsbury and Hall to block conduction in the spinal cord. This technique utilizes 23 gauge syringe tubing through which is circulated cold methanol at $0^{o}C$. He presented evidence that when these cold probes were placed on the dorsal columns conduction from the spinal cord to the dorsal column nuclei was blocked reversibly. The technique could be repeated multiple times. Dr. Schmidt asked if the block could be made to be complete. Dr. Apkarian's answered "sometimes". The implications are that this cold-block technique can be used to determine the tracts which contain the axons of various ascending and descending systems.

Dr. Hand presented a technique by which local blood flow and metabolic labeling could be performed and distinguished in the same brain. To do this he injected C^{14} labeled 2-deoxyglucose to rats exposed to a controlled somatic stimulus, such as stroking one skin area, and I^{123} labeled antipyrine given before somatosensory stimulation of another skin region. The brain subsequently is removed and frozen and autoradiography is done. Since the labels are of two energies and different half lives, they can be demonstrated selectively in different autoradiograms. Dr. Hand demonstrated that the antipyrine label (which measures blood flow quantitatively) was found in exactly the same location in the cortex as the 2-deoxyglucose label (which labels metabolic activity quantitatively) following stimulation applied to a single whisker in a rat.

The implications of this technique are that the labeling produced by two different stimuli (differing in location or modality) can be demonstrated in the same animal, allowing direct comparisons to be made. The most serious problem with the technique is the need for very rapid removal and freezing of the brain. He also noted that I^{123} should be handled with caution because of its affinity for the thyroid.

Dr. Koerber demonstrated the technique of stimulating single dorsal root ganglion cells in vivo and recording the resulting field potentials in the spinal cord by using averaging techniques. This technique demonstrated that the spinal cord potential evoked by stimulating a single low-threshold dorsal root ganglion cell was decreased by a preceding stimulus of the same cell. However, when a single spike was induced in a myelinated nociceptor (high threshold mechanoreceptor) dorsal root ganglion cell, a preceding spike in the same cell actually enhanced the potential. Dr. Koerber also demonstrated the technique of stimulating a single nociceptive dorsal root ganglion cell and recording extracellulary and intracellularly in a lamina I and lamina V cell. He demonstrated that a single spike in a nociceptive primary afferent produced EPSP's in lamina I and V cells, but that 2 closely timed spikes were usually necessary to evoke a discharge in the lamina I and V cells.

This technique can be used to show how specific primary afferent inputs are processed by specific neurons in the dorsal horn. Thus, alterations in the normal pattern following injury can be assessed.

Dr. Kruger demonstrated the use of an antibody to calcitonin gene-related peptide (ACGRP) to label presumed nociceptive nerve terminals using immunocytochemistry. He showed examples of terminal labeling both in the periphery and in the central nervous system. He pointed out that pathways other than nociceptive pathways were also labeled in some brain locations. He demonstrated that this antibody labeled over 50% of the dorsal root ganglion cells and that colchicine was not required for labeling. Both cells with unmyelinated and cells with fine myelinated axons were labeled. Dr. Kruger showed that the technique worked on decalcified tissue and could be carried to the electron microscopic level. He demonstrated nerve endings in periosteum, mesenteric whole mounts, teeth, tympanic membrane, skin, and cornea.

Dr. Burton remarked that very few terminals were labeled in the cornea when many should be labeled. Dr. Kruger answered that possibly most terminals in the cornea don't have CGRP antigen.

The implications of this technique are that it can be used to label, in a Golgi-like fashion, the nerve terminals of large numbers of nociceptors in both the periphery and central nervous system. These terminals can be examined with both the light and electron microscopes. Thus, this technique could be used to assay changes in these endings following injury.

Dr. Rassmusen demonstrated the use of specific receptor binding techniques to assay changes in receptor binding following injury. He used tritiated QNP to demonstrate that glutamate receptors were up-regulated in a particular region of the raccoon cortex following amputation of a digit. However, he has not been able to replicate this observation, presumably for technical reasons.

VI
POSTER ABSTRACTS

Effects of Injury on Trigeminal and Spinal Somatosensory Systems, page 477

RESPONSE OF SKIN NERVES TO NOXIOUS STIMULI: ELECTRICALLY EVOKED AXON REFLEX FLARE IN MAN.

R.A. Westerman*, W. Magerl, J. Szolcsanyi, H. Handwerker, A. Low*, A. Pratt*, R. Widdop**.

II Physiological Institute, University of Heidelberg, & *Physiology Department, & **Pharmacology Department, Monash University.

Direct stimulation of intact forearm skin affects adjacent microvascular blood flux. Current pulses, effective in activating C-fibres, were applied over a period of 1-16s at 2 Hz using transcutaneous stimulation. An increase in skin microvascular blood flux up to 50% was observed. The increased blood flux correlated well with increasingly painful sensations. Some subjects responded to one or two pulses at 2 Hz, 0.5ms duration and 150 V. Response onset latency of 4-15s, lasting up to 5 min was recorded. At higher frequency (4-8 Hz) and total stimulus pulses (16-32) vasoconstriction was often observed just preceding the usual flux increase. After administration of local anaesthetic (2% lignocaine) the skin resting blood flux increased, but electrical stimulation still produced vasodilatation. The local cutaneous flare response to electrical stimulation was abolished or greatly reduced by capsaicin pretreatment. Excitation of small intracutaneous forearm nerve C-fibres produces increased microvascular blood flux which is dependent on local release of vasodilator substances. The neurogenic flare (axon reflex) may have a physiological role in regulating skin microvascular blood flow, and nociceptor function may be measured by applying the above mentioned transcutaneous electrical stimulation.

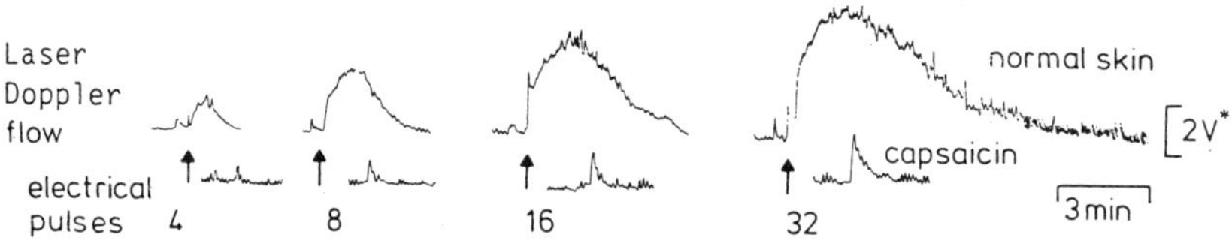

Effects of Injury on Trigeminal and Spinal Somatosensory Systems, page 479

THE IMPACT OF ABNORMAL INNERVATION ON THE DIFFERENTIATION OF THE PELAGE

Terrell E. Jones and Bryce L. Munger

Department of Anatomy, The Pennsylvania State University College of Medicine, Hershey, Pennsylvania 17033

The present study has focused on the impact of altered cutaneous sensory innervation on the development of hairs. We have found that hair growth is abnormal, both precocious and retarded, in the skin associated with lesions involving cutaneous afferent nerves. Normal development of peripheral cutaneous derivatives such as the sequencing of hair growth is altered following disruption of the pattern of normal innervation. Postoperative responses of the pelage covering lumbar spinal cord were evaluated following surgical deletion of associated segments of spinal cord and dorsal root ganglia in the neonate opossum (Monodelphis domesticus) pup. Eight days following the operative procedure abnormal hairs developed in the region of the lesion. The abnormal hairs corresponded to developmental stages seen only in twelve or thirteen day sham and normal animals. In other areas of skin devoid of sensory nerves, hairs failed to develop in a normal sequence. An abnormally dense invasion of neural elements into the area of skin above a neural lesion has previously been reported (Jones and Munger, 1966, Anat. Rec., 214(3):62A). Our results indicate that the normal development of skin and its derivatives are dependent on normal development of their associated afferent innervation.
Supported in part by USPHS grant NS19462.

Effects of Injury on Trigeminal and Spinal Somatosensory Systems, page 481

FREEZE FRACTURE ASPECTS OF SENSORY TERMINAL MEMBRANE IN THE FROG MUSCLE SPINDLE AFTER DENERVATION

N. Fujitsuka and F. Ito

Department of Physiology, Nagoya University
School of Medicine
Nagoya 466, Japan.

The size and population density of intramembrane particles in the non-myelinated sensory nerve terminals of frog muscle spindle were studied in comparison with changes in discharge patterns from the sensory terminals during stretch 1 - 28 days after denervation. The sciatic nerve in the right leg was cut at the dorsal part of hip joint. Spindle receptors in the left leg were used as a control. Muscle spindles were isolated from semitendinosus and iliofibularis muscles. The mean density of particles, which occurred mainly on the protoplasmic (P) face, declined rapidly to 60 % of the control values 2 days after denervation, 30 % after 4 days and to less than 10 % 7 days. The mean diameter of particles changed from 8.0 + 1.5 nm in the control to 12.8 + 2.5 nm 7 days after denervation. No significant difference between the results for the trunks (>2 μm in diameter) and the branches (<0.5 μm) of the non-myelinated axon was observed. The peak rate of afferent discharges during a ramp-and-hold stretch survived up to 4 days after denervation, whereas the static component disappeared after 3 days. It is suggested that the decline to less than 20 % of the control density of particles removes the mechanosensitivity of the sensory endings.

Effects of Injury on Trigeminal and Spinal Somatosensory Systems, page 483

DYNAMIC AND STATIC RESPONSIVENESS OF SAI RECEPTORS IN HYPOTHYROID RATS

M.S. Leung

Department of Physiology, Faculty of Medicine,
The Chinese University of Hong Kong,
Shatin, New Territories, Hong Kong.

It has previously been shown that the responsiveness of slowly adapting type I cutaneous mechanorecetor (s.a.I) in the rat is reduced by 10-15% in the hypothyroid (HT) state. The present analysis differentiates between interspike time intervals during dynamic & static phases in nervous responses during mechanical stimulation of s.a.I receptors in HT & control rats. After weaning, HT rats were given 0.5% (w/v) Methimazole in drinking water (ad lib.) for 3 months. Treated rats showed a slower growth rate. After 3 months of treatment, single unit recordings were made from afferent nerve fibres supplying s.a.I receptors in the gluteal skin. Mechanical stimuli with constant force of 20 mN were applied through a nylon probe (spherical tip, 1 mm). Individual stimuli rose over 0.2s (dynamic phase) to a force of 20 mN and were kept constant at this level for 2s (plateau phase). Interspike interval histograms for the dynamic phase were similar for both groups of rats with the highest incidence in the class of 4 ms. The median was in 5 ms & 4 ms class for the HT & controls rats, but the 90% percentile was in the 10 ms & 8 ms class for the HT & the control rats respectively. During the last second of the plateau phase (1.2-2.2s of the stimulus), the median was in 8 & 9 ms class for the HT & controls but the 90% percentile was in the 23 ms & 20 ms class for the HT & the control rats. Interspike intervals during both dynamic and static phases were affected almost to the same extent.

Effects of Injury on Trigeminal and Spinal Somatosensory Systems, page 485

CHRONIC PAIN FROM THE PERIPHERY: THE ROLE OF NEUROMAS

Lisa C. Russell and Kim J. Burchiel

Veterans' Administration Medical Center
Seattle, Washington 98108

Ectopic activity from a neuroma may not be the primary cause of chronic pain of peripheral origin. We have modified the microfilament recording technique such that averaged signals from 2 recording sites are used to determine the origins of spontaneous impulses and conduction velocities. In 32 Sprague-Dawley rats the saphenous nerve was sectioned in the distal thigh and in 7-10 days, recordings were made in the nerve. Most spontaneous discharges originated in potentially nociceptive fibers ($p<0.001$, $t=4.24$, $df=62$). In these rats, we recorded spontaneously active C-fibers from fascia ($n=3$, $cv=0.82 \pm 0.67$ m/s), blood vessels ($n=2$, $cv=0.93 \pm 0.33$ m/s), and skin ($n=2$, $cv=1.93 \pm 0.03$ m/s). In a second group of 28 rats without prior saphenous section we found C-fiber discharges from hairy skin ($n=9$, $cv=1.01 \pm 0.24$ m/s), glabrous skin ($n=7$, $cv=1.04 \pm 0.24$ m/s), and joints ($n=2$, $cv=1.28 \pm 0.46$ m/s), but no spontaneously active C-fibers from neuromas. Analysis of data from rat saphenous neuromas ($n=23$) recorded before and after gallamine produced a 1275% increase in the incidence of spontaneously active axons. Conclusions: (1) Neuromas not exposed to potassium channel-blocking agents manifested minimal spontaneous electrical activity, (2) A-delta and C-fiber activity recorded in saphenous neuroma preparations are derived form vascular, fascial and other receptive fields, and (3) these data are consistent with clinical observations that neuromas are usually not spontaneously painful.

Effects of Injury on Trigeminal and Spinal Somatosensory Systems, page 487

MORPHOLOGICAL BASIS FOR 'EPHAPTIC' EXCITATION IN NEUROMA NERVES

Christiane Vahle-Hinz, Kay-Michael Gottschaldt† and Harald Kräft

Physiologisches Institut der Universität, D-8700 Würzburg, and MPI für Biophysikalische Chemie, D-3400 Göttingen, FRG

Afferent activity can be elicited by antidromic stimulation of neuroma nerves in 25% of the fibers (Blumberg & Jänig, Exp. Neurol., 1982). This phenomenon could be due to ephaptic coupling within the neuroma or to retrograde axon sprouting. To test the latter hypothesis, fiber counts and morphometric measurements at regular intervals along the superficial peroneal nerves of cats were compared from normal nerves, neuroma nerves, and neuroma nerves cut several days prior to fixation at the proximal end of the neuroma. Cutting a neuroma nerve should result in a marked anterograde degeneration of retrogradely sprouting axons all along the nerve, if present.

The data show that the number of myelinated and unmyelinated fibers increases from proximal to distal in the neuroma nerves, while their axon diameter decreases in the same direction. This indicates that the fibers branch along the nerve and grow towards the neuroma. In cut neuroma nerves the degeneration of unmyelinated fibers is confined to the distal parts of the nerve stump. Thus, the morphometric analysis showed that retrograde axon sprouting over long distances is not prominent in neuroma nerves. Close appositions of axon profiles were found inside the neuromas as well as in the neuroma nerves, which may be the areas of electrical coupling between different fibers. Afferent activity after antidromic stimulation in neuroma nerves therefore seems to have its source in ephaptic excitation of the fibers via the axon appositions.

Supported by SFB 33 of the Deutsche Forschungsgemeinschaft.

Effects of Injury on Trigeminal and Spinal Somatosensory Systems, page 489

A PERIPHERAL STIMULUS INITIATES THE COLLATERAL REINNERVATION OF CAT TEETH

Peter P. Robinson

Department of Physiology, The Medical School, University of Birmingham, Birmingham B15 2TJ

Experiments in adult cats have shown that when the inferior alveolar nerve is sectioned and regeneration prevented, the denervated teeth receive a collateral reinnervation from neighbouring ipsilateral and contralateral nerves. The stimulus which initiates collateral reinnervation from sensory nerves is not known and may be located either peripherally or centrally. The present experiments have investigated whether removing the central terminals of a nerve prevents its peripheral branches from sprouting to form a collateral reinnervation.

In four anaesthetized cats a left trigeminal rhizotomy was carried out and the right inferior alveolar nerve was sectioned and regeneration prevented. Twelve weeks later electrophysiological recordings were made to determine the sources of innervation of the lower canine and incisor teeth. These recordings revealed an extensive collateral reinnervation of the teeth on the right side from nerves on both the ipsilateral and contralateral sides. The left inferior alveolar, lingual and mylohyoid nerves contained fibres supply the pulps of teeth on the right side, significantly more than have been found in normal animals. As rhizotomy did not prevent the development of this transmedian collateral reinnervation it appears that central terminals are not essential for this nerve to respond to the stimulus which initiates sprouting. This suggests that the stimulus must be located peripherally.

Supported by the MRC (U.K.).

Effects of Injury on Trigeminal and Spinal Somatosensory Systems, page 491

PERIPHERAL FACTORS EFFECTING THE CODING OF TACTILE INFORMATION AFTER CUTANEOUS REINNERVATION

B.G. Turnbull and J.K. Terzis

Department of Physiology & Biophysics
Dalhousie University, Halifax, NS and the
Microsurgical Research Centre, Eastern
Virginia Medical School, Norfolk, VA

Cutaneous reinnervation was studied in the hairy skin of the rabbit ear using single fibre and whole fascicle recordings of the greater auricular (GA) nerve. The detailed examination of single fibre receptive fields (RFs) showed that: 1) the number of receptors reinnervated by single fibres was chronically reduced to half the number innervated by normal fibres (up to 20 months post-op); 2) the spatial organization of reinnervated receptors was more scattered and diffuse; and 3) single fibres could reinnervate 2 or more areas of skin (multiple RFs). The responses of fibres to high frequency stimulation with vibrating tuning forks was diminished. However, stimulation of hair follicles with an electromechanical stimulator showed receptor function to be nearly normal. The spatial distribution of mechanosensory fibres to the skin was also examined using whole fascicle recordings. Following cutaneous reinnervation, the spatial patterns of fascicular RFs were grossly altered: 1) the skin area served by each fascicle was markedly enlarged; 2) the topographic relationship between the fascicle location and the area of skin served was lost; 3) the normal pattern of innervation density was lost, and replaced with an irregular and patchy pattern of innervation.

Effects of Injury on Trigeminal and Spinal Somatosensory Systems, page 493

CHANGES IN AXONAL COUNTS PROXIMAL TO LESIONS OF THE INFERIOR ALVEOLAR NERVE IN THE CAT

G.R. Holland and P.P. Robinson*

University of Alberta, Edmonton, Alberta, Canada, *University of Birmingham, U.K.

Damage to peripheral branches of the trigeminal nerve results in central changes which have been observed in the trigeminal ganglion and brainstem. The severity of these central changes is probably related to the nature, extent and position of the nerve lesion and may also be reflected by changes in the peripheral nerve proximal to the injury. There is little information on the changes occurring in the nerve trunk proximal to peripheral nerve lesions in adult animals. The present study has been carried out to determine the effect of various types of inferior alveolar nerve injury on the number of myelinated and non-myelinated fibres proximal to the lesion.

In 12 adult cats the inferior alveolar nerve was either; sectioned and reapposed, sectioned and regeneration impeded by covering the central stump with acrylic, or sectioned and regeneration prevented by sealing the central stump inside a nylon tube. Counts of myelinated and non-myelinated axons were made from the proximal stump of operated nerves and compared with counts from unoperated controls.

After reapposition, counts central to the section were similar to those of controls. Impeding regeneration resulted in a loss of non-myelinated fibres, whereas preventing regeneration caused an increase in axonal numbers similar to that found in a neuroma.

Changes in the axon population in the proximal stump are clearly related to the type of nerve lesion.

Supported by the Alberta Heritage Foundation for Medical Research, M.R.C. (Canada) and M.RC. (U.K.).

Effects of Injury on Trigeminal and Spinal Somatosensory Systems, pages 495–498

PARTIAL DEAFFERENTATION OF THE SPINAL DORSAL HORN DOES NOT INDUCE CHANGES OF SYNAPTIC CONNECTIVITY AS REVEALED BY RECORDING CORD DORSUM POTENTIALS IN ADULT AND NEWBORN CATS

M. Zimmermann and R.A. Westerman

Department of Physiology, University of Heidelberg, Heidelberg, FRG, and Department of Physiology, Monash University, Clayton/Vic., Australia

INTRODUCTION

Degeneration of part of the presynaptic terminals to a neuron has been suggested to modify the connectivity of the remaining synapses, or to initiate the formation of new synapses by collateral sprouting (Liu and Chambers, 1958; Goldberger and Murray, 1974). To test whether such phenomena occur in the spinal dorsal horn following deafferentation, we have cut some of the lumbar dorsal roots in kitten and cats unilaterally. Weeks or months later, cord dorsum potentials were recorded as indicators of synaptic connectivity in the dorsal horn and analyzed for changes in the region of partial deafferentation.

METHODS

In anesthetized kittens (2 weeks old) or adult cats one or several lumbar dorsal roots were transected under sterile conditions. Four months (kitten) or 1 to 6 weeks (cats) later animals were reanaesthetized (pentobarbital) and spinal cords exposed by laminectomy and covered by paraffin oil. Cord dorsum potentials were recorded upon stimulation of cutaneous nerves or dorsal rootlets, at strengths supramaximal for the A-beta-fibers. Potentials were systematically mapped along the cord (for details see Brinkhus et al., 1983).

RESULTS

The N-wave (negative) recorded from the cord dorsum (Fig. 1) reflects the compound postsynaptic currents of dorsal horn neurons elicited by the afferent volley. The spatial distribution of the amplitude of the N-wave along the cord shows a maximum near the site of major afferent input from the stimulated nerve or root (Fig. 1, 2). The mappings were performed at symmetric positions on the normal and deafferented sides, with the same stimulation parameters applied to nerves or dorsal rootlets on either side. N-waves appear several segments above and below the site of major input, which is in line with the fact that collate-

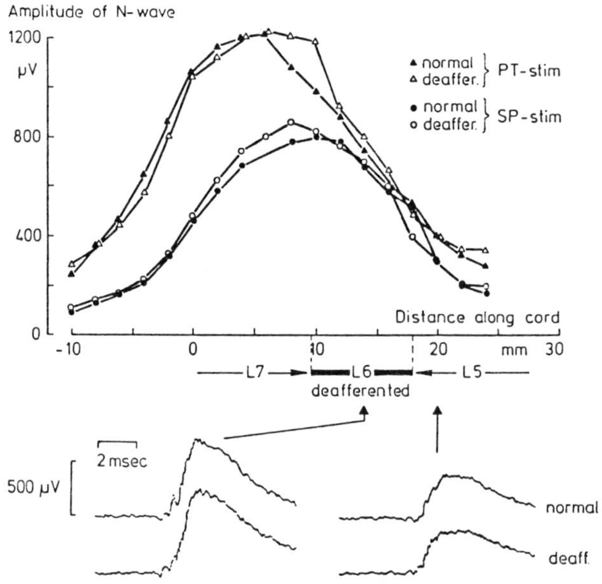

Figure 1. Spatial distribution of the amplitude of the N-wave component of the cord dorsum potential along the spinal cord, following stimulation of the posterior tibial (PT) or superficial peroneal (SP) nerves. On the left side the L6 dorsal root had been transected 22 days before (deafferented). The specimen records below show examples of N-waves recorded at the sites indicated by arrows. (From Brinkhus and Zimmermann, 1983).

rals of the dorsal root fibers extend in rostral and caudal directions over several segments (Brown, 1981). However, N-wave amplitudes show decrements with increasing distance from the segment of dominant input. The main finding was that no difference existed between normal and deafferented sites of the longitudinal distribution of the amplitudes of N-waves, including the zones of deafferentation. This was true for animals in which the dorsal root sections were performed in the early postnatal state 3 to 4 months before the electrophysiological analysis (Fig. 2) as well as for animals deafferented in the adult state 11 to 45 days before recording (Brinkhus and Zimmermann, 1983) (Fig. 1).

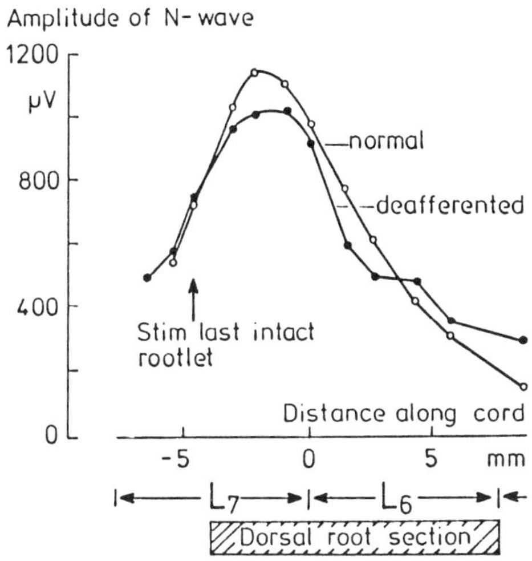

Figure 2. Longitudinal distribution of the N-wave component of the cord dorsum potentials following electrical stimulation of a rootlet in the L7 segment, as indicated by arrow. On the left side dorsal root transection had been performed of L6 and half of the L7 roots, as indicated, 90 days before in the early postnatal state of the animal. On the deafferented side the next intact rootlet adjacent to the zone of root section was used for stimulation, and the corresponding rootlet was stimulated on the right side.

DISCUSSION

Absence of changes of the longitudinal distribution of the N-wave in partially deafferented cord segments indicates that no reactive changes have occurred in the synaptic connectivity of the remaining synapses, irrespective of whether the deafferentations were performed in kittens or in adult cats. Therefore, the stability of synaptic transmission does not support the assumption that the persisting fibers increased their connectivity by collateral sprouting (increasing number of synapses per afferent fiber) or by increasing the gain or sensitivity of synaptic contacts. This finding is in agreement with part of previous results (e.g., Kerr, 1983) and assumptions, and in disagreement with others (e.g., Basbaum and Wall, 1976).

REFERENCES

Basbaum AI, Wall PD (1976). Chronic changes in the response of cells in adult cat dorsal horn following partial deafferentation: the appearance of responding cells in a previously non-responsive region. Brain Res 116: 181-204.

Brinkhus HB, Zimmermann M (1983). Characteristics of spinal dorsal horn neurons after partial chronic deafferentation by dorsal root transection. Pain 15: 221-236.

Brown A (1981). Organization in the spinal cord: the anatomy and physiology of identified neurones. Berlin, Heidelberg, New York: Springer

Goldberger ME, Murray M (1974). Restitution of function and collateral sprouting in the cat spinal cord: the deafferented animal. J comp Neurol 158: 37-54.

Kerr FWL (1983). Central nervous system changes and deafferentation pain: the role of reorganization and gliosis. In Bonica JJ, Lindblom U, Iggo A (eds): "Advances in Pain Research and Therapy, vol 5," New York: Raven, pp 663-675.

Liu CN, Chambers WW (1958). Intraspinal sprouting of dorsal root axons. Development of new collaterals and preterminals following partial denervation of the spinal cord in the cat. Arch Neurol Psychiat (Chic) 79: 46-61.

Effects of Injury on Trigeminal and Spinal Somatosensory Systems, page 499

NEURAL RECONNECTIVITY IN THE SPINAL CORD AFTER ANTEROLATERAL CHORDOTOMY

Elizabeth Bullitt, William D. Stofer, Charles J. Vierck, and Edward R. Perl
Department of Physiology (E.B.,E.R.P.) University of North Carolina, Chapel Hill, N.C. 27514; University of Pittsburgh (W.D.S.), Pittsburgh, Pa; University of Florida College of Medicine (C.J.V.), Gainesville, Fla.

A primate model has been used to explore the possibility that recovery of sensory function following ventrolateral chordotomy may be related to intraspinal sprouting or rearrangements of primary afferent nerve terminals. Monkeys were trained to terminate a noxious electrical stimulus and to differentiate it from innocuous stimulation. Behavioral testing after chordotomy was used to evaluate the presence of sensory recovery or its absence. At the terminal experiment, lumbar dorsal rootlets were labelled with HRP. The distribution of labelled synaptic complexes was then determined within the spinal dorsal horn by light level microscopic examination.

Six normal controls (12 roots), 12 monkeys that had undergone chordotomy (20 contralateral, 11 ipsilateral roots), and 2 monkeys that had received diffuse spinal cord lesions (3 contralateral, 4 ipsilateral roots) were studied. When compared to controls, animals undergoing chordotomy showed a loss of terminals in the superficial dorsal horn and an increase in synaptic complexes in deeper layers. Effects were bilateral, but most pronounced on the side contralateral to chordotomy. Animals with diffuse spinal lesions showed a completely different terminal redistribution pattern, with a bilateral increase of synaptic terminals within the superficial dorsal horn and a loss of terminals in deeper layers. No correlation was established between postsurgical terminal distribution and behavioral recovery.

Supported by grants NS 14899 and NS 01006 from the National Institute of Neurological and Communicative Diseases and Stroke of the National Institute of Health.

Effects of Injury on Trigeminal and Spinal Somatosensory Systems, page 501

NEUROPHYSIOLOGICAL CHARACTERISTICS OF TRIGEMINAL SENSORY UNITS AFTER NERVE REGENERATION IN THE CAT

Y. Tsuiki, K. Tabuchi, Y. Dateoka, T. Shimosato,
K. Tsuru, and Y. Shigenaga
Department of Oral Anatomy, and Oral-Maxillofacial Surgery (2nd division), Hiroshima University School of Dentistry, Hiroshima, JAPAN

The process of functional neural recovery was studied with the single-fiber recording technique. Following transection of the inferior alveolar nerve six cats were investigated 3 and 6 months after the nerve suture.

Observations at 3 months showed that three types of low-threshold mechanoreceptive units (SAI, 21; SAII, 1; FAI, 52), nociceptive (n=3) and cold fibers (n=2) were isolated. At 6 months the ratio of cold (n=7), nociceptive (n=7) and SAII (n=9) units showed a tendency to be increased. The functional disorders of the regenerated fibers were represented in especially low-threshold mechanoreceptive afferents (L-SMA). The results showed that a significant reduction of conduction velocity recognized in the L-SMA at 3 and 6 months (it was more prominent in cases of 3 months), but not in nociceptive and cold fibers. Other distortions were found in the response profiles of SAI units at 3 months. The intensity function of the SAI fibers with high-threshold showed a non-linear relationship between cumulative impulse count over a period of one second of stimulation and amplitude of indentation. Furthermore, the discharge pattern of the static or tonic component of these SAI fibers also showed abnormal firing characterized by very irregular, intermittent, and augmenting or recruiting profiles. At 6 months, the response profile of most SAI units recovered to the normal pattern except for a reduction of conduction velocity.

Similar to the responses of control experiments, most FA fibers examined at 3 and 6 months had gentle U-shaped tuning curves responding optimally to vibratory stimuli with frequencies of 10-40 Hz.

Effects of Injury on Trigeminal and Spinal Somatosensory Systems, page 503

CENTRAL ARBOR MORPHOLOGY OF PERIPHERALLY TRANSECTED INFRA-ORBITAL (IO) PRIMARY AFFERENTS

William E. Renehan, Robert W. Rhoades, Richard D. Mooney and Mark F. Jacquin

Department of Anatomy, University of Louisville (WER); University of Medicine and Dentistry of NJ (RWR and RDM); Department of Neuroscience, New York College of Osteopathic Medicine (MFJ).

We have previously shown that IO nerve section in the adult rat results in abnormal receptor reinnervation (Renehan and Munger, J. Comp. Neurol., in press) and altered primary afferent receptive fields (Renehan et al., Anat. Rec., 1986, 214:107A). In the present study, we have used standard intra-axonal recording and HRP injection techniques to label IO primary afferents 90-120 days subsequent to peripheral transection to examine the relationship between peripheral connectivity and central arbor morphology in the trigeminal brainstem nuclear complex (TBNC). Vibrissa afferents, which normally exhibit circumscribed arbors, were frequently found to have widespread and topographically inappropriate terminations. Similarly, nociceptive units, which have widespread arbors terminating primarily in laminae I, II and V of normal animals, frequently had very circumscribed arbors. Although anterograde HRP labelling experiments in adult-lesioned rats have suggested a nearly normal primary afferent pattern in the TBNC, our intra-axonal results suggest that regenerate IO axons may have abnormal central arbors in subnuclei interpolaris and caudalis. Thus, while peripheral nerve transection in the adult animal may leave the overall central termination pattern essentially unchanged, structure-function relationships for individual primary afferents are apparently altered. Supported in part by DE06528, NRSA NS07444 and the AOA.

Effects of Injury on Trigeminal and Spinal Somatosensory Systems,
page 505

FUNCTIONAL PROJECTIONS OF SINGLE IDENTIFIED CUTANEOUS AFFERENTS IN INTACT AND "SPARED ROOT" PREPARATIONS

H. Richard Koerber and Lorne M. Mendell

Department of Neurobiology and Behavior
SUNY, Stony Brook, NY 11794

We have constructed maps of functional spinal projections of single afferent fibers in the L7 DRG of the cat. These cells were impaled, characterized as to modality and receptive field, and stimulated through the intracellular electrode. Cord dorsum potentials (CDPs) were averaged simultaneously at 4 sites and up to 40 afferents were so characterized in a single experiment. We found that in response to 18 Hz stimulation, CDPs consisted of a monophasic monosynaptic (0.4-0.8 ms central latency) component followed by a complex slow wave which were both maximal at one site in strict accordance with receptive field location. CDPs were largest for afferents with the larger axons and among this group SAI afferents produced larger monosynaptic waves than hair follicle afferents. At .67 Hz stimulation the slow wave became more prominent and less focused for all afferents. HTMR afferents differed from all other receptor types in their response to conditioning-testing (C-T) pairs of stimuli. At C-T intervals of 30-100 ms, HTMRs exhibited facilitation of the second response in contrast to all others which showed depression. Preliminary results for afferents in chronically spared roots employing 18 Hz stimulation reveal that their functional projections can differ. These include: 1) monosynaptic CDPs at two discrete locations; 2) enhanced security of polysynaptic inputs such that the monosynaptic waves are not always monophasic; 3) polysynaptic slow waves can be present without being preceeded by a monosynaptic wave. These results suggest possible emergence of novel monosynaptic inputs and strenthening of polysynaptic inputs in the "spared root" preparation. Supported by NS 14899 and NS 16996.

Effects of Injury on Trigeminal and Spinal Somatosensory Systems, page 507

THE EFFECTS OF 4-AMINOPYRIDINE, STRYCHNINE AND PICROTOXIN ON RAT SPINAL CORD SOMATOTOPY FOLLOWING ACUTE SCIATIC NERVE LESION

Howard Markus and Bruce Pomeranz
Department of Zoology
University of Toronto
Toronto, Ontario M5S 1A1
Canada

Previous studies have shown that immediately following sciatic nerve lesion, the dorsal horn cells in the lumbar cord were deafferented and did not respond to mechanical stimulation of the hindlimb. However, 3 weeks after sciatic nerve lesion the dorsal horn cells in the deafferented area of the spinal cord responded to cutaneous stimulation. However these responses were elicited from areas of the hindlimb outside the cells' normal receptive fields. Other investigators have suggested that new connections in the spinal cord are not due to collateral sprouting but to the expression of latent synapses. To determine whether the appearance of novel receptive fields following chronic nerve lesion was due to the strengthening of latent synapses, chemicals which facilitate synaptic transmission were administered to the acutely denervated rat. Following administration of these chemicals, dorsal horn cells in the deafferented area of the cord responded to cutaneous stimulation of the hindlimb. However, the size of the deafferented cord which exhibited responses was smaller in these animals than in chronically denervated animals. These results indicate that although latent synapses are present, some time dependent factors may be involved in their functional expression.

Effects of Injury on Trigeminal and Spinal Somatosensory Systems, page 509

ALTERATIONS WITHIN THE FELINE TRIGEMINAL GANGLION FOLLOWING APPLICATION OF RICIN TO TOOTH PULP

Michael A. Henry, Lesnick E. Westrum, Lonnie R. Johnson, and Robert C. Canfield

Univ. of Florida, Gainesville, FL (M.A.H.), Univ. of Washington, Seattle, WA (L.E.W., R.C.C.), and Univ. of Colorado, Denver, CO (L.R.J.)

The application of the neurotoxin ricin, to peripheral nerves has recently been shown to be a highly effective method for producing central axonal and terminal alterations (thus transganglionic degeneration). The purpose of this study is to examine the axonal and cell body changes within the trigeminal ganglion associated with the application of ricin (RCA 60; E.-Y. Labs) to the pulpal chambers of unilateral maxillary and mandibular posterior teeth and cuspids in the adult cat. Following survival times ranging from 6-10 days, the animals were sacrificed and the trigeminal ganglion processed for EM. Examination of the ipsilateral trigeminal ganglion reveals striking axonal and cell body changes. Altered large myelinated axons are characterized by a fragmentation, compartmentalization or loss of axoplasm (all electron- lucent), while altered smaller myelinated and unmyelinated axons appear to be undergoing either electron-dense or lucent degeneration. The cytoplasm of altered cell bodies contains numerous electron-lucent degenerating mitochondria, decreased numbers of ribosomes but an increased number of neurofilaments. The action of ricin appears to be specific, as isolated altered elements are surrounded by normal profiles. In conclusion, this study demonstrates the specificity of the degenerative changes induced by ricin and its effectiveness on a wide range of different types and sizes of axons.

Supported by NIH Grants DE 04942, NS 07144 and NS 20482.

Effects of Injury on Trigeminal and Spinal Somatosensory Systems, page 511

CELLS OF ORIGIN OF THE SPINOTHALAMIC PATHWAY WHICH BRANCH TO TERMINATE IN MULTIPLE THALAMIC SITES.

R.T. Stevens, A.V. Apkarian and C.J. Hodge, Jr.

Neurosurgery Dept., SUNY Health Science Center at Syracuse, Syracuse, New York 13210

The spinothalamic tract (STT) terminates in various thalamic nuclei. Yet, it is uncertain to what extent cells of the STT branch to terminate in multiple thalamic nuclei. This study investigates the branching of the STT to the ventral posterolateral n. (VPL), the central lateral n. (CL) and n. submedius (SM).

Cats were injected with two dyes (Evans blue and granular blue) into 2 of the 3 following thalamic nuclei: VPL, CL or SM. Thus, retrogradely labeled lumbar spinal cord cells projecting to both nuclei could be identified.

On the average 10% of all labeled cells in the lumbar cord were double labeled. However, there was a larger number of double labeled cells projecting to VPL and SM than to CL and SM or CL and VPL ($p<.01$). Most double labeled cells were in laminae I & VIII. Lamina I cells with branching axons were most often found projecting to VPL and SM ($p<.03$) while cells of lamina VIII branched equally to VPL, CL and SM. Single labeled lamina I cells projected mainly to VPL or SM ($p<.004$), while single labeled lamina VIII cells projected mainly to CL or SM ($p<.002$).

Cells with branching axons constitute a small but significant portion of the STT. The termination sites of these cells correlate with their laminar locations. Since cells of lamina I constitute the dorsolateral STT while deeper laminae constitute the ventrolateral STT, these two pathways have distinct termination regions as well as regions where their terminations overlap.

Effects of Injury on Trigeminal and Spinal Somatosensory Systems, page 513

THALAMIC TERMINATIONS OF THE DORSOLATERAL AND THE VENTROLATERAL SPINOTHALAMIC PATHWAYS.

A.V. Apkarian, C.J. Hodge, Jr., M.W. Jones and R.T. Stevens
Neurosurgery Dept., SUNY Health Science Center at Syracuse, Syracuse, New York 13210

Recently we have reported the existence of two distinct spinothalamic pathways, a dorsolateral spinothalamic pathway (DSTT) which originates in the contralateral lamina I, and a ventrolateral spinothalamic pathway (VSTT) which originates in the contralateral laminae IV-X. Both tracts appear to be involved in nociception, hence the DSTT is probably the pathway responsible for return of pain sensation following cordotomy in humans. In this study the thoracic termination sites of the DSTT and the VSTT were investigated.

Anterograde transport of WGA-HRP from the lumbar spinal cord was used to map terminal sites in the thalamus. Thoracic spinal cord lesions were used to isolate either the DSTT or the VSTT.

In the lateral thalamus, the terminations of the DSTT and the VSTT overlap along the ventral border of VPL, whereas only the VSTT projects more anteriorly to caudal VL. In the medial thalamus, the DSTT terminates in n. submedius, the VSTT terminates in n. centralis lateralis, and both tracts have terminations within n. reuniens.

These results demonstrate that both the DSTT and the VSTT innervate thalamic structures implicated in nociception. The segregation of DSTT and VSTT into distinct cells of origin, pathways, and termination sites, suggests separate functional roles for these two pathways in coding nociception.

Effects of Injury on Trigeminal and Spinal Somatosensory Systems, page 515

TWO SEPARATE OUTPUT SYSTEMS OF TRIGEMINAL SENSORY INPUTS IN CAT CEREBRAL CORTEX

Rhyuji Sumino, Hiroshi Itoga, Hiroyuki Muramatsu, and Koichi Iwata
Department of Physiology, Nihon University School of Dentistry
1-8-13 Kandasurugadai, Chiyoda-ku, Tokyo 101
Japan

Number of researchers, using intra-cortical microstimulation (ICMS), investigated the cortical motor topography in the cats. These studies were centered on the cortical functions in relation to limb muscles and limb movements. The representation of jaw and oro-facial musculature in the cat's cerebral cortex has not been accurately determined. In the present experiment, input output relations of orofacial sensorimotor cortex were studied by ICMS and recording single neuronal activities in the lightly anesthetized cat. Jaw and orofacial motor effects were evoked by ICMS ($<30\mu A$) delivered to anterior part of the coronal and lateral sigmoid gyri (C area), and the anterior part of the orbital gyrus (O area). Different patterns of movements in the jaw and oro-facial regions were evoked from these two areas. In C area one or, at most, two types of simple movement were produced by ICMS to one location, while in O area more coordinated movements than those in C area were produced. Cytoarchitectonically the jaw and oro-facial motor areas were restricted to areas 3a, 4γ, and 6aβ in C area, and to area 6aβ and 43 in O area. Ablation of C area produced obvious changes in patterns of movements which were produced by ICMS to C area, while that of O area did few changes in patterns of C area. Cortical cells in C area received cutaneous inputs from orofacial regions, while those in O area received no cutaneous inputs. Retrograde transport of HRP represented cortico-cortical relation between two areas, thus C area and O area were reciprocally connected, and projection from O area to C area was found to be more dominant than that from C area to O area.

Effects of Injury on Trigeminal and Spinal Somatosensory Systems, page 517

DIFFERENT LESIONS IN THE ASCENDING PATHWAYS OF PRIMATE SPINAL CORD LEAD TO DIFFERENT PATTERNS OF METABOLIC LABELING.

S.L. Juliano*, C.J. Vierck+, B.Y. Cooper+;

*USUHS, Bethesda, MD, USA; +U. Florida,

Gainsville, FL, USA.

Earlier studies have indicated that lesions of the ascending pathways in primates can lead to specific discriminative deficits. Experiments were undertaken to ascertain if the behavioral changes observed following lesions of the ascending pathways in the spinal cord of primates had underlying structural correlates which might be detected using histochemical or metabolic mapping techniques. Two types of spinal cord lesion in Macaca spesiosa were evaluated including (i) the interruption of the gracile fasciculus (GF) unilaterally and (ii) the severing of the dorsolateral column on one side and the anterolateral column on the other, i.e., a dorsal column isolation (DCI). Four months to 1 year following the lesions, the animals underwent a 2-deoxyglucose (2DG) experiment in which they received a tactile stimulus. Following this procedure the brains were processed for autoradiography and reacted for cytochrome oxidase activity (CO). Different patterns of labeling were found in the somatosensory cortex for both CO and 2DG for the 2 different lesion types. The DCI lesion produced a distinct patchiness in the pattern of CO labeling which was not present in the distribution of CO following a lesion of the GF. Both lesions produced a decrease in the 2DG activity, although the GF lesion lead to an unusual laminar pattern of 2DG labeling which was inversely correlated with the CO activity. No concrete relationship was observed between the CO and 2DG labeling in the animals with the DCI lesion.

Effects of Injury on Trigeminal and Spinal Somatosensory Systems, page 519

SI CORTEX REORGANIZATION AFTER SPINAL TRANSECTION IS AGE-DEPENDENT IN CATS

P.A. McKinley, J.L. Smith and L. Swyter

Department of Kinesiology, UCLA, Los Angeles, CA 90024 USA

Primary somatosensory (SI) cortex was mapped in spinal cats that sustained complete cord transection at T-12 at two different periods of postnatal development, 2 weeks and 6 weeks of age. SI was mapped sequentially from 3 weeks to 4 months post-transection. At 4 months post-transection, there was extensive reorganization of the deafferented hindlimb cortex in cats spinalized at 2 weeks that resulted in a second, somatotopically arranged representation of intact tactile input from the trunk and forelimb. In contrast, cortical reorganization in the cats spinalized at 6 weeks of age was limited. Trunk afferent input alone expanded into the deafferented hindlimb region but did not fully occupy it, although the input was topologically organized. This is strikingly different from representations at 3 weeks post-transection in these animals, where the deafferented region was fully occupied by trunk receptive fields, but poorly organized.

These observations provide further evidence that SI cortex organization changes to reflect alterations at the periphery and demonstrate that reorganization can occur across somatotopic boundaries. The character of the response, however, is age-dependent. Additionally, the process of reorganization in young animals occurs in two steps: an initial general expansion into the deafferented zone followed by retraction and topological shaping of receptive fields.

Effects of Injury on Trigeminal and Spinal Somatosensory Systems, page 521

RESPONSES OF CORTICAL NEURONS DRIVEN BY INTRA-PULPAL APPLICATION OF BRADYKININ IN THE CAT

Koichi Iwata, Hiroshi Itoga, Hiroyuki Muramatsu, Aiko Suzuki and Rhyuji Sumino
Department of Physiology, Nihon University School of Dentistry
1-8-13 Kandasurugadai, Chiyoda-ku, Tokyo 101
Japan

A recent histological and electrophysiological studies have indicated that there are three components of nerve fibers (Aβ, Aδ and C fibers) concerned in pulpal sensory mechanisms. It is still unclear, however, which group of pulpal nerve fibers conbeys intra-pulpal nociceptive information to the somatosensory cortex, because it is difficult to activate selectively intradental small fibers such as Aδ and C fibers by electrical stimulation of the tooth pulp. In the present experiments, single neuronal activities driven by electrical stimulation of the tooth pulp (TPNs) were recorded from anterior and middle parts of the coronal gyrus and the properties of TPNs responded to intra-pulpal application of bradykinin were studied in the cat anesthetized with ketamine-HCL (50mg/kg,i.m.) and immobilized with pancronium bromide (1mg/kg,i.v.). A total of 165 TPNs were recorded in this area, 26 TPNs increased firing after application of bradykinin (fa.BK-TPNs). On the other hand, 139 TPNs were insensitive to bradykinin (non.BK-TPNs). Stimulus threshold of fa.BK-TPNs were higher than those of non.BK-TPNs to electrical stimulation of the pulp. Peak latency of fa.BK-TPNs were longer than those of non.BK-TPNs. All fa.BK-TPNs were located in the deep layers of the area 3b of the anterior part of the coronal gyrus, while non.BK-TPNs were in the area 3a and 3b. 80% of fa.BK-TPNs received inputs not only from low threshold cutaneous afferents but also high threshold nociceptive ones. These findings suggest that fa.BK-TPNs in this cortical area may be involved in sensory processing of noxious information from trigeminal regions.

Effects of Injury on Trigeminal and Spinal Somatosensory Systems, page 523

ACUTE EFFECTS OF PERIPHERAL DEAFFERENTATION ON ADULT RACCOON SI CORTEX

B. G. Turnbull and D. D. Rasmusson

Department of Physiology & Biophysics
Dalhousie University
Halifax, Nova Scotia
Canada B3H 4H7

The immediate effects of deafferentation on the SI forepaw cortex of adult, chloralose-anesthetized raccoons were studied using multiunit recording techniques. Deafferented cortex was found to receive predominantly excitatory or inhibitory inputs, depending on whether a digit was partially or totally denervated. Following transection of ventral digital nerves, the deafferented cortex was responsive to mechanical stimulation of skin that normally drives neurons in adjacent cortex and the unmasked inputs were predominantly excitatory. The "expansions" involved cortical surface distances of 1 to 3 mm and were not topographically consistent, since local map reversals and discontinuities were seen. In many cases, multiunit receptive fields were exceptionally large, covering up to two-thirds of the forepaw. Similar receptive fields were seen within palmar cortex.

The inputs remaining after denervation of a whole digit (by amputation) were inhibitory, with units responding only to stimulus offset. Thus, graded disruptions of normal input to SI reveal different levels of converging excitatory and inhibitory inputs. The patterns and properties of these inputs suggest that the "expansion" of adjacent cortical representations seen in acutely deafferented cortex may be mediated by intracortical circuitry.
Supported by MRC of Canada.

Effects of Injury on Trigeminal and Spinal Somatosensory Systems, page 525

AUTOMATED TESTS OF FACIAL SOMATIC SENSATION IN THE AWAKE, MINIMALLY-RESTRAINED RAT. APPLICABILITY FOR USE IN LONG-TERM DEAFFERENTATION STUDIES

J.G. Broton and J.P. Rosenfeld

Department of Psychology, Northwestern University, Evanston, Illinois 60201 (J.P.R.), and Faculty of Dentistry, University of Toronto, Toronto, Canada M5G 1G6 (J.G.B.)

For several years, we have used a portable device to deliver noxious thermal stimuli to facial skin. The heat source is a small resistor. Current (250 mA, DC) passed through the resistor increases its temperature. When the resistor becomes noxiously hot, rats execute a face-rubbing (FR) response to terminate the stimulus. In the present study, less current (200 mA) was used, the surface temperature of the resistor increased more slowly, and thermal stimulus detection was assessed. Also, air puff stimuli were delivered to the same discrete areas of facial skin by means of another similarly-constructed portable device. For each test, stimulus detection was defined as a change in the monitored cortical EEG from high-amplitude, low-frequency waves to lower-amplitude activity indicating cortical arousal. The fixed stimuli and the rat's responses to them were automatically controlled and recorded. The latencies to stimulus detection (DL) were less than one sec for the air puff, and 1.0-5.0 sec for the thermal stimulus. Response latencies did not significantly change with repeated (once/day) testing. Rats always executed a FR response 1.0-4.0 sec after thermal detection; therefore we consider the thermal DL to be a measure of non-noxious thermal sensation. Together, these three measures provide a battery of tests of somatosensory responsiveness which can be used in long-term studies involving peripheral or central deafferentations.

Effects of Injury on Trigeminal and Spinal Somatosensory Systems, page 527

Demyelination-Induced Deficits in Vibrotaction: Differential Effects on Frequency and Amplitude Sensitivity.

Andrew M. Kelahan, Michael J. Buckley and Bruce A. Cohen
Department of Neurology, Northwestern University Medical School, Chicago, IL 60611

Sensitivity of the skin of humans and rats to vibrotactile stimulation was studied to determine if axonal demyelination - such as occurs in multiple sclerosis (MS) - can produce frequency-specific deficits, or if generalized deficits occur. These studies were undertaken using a stimulator designed to allow the independent quantification of detection thresholds for vibratory frequency and amplitude.

Tests conducted on a group of 24 normal adult humans (20-55 yrs. of age) showed that at an amplitude of 0.05 um (approx. 2x threshold at 128 Hz) subjects reliably detected vibrations between 50 and 280 Hz. Similar testing of 12 chronic MS patients (> 3 yrs. duration) showed that 33% had significantly reduced high-frequency sensitivity (up to 100 Hz less than normal) while amplitude thresholds were within normal limits as tested by either the stimulator or tuning forks. Testing of high-frequency sensitivity may be of even greater value in the diagnosis of acute MS when demyelination is less pronounced.

The vibratory sensitivity of 10 rats was tested using a conditioned emotional response (CER) paradigm. The conditioned stimulus (CS) was a 60 sec. constant frequency, constant amplitude vibration; the unconditioned stimulus was a 500 msec. foot shock delivered at CS offset. Endpoints for frequency detection at several amplitudes as defined in the CER paradigm are as follows: a) 50+200 Hz at 0.32 um; b) 50+240 Hz at 0.40 um; and c) 50+400 Hz at 0.50 um. Retesting of the same rats following cervical spinal cord demyelination is presently underway.

(Supported by grants from the Hearst Found., Inc. & the J.D. and Iva Leiper Trust)

Effects of Injury on Trigeminal and Spinal Somatosensory Systems, page 529

EVIDENCE THAT SENSORY FEEDBACK IS REGULATED BY THE PYRAMIDAL TRACT DURING LOCOMOTION

Joyce Keifer and Katherine Kalil

Neurosciences Training Program and Department of Anatomy, University of Wisconsin, Madison, WI 53706 USA

The pyramidal tract (PT) of the hamster projects from the sensorimotor cortex to all segments of the spinal cord where it terminates primarily within the dorsal horn. In order to understand the role of the PT in behavior, a kinematic analysis was performed on the movements of the forelimb and hindlimb during locomotion of normal adult hamsters and of those with lesions of the PT. To test the hypothesis that the PT is important in behaviors that require sensory feedback, locomotion on two types of terrain was filmed, smooth terrain, on which the locomotor rhythm is relatively automatic, and rough terrain, on which the movement must be constantly modified by sensory feedback during its execution. The analysis revealed that following a lesion of the PT animals failed to express a yield during the stance phase of locomotion, and that this deficit was more pronounced during locomotion on rough terrain than on smooth. From these results we propose that the PT regulates the stiffness of the limb through the modulation of sensory feedback during movements that require continual adjustment during their performance.

Although hamsters that received lesions of the PT as adults did not demonstrate behavioral recovery, infant lesioned hamsters exhibited nearly normal locomotor function, which is well correlated with the regrowth of severed PT axons to their normal sites of termination in the spinal cord. However, control of the yield phase during movements of the forelimb is permanently impaired. This suggests that the control of the forelimb requires a precision of neural input for which regrowing PT axons or other descending systems cannot compensate.

Supported by NSF Grant BNS-8311517 and NIH Grant NS 14428.

Index